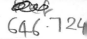

Level 2

hairdressing

Level 2
hairdressing

Rachel Gould and Martyn Wady

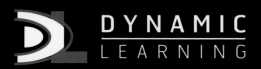

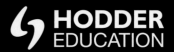

Orders: please contact Bookpoint Ltd, 130 Milton Park, Abingdon, Oxon OX14 4SB. Telephone: (44) 01235 827720. Fax: (44) 01235 400454. Lines are open from 9.00–5.00, Monday to Saturday, with a 24-hour message answering service. You can also order through our website: www.hoddereducation.co.uk

If you have any comments to make about this, or any of our other titles, please send them to educationenquiries@hodder.co.uk

British Library Cataloguing in Publication Data
A catalogue record for this title is available from the British Library

ISBN: 978 1 444 112 023

First Published 2010
Impression number   10 9 8 7 6 5 4 3 2 1
Year   2012 2011 2010

Copyright © 2010 Rachel Gould and Martyn Wady

Hachette UK's policy is to use papers that are natural, renewable and recyclable products and made from wood grown in sustainable forests. The logging and manufacturing processes are expected to conform to the environmental regulations of the country of origin.

Cover photo © Hair: HOB Salons Creative Team; Photography: John Rawson
Typeset by Fakenham Photosetting Ltd, Fakenham, Norfolk
Printed in Italy for Hodder Education, An Hachette UK Company, 338 Euston Road, London NW1 3BH

Contents

Section 3: With the team

Introduction

Congratulations! You've chosen a great career. You are now part of a vibrant industry, packed with creative and style-conscious people like you. This is an industry where you can work behind the camera or in front of it, where you can travel, be your own boss, perform for an audience of thousands, make your fortune, transform your clients' looks (and occasionally their lives) and express your creativity every day. Studying the theory, practising hard and developing a passion for great hairdressing will help you to achieve the skill and the confidence to carry out your chosen career ... anywhere from a top London salon to a beach hut in Thailand.

Hairdressing will give you lots of things, but above all it will give you choice: your choice of speciality and the training available to change your mind; the skills to choose where and how much you work; the opportunity to commit to becoming a great freelance hairdresser or the next British Hairdresser of the Year. Few professions can promise you the potential that hairdressing does, so be excited because you are about to embark on an adventure that should last you a lifetime!

Case study

Hairdressing as a career: where it can take you

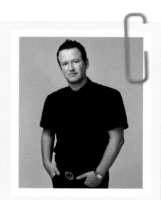

'I have built up a successful business in Mansfield and think I have proved that you definitely don't have to be in London to be a star hairdresser. Many of my team members are respected throughout the industry and have won awards, including Eastern Hairdresser of the Year and Newcomer of the Year. They are also regularly featured as experts in the hair trade and consumer press.'

'Like many of my peers, I've worked non-stop to develop my skills and over the years I've won many amazing awards – to be in the British Hairdressing Hall of Fame is a truly fantastic achievement.'

'Hairdressing can take you wherever you choose. Your drive and goals will determine which path your career takes, but nothing is impossible. Continually train and push yourself to be the best, you never stop learning. Take inspiration from everything around you and remember, you're an artist!'

Mark Leeson, Mark Leeson Hair, Body & Mind, Mansfield

Case study

Focus on your future

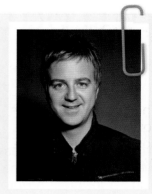

Mark Woolley is an award-winning owner of salons based in London and the South. He is also one of the hair industry's rising stars with a strong vision for the future of his business.

'I grew up in North Yorkshire and did hairdressing at 15 for work experience. I was inspired and made the decision to get started in the industry when I left school. I joined the SAKS group, which gave me a great grounding but I knew that I wanted to own my own business. By 21, I had my first franchise and I added six more over the next seven years. After a while, I began to plan for my very own brand and in 2008 I opened my first Electric Hairdressing salon in Brighton. Electric is all about great quality hairdressing in beautiful settings. It's about a personal service that gives every client one-to-one time with a first-class hair professional. My staff are so committed and I invest a lot in them. We have bi-annual Electric Sessions, which combine plenty of fun with inspirational learning. We have our own training programme and I've created a partnership programme which will allow my management staff to own a chunk of the business they help to create. We've won awards and recognition from key people in the industry. I've even been named Hair Magazine Salon Stylist of the Year. I have an ambassador role with Denman professional tools and myself and my artistic team travel the world for photographic shoots, shows and seminars. The future looks amazing with more Electric Salons and a whole range of Electric products.'

'This industry is so inspirational and every day brings new challenges. I never forget that I was a trainee once and I encourage my staff to have a vision for their future. Hairdressing is packed with opportunity but they are opportunities that can only be taken if you plan to do so. My staff create their own goals for the next three months, one year and five years and they constantly review it. I'd encourage everyone to do the same!'

Mark Woolley, Owner and Creative Director, Electric Hairdressing

How to use this book

These pages are packed with the technical and practical knowledge you will need to achieve NVQ Level 2, and every new skill is set in the context you will experience in the real world.

We have divided all the NVQ standards into three sections:

> In the salon
> With the client
> With the team.

'In the salon' looks at the knowledge required to be a part of a well-functioning salon. 'With the client' takes in all the key hairdressing skills, duties, techniques and services that you will need to give your clients a great hairdressing experience. 'With the team' explores ways in which you can be a positive member of a successful salon team.

Each section of the book contains advice, comments and case studies from real hair professionals, offering you first-hand experiences from the people that matter – your industry colleagues.

There are lots of useful tips and activities to help bring your new skills to life. We have also added chapter summaries and a glossary to give you a quick reference guide. Plus there is a host of digital resources retained by your college tutor to enrich your learning experience.

This book is your handbook and your user guide to becoming a fully fledged hair professional. Whether you are salon trainee or a full-time student, this book will be a positive asset, and will help you as you work towards a successful outcome from all the time and effort you are investing. Enjoy!

Acknowledgements

Many of the photographs in this book were taken by Paul Gill at HOB Salons. This photography work could not have been done without the help of the authors and the team at HOB. The publishers are grateful to everyone involved for their hard work, without which this book would be much poorer.

The publishers would particularly like to acknowledge the following people for their work.

The hairdressing team at HOB Salons were:

> Darren Bain
> Carrie Henry
> Andrea Martinelli
> Abby Smith
> Christel Lundqvist
> Mary Roberton

The models on the photo shoot were:

> Laura Adaken
> Chloe Backler
> Jennifer Brewer
> Myles Davis
> Jade Dorsett
> Siobhan Entwistle
> Simone Gordon
> Charlotte Hodson
> Rachael Lyons
> Andrea Martinelli
> Mary Roberton
> Kate Short
> Matthew Smith
> Jade Taylor
> Isobel Rose Thompson
> Gabriela Veresova
> Magda Wallmont
> Natalie Willcox.

In addition, the publishers would like to thank Katie Pearson and Amrit Sagoo at HOB Salons for organising the photography, and Lucy Flower for her expert make-up skills.

Special thanks to **Joshua Galvin @ Central Training Group**'s Head of Internal Verification, Rani Juttla, for her help and guidance in producing the photography for this publication. Central is the largest hairdressing training organisation in the United Kingdom and works alongside the **HOB** Team and most of London's other top hairdressing salons to ensure their learners achieve both the in-salon and college-based training they need to exceed their expectations. For further information, please visit www.centraltraininggroup.com.

The authors and publishers would also like to thank the following individuals and companies for supplying photos for use in this book: Alison Jameson Consultants, City Boy, Denman, Corioliss, Electric Hairdressing, Goldwell, Great Lengths, Mackinder Hair, Procare, Takara Belmont and Tigi.

About HOB Salons

Home to the 2008 and 2009 British Hairdresser of the Year, 2009 London Hairdresser of the Year, and 2008 and 2009 Artistic Team of the Year, HOB Salons have secured a reputation as one of the UK's leading hairdressing groups.

With a chain of successful salons located throughout London, Hertfordshire, Middlesex, Essex, Leeds and Buckinghamshire, HOB Salons are renowned for the highest of hairdressing standards and firmly site ongoing training and education as the bedrock of their success and the key to their growth.

The HOB Academy not only serves as a training centre for the company's staff and growing franchise network, but also delivers a full range of courses to hairdressers from around the globe, taught by the award-winning HOB Creative Team. Situated in the hub of London's vibrant and fashionable Camden Town, the HOB Academy is an inspired place to learn.

Believing that education is the route to a rewarding and successful career, HOB Salons are proud to be supporting Hodder Education on this project.

For more information on HOB Salons visit www.hobsalons.com.

Picture credits

Every effort has been made to trace the copyright holders of material reproduced here. The authors and publishers would like to thank the following for permission to reproduce copyright illustrations:

p.vii Mark Leeson; p.viii Mark Woolley; p.1 Electric Hairdressing; p.3 Barrie Stephen; p.4 courtesy of (top L) RUSH London, (top R) Cutting Room Creative Leeds, (bottom) Hooker & Young; p.5 PurestockX.com; p.6 Francesco Group; p.8 Shortcuts www.shortcuts.co.uk; p.10 Francesco Group; p.13 Pali Rao/iStockphoto; p.14 courtesy of RUSH London; p.17 Electric Hairdressing; p.20 (top) Anatoly Repin/iStockphoto.com, (bottom) Stockbyte/Getty Images; p.21 (top) Edward Hemmings; p.23 Shortcuts www.shortcuts.co.uk; p.24 courtesy of (bottom L) Great Lengths, (bottom centre) Denman, (bottom R) John Rawson Partnership; p.25 Francesco Group; p.27 Hodder Education; p.30 Errol Douglas; p.32 Edward Hemmings; p.33 courtesy of Cutting Room Creative Leeds; p.34 (R) Getty Images/Glowimages; p.37 (R) Ken Ng – Fotolia.com; p.38 (top) STEVE HORRELL/SCIENCE PHOTO LIBRARY, (bottom) Mark Richardson – Fotolia.com; p.39 (top) James Steidl – Fotolia.com; p.40 Paul Gibbings – Fotolia.com; p.42 (L) DK Limited/Corbis, (R) Ian Miles–Flashpoint Pictures/Alamy; p.44 courtesy of (top, middle) RUSH London, (bottom) Cutting Room Creative Leeds; p.45 Scott Tilley/Alamy; p.46 (top) Patricia Hofmeester – Fotolia.com, (middle) www.skinmatebeauty.com, (bottom L) Renscene Ltd, (bottom middle) STEVE PERCIVAL/SCIENCE PHOTO LIBRARY, (bottom R) Jamie Grill/Getty Images; p.47 courtesy of (top, L–R) Denman, John Rawson Partnership, Denman (combs), Great Lengths, Denman, (bottom, L–R) Goldwell (bowl, trolley, apron), Denman, Corioliss; p.48 courtesy of (top L) Denman, (others) Goldwell; p.51 (bottom) Health and Safety Executive; p.61 Anya Dellicompagni; p.64 Francesco Group; p.65 courtesy of Goldwell; p.67 (centre L) Jupiterimages/Getty Images, (centre R) Ingram Publishing Limited, (bottom L) Steve Debenport/iStockphoto.com, (bottom R) Robert Kneschke – Fotolia.com; pp.71–2 courtesy of Great Lengths; p.77 (top) STEVE GSCHMEISSNER/SCIENCE PHOTO LIBRARY, (bottom) POWER AND SYRED/SCIENCE PHOTO LIBRARY; p.83 (top) University of Aberdeen/Mediscan, (bottom) DR P. MARAZZI/SCIENCE PHOTO LIBRARY; p.84 (top two) DR P. MARAZZI/SCIENCE PHOTO LIBRARY, (third) CNRI/SCIENCE PHOTO LIBRARY, (bottom) ST BARTHOLOMEWS HOSPITAL/SCIENCE PHOTO LIBRARY; p.85 (top two) SCIENCE PHOTO LIBRARY, (bottom two) DR P. MARAZZI/SCIENCE PHOTO LIBRARY; p.86 (top) Mediscan, (second) KLAUS GULDBRANDSEN/SCIENCE PHOTO LIBRARY, (third) DR P. MARAZZI/SCIENCE PHOTO LIBRARY, (bottom) Mediscan; p.87 (top) DR P. MARAZZI/SCIENCE PHOTO LIBRARY, (second) Wellcome Images, (third) DR P. MARAZZI/SCIENCE PHOTO LIBRARY, (bottom) DR HAROUT TANIELIAN/SCIENCE PHOTO LIBRARY; p.88 (top two) DR P. MARAZZI/SCIENCE PHOTO LIBRARY, (third) ST BARTHOLOMEWS HOSPITAL/SCIENCE PHOTO LIBRARY, (bottom) Mediscan; p.89 (top) DR P. MARAZZI/SCIENCE PHOTO LIBRARY, (second) SCIENCE PHOTO LIBRARY, (third) DR TONY BRAIN/SCIENCE PHOTO LIBRARY; p.90 (top) STEVE GSCHMEISSNER/SCIENCE PHOTO LIBRARY, (middle) Wellcome Images, (bottom) i love images/Alamy; p.94 courtesy of (top L) Cutting Room Creative, (top R) Leo Bancroft, (bottom) RUSH; p.95 courtesy of Aston & Fincher; p.96 courtesy of (top) Goldwell, (bottom L) Tigi, (others) Goldwell; p.97 (top) reproduced by kind permission of Cengage Learning, from *Hairdressing: The Foundations* 6th ed., Leo Palladino & Martin Green (2009: p.161); p.98 (top) courtesy of Goldwell; pp.99–100 courtesy of Goldwell; p.101 (top) Doug Steley A/Alamy, (bottom L) INSADCO Photography/Alamy, (bottom middle) DR TONY BRAIN/SCIENCE PHOTO LIBRARY, (bottom R) Greg Ceo/Getty Images; p.102 (top L) DR P. MARAZZI/SCIENCE PHOTO LIBRARY, (top middle) ST BARTHOLOMEWS HOSPITAL/SCIENCE PHOTO LIBRARY, (top R) DR P. MARAZZI/SCIENCE PHOTO LIBRARY; p.103 Anatoly Repin/iStockphoto.com; p.111 (bottom) Micro Mist, courtesy of Takara Belmont; p.112 courtesy of Goldwell; p.114 hair by Lisa Shepherd; p.115 (L) ACE STOCK LIMITED/Alamy, (middle) David Burton/Alamy, (R) Domen Colja/Alamy; p.117 (top) Image Source/Alamy, (bottom) vincent abbey/Alamy; p.118 (L) Christine Kublanski/iStockphoto, (R) courtesy of Goldwell; p.120 (top) courtesy of Goldwell, (bottom) Image Source/Alamy; pp.125–6 courtesy of Goldwell; p.128 (L) Image Source/Alamy, (middle) Gabe Palmer/Alamy, (R) Andres Rodriguez/Alamy; p.129 (bottom R) Martyn f. Chillmaid, (others) courtesy of Denman; p.130 (top L) courtesy of Denman, (top R) Paul Gill/Hodder Education/courtesy of Denman, (bottom L two) courtesy of Goldwell, (third) Alphavisions/iStockphoto, (fourth) courtesy of Procare; p.131 (top L) courtesy of Goldwell, (top middle) Indola, (top R) Paul Gill/Hodder Education/Fanci-Full Clean Touch Gentle Skin Cleanser, (middle) courtesy of Goldwell, (bottom L) www.cowens.co.uk, (bottom middle) courtesy of Denman, (bottom R) courtesy of Goldwell; p.132 (top) Paul Pedersen/Papsnap/Picture-That, photographersdirect.com/image used with the permission of D Macintyre & Son Ltd, (middle L) Francesco Group, (middle R) Tony Rusecki/Alamy, (bottom) courtesy of Takara Belmont; p.135 Charlotte Nation/Getty Images; p.141 Itani101/Alamy; p.147 courtesy of Procare; p.150 Mackinder Hair; p.151 (top L, middle) Mackinder Hair, (top R) City Boy, (middle) Mackinder Hair, (bottom) City Boy; p.154 (top) City Boy, (middle) David Sacks/Getty Images, (bottom) City Boy; p.155 Mackinder Hair; p.157 City Boy; p.164 hair by Mark Leeson; p.166 Andreas Kuehn/Getty Images; p.167 (top L) Smith Collection/Getty Images, (top middle) Paul Falltrick Hairdressing, (top R) Ragnar Schmuck/Getty Images, (middle) Mark Woolley, (bottom) Mark Woolley for the Five Point Alliance; p.168 (top) reproduced by kind permission of Cengage Learning, from *Hairdressing: The Foundations* 6th ed., Leo Palladino & Martin Green (2009: p.230), (middle) courtesy of Goldwell, (bottom) courtesy of Tigi; p.169 (top) Andre Thijssen/Getty Images, (bottom) Adams Picture Library t/a apl/Alamy; p.170 Akin Konizi for the Five Point Alliance; p.171 courtesy of (top, bottom) Goldwell, (middle) Tigi; p.172 courtesy of (middle R) Tigi, (others) Goldwell;

pp.173–4 courtesy of Denman; p.175 (fourth from top) Xuejun li – Fotolia.com, (others) courtesy of Denman; p.176 courtesy of Corioliss; p.177 (top) Aleksandr Ugorenkov/Alamy, (bottom) courtesy of Corioliss; p.178 (top) Kerioak – Fotolia.com, (second) Mode Images Limited/Alamy, (third) Paul Pedersen/Papsnap/ Picture-That, photographersdirect.com, (fourth) Luis Albuquerque/iStockphoto.com; p.179 (top) Michele Constantini/Getty Images, (others) courtesy of Denman www.denmanbrush.com; p.180 Michele Constantini/Getty Images; pp.182–6 courtesy of Denman; pp.187–8 courtesy of Corioliss; p.189 Andreas Kuehn/Getty Images; p.197 hair by Mark Leeson; p.198 Image Source/Alamy; p.206 Thomas Northcut/Getty Images; p.207 (top) DR P. MARAZZI/SCIENCE PHOTO LIBRARY; p.212 Catchlight Visual Services/Alamy; pp.213–14 courtesy of Great Lengths; p.215 Balmain Hair/Color Fringe; pp.218–21 courtesy of Great Lengths; p.226 courtesy of (top) Tigi, (bottom) Goldwell; p.227 hair by Errol Douglas; p.229 (L) Ronand Durmont/Getty Images, (middle) Michael Ochs Archives/Getty Images, (R) Col Pics/Everett/Rex Features; p.230 Mark Hayes; p.232 (top) Five Point Alliance, (middle) Butch Martin/Alamy, (second from bottom) spellermilner design, photographersdirect.com, (bottom) Picture Partners/Alamy; p.233 (top) Andrew Wakeford/Getty Images, (bottom) Image Source/ Alamy; p.234 (middle) Linda Matlow/Alamy, (bottom) Five Point Alliance; p.236 courtesy of John Rawson Partnership; p.237 (middle, bottom) courtesy of John Rawson Partnership; p.238 (bottom) courtesy of Denman; p.256 courtesy of Tigi; p.257 hair by Stephen Mackinder; p.259 Illustrated London News Ltd/Mary Evans Picture Library; p.260 courtesy of Great Lengths; p.261 (L) Five Point Alliance, (middle) Image Source/Alamy, (R) courtesy of Great Lengths; p.262 (top L) reproduced by kind permission of Cengage Learning, from *Hairdressing: The Foundations* 6th ed., Leo Palladino & Martin Green (2009: p.421), (bottom) Wella Professionals Soft & Lasting; p.268 (L) courtesy of Great Lengths, (middle) Bambu Productions/Getty Images, (R) Lori Andrews/Getty Images; p.270 (top) courtesy of Denman, (second) Timur Arbaev/iStockphoto, (third) Paul Gill/Hodder Education/Wella Professionals, (fourth) Paul Pedersen/Papsnap/Picture-That, photographersdirect.com, (bottom L) Gino Santa Maria/Fotolia, (bottom R) Indola; p.271 (top) courtesy of Denman, (second) Paul Pedersen/Papsnap/ Picture-That, photographersdirect.com/image used with the permission of D Macintyre & Son Ltd, (third) Tony Rusecki/Alamy, (fourth, fifth) courtesy of Goldwell, (bottom L) courtesy of Denman; p.272 (top) Francesco Group, (bottom) courtesy of Takara Belmont; p.273 courtesy of Goldwell; p.288 courtesy of Goldwell; p.290 Anthony Mascolo; p.293 Getty Images/Image Source; p.294 (top L) Cultura/Alamy, (second) Manabu Ogasawara/Getty Images, (third) blick-winkel/Alamy, (R) UpperCut Images/Alamy, (bottom L) ANK/Fotolia, (R) dk/Alamy; p. 295 (top L) Cultura/Alamy, (second) Manabu Ogasawara/Getty Images, (third) blickwinkel/Alamy, (R) UpperCut Images/Alamy, (bottom L) IMAGEMORE Co., Ltd/Getty Images, (R) Image Source/Alamy; p.296 (L) Somos/Veer/Getty Images, (R) Shalom Ormsby/Getty Images; p.298 (top) courtesy of Denman, (middle L) John Lee/Fotolia, (middle R) Paul Pedersen/Papsnap/Picture-That, photographersdirect.com, (bottom two) courtesy of Denman; p.299 courtesy of (bottom) Goldwell, (others) Denman; p.200 (L) Andrew Wakeford/Getty Images, (middle) DX/Fotolia, (R) Mediscan; p.301 Meonshore Studios Limited/Photographersdirect.com/Sebastian Professional; p.303 Scott Tilley/Alamy; p.306 (top L) Glowimages/Corbis, (top R) Pavel Sazonov/Fotolia, (bottom L) Lordsbaine/Fotolia, (bottom R) Eric Tormey/Alamy; pp.310–16 courtesy of City Boy; p.318 courtesy of Denman; p.320 Martyn f.Chillmaid/Wella Professional High Hair; pp.336–7 Adam Sloan at Big Yin Academy; p.327 Andres Rodriguez/Fotolia; p.334 Sally Brooks; p.335 Michael van Clarke salon team; p.337 Michael Van Clarke; p.340 (top L) Hodder Education, (top R) Ingram Publishing Limited, (bottom L) PurestockX.com, (bottom R) Robert Kneschke – Fotolia.com; p.342 Jamie Stevens, Errol Douglas and Karine Jackson, Karine Jackson Hair and Beauty; p.347 Debbie G; p.357 courtesy of Goldwell; p.358 courtesy of RUSH London; p.359 (L) courtesy of Great Lengths, (R) Francesco Group; p.361 Julie Eldrett; p.363 courtesy of Great Lengths; p.366 hair by Ross Taylor, Paul Falltrick Hairdressing; p.368 Akin Konizi.

All other photographs in this book are by Paul Gill and illustrations by Simon Tegg. Crown copyright material is reproduced with the permission of the Controller of HMSO and the Queen's Printer for Scotland.

Section 1
In the salon

Understanding the way a salon functions is essential to fully grasping your role within it. This section starts at reception – the first and last place a client will experience your salon in person. We begin by looking at the many ways in which a great reception service can positively influence the client journey and the overall salon business. We demonstrate how important reception duties are to the smooth running of the working day, and show you ways in which you can cultivate good reception habits. 'In the salon' goes on to illustrate that you only get one chance to make a great first impression, and provides you with lots of helpful tips and information on how to make it happen. This section finishes with health and safety – a hot topic in a profession that routinely handles sharps and chemicals, and where staff are constantly exposed to small but real risks. Learning health and safety procedures well now will lay a firm foundation for your career ahead.

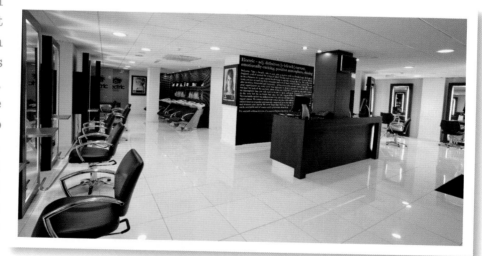

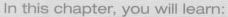

In this chapter, you will learn:

> **the skills to receive and welcome people as they enter your salon**
> **how to handle enquiries**
> **how to make appointments**
> **how to deal with client payments**
> **how to maintain a perfect reception area.**

You will be assessed against your knowledge and ability to:

1 Know your salon's services, products and pricing. Understand what your salon offers and the timing and pricing of services. Understand product literature, products and product offers.

2 Maintain the reception area. Keep it clean, stocked and ready to welcome clients, according to your salon policy.

3 Attend to clients and enquiries. Be prompt, polite and clear. Handle the needs of a number of people efficiently and ask relevant questions to identify their needs. Record messages, confirm appointments, be discreet and ask for help if required.

4 Communicate well. Understand the importance of great communication and know best practice. Adjust your communication and your attention to meet your audience needs.

5 Make appointments for salon services. Be fast, efficient and accurate. Balance the needs of the client, business and stylist effectively.

6 Make appointments. Follow correct policy and procedures and typical methods of taking appointments.

7 Calculate and process payments. Know the different methods of payment and how to handle them. Understand how to spot potential fraud, calculate payments and tackle client interactions on money-related issues.

8 Handle payments from clients. Be courteous and careful when handling payment, stick to your salon policies and keep good records. Handle rejected payments with tact.

9 Know your salon and legal requirements. Familiarise yourself with all relevant salon policies and government legislation. Handle data accurately.

Case study
More than meet and greet

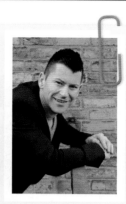

Barrie Stephen has four busy salons in the Leicester area, offering a premium standard of hairdressing in both city-centre and market-town settings.

'Experience has taught me that fabulous reception services are absolutely central to the success of a salon business. The job title "receptionist" implies someone that answers the phone so I've done away with the title and instead employed "Salon Coordinators". I've intentionally recruited people in this role with experience in restaurants and hotels because I think it's a great comparison for the kind of approach a salon should have to its clients.'

'My Salon Coordinators take their role very seriously and help the rest of my teams understand their own responsibilities toward the reception service. Every client or potential client that steps through my door will be greeted warmly by a member of my team. A stylist would never dream of leaving a client unattended if the Salon Coordinator was busy. All the stylists are familiar with the functions and processes required to run the reception area. The phones are answered with a warm corporate greeting, the waiting area is kept spotless and all the literature we need is kept orderly and close to hand. Equally my Salon Coordinators provide a crucial level of support to the stylists, helping them plan their day, organise their time and equipment and answer client queries, as well as supporting the retailing process by educating clients about products and securing that crucial rebooking of the appointment. Without doubt, great reception services have helped my business grow because my whole team have given it the focus and respect it deserves.'

Barrie Stephen, Managing Director, Barrie Stephen Hairdressing

Salon success starts here. The reception is the first (and the last) place your client will experience your salon and it's usually the hub of a bustling business. While your salon is likely to have dedicated reception staff, it's absolutely essential that, as a fully fledged team member, you are knowledgeable about all the processes and procedures required at reception and confident about running the desk and answering the phone.

Reception is the place where clients are first greeted, either in person or by phone, where clients wait to be seen, where lots of information is exchanged and records established and updated, where coats are taken and gowns put on, where retail is sold, where bills are paid, where tips are collected, where rebookings are made and where, finally, after what should have been the best salon experience they've had, the client is thanked before they leave. A cleanly kept, well-functioning and friendly salon reception will go a long way towards making a positive impression on clients and have a huge impact on the business, so never underestimate its value.

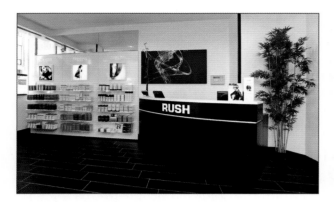

Spotless receptions make a difference

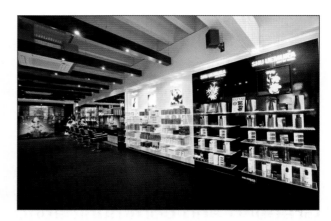

Well-kept retail units promote sales

Keep it clean

Like the rest of your salon, the reception should be spotless. You should pay attention to the following.

Floors and waiting area

Make sure that the floor is kept dry and clean. When the weather is bad this might be difficult, but mop and sweep throughout the day, as required, and put out safety signs if the floor becomes slippery. Keep the seating free of dirt and litter. Keep the coffee table clean of empty cups and glasses. Tidy and reorganise books and magazines regularly.

Retail area

Keep shelves free from dust and dirt. Dispose of bottles that have been tampered with or opened – unless of course it's a tester sample. Maintain the product display by making sure labels face outwards, spacing bottles evenly, bringing products to the front of the shelf and maintaining 'shelf talkers' (small price labels and product descriptions that are often clipped to the edge of the shelf).

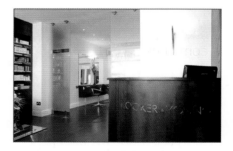

Reception desk

Reception desk

Keep the desk clean and orderly. This includes the staff surface, as well as the area of the desk used by clients. Keep polished surfaces clean of smudges.

Gown and coat cupboards

When you gown a client, check that the gown you are putting on them is fresh, and always place gowns that you take off clients in the salon laundry. If your salon runs a ticket system for the cloakroom, place each client's coat on a hangar and give them their ticket. If your salon offers secure storage for client belongings, store any items and give the key to the client. Should your client have a wet umbrella, store this somewhere where it will not cause the floor to become slippery.

Doors and windows

Make sure that glass doors and windows and all door handles are free of dirt and smears. If your salon has window displays, dust and check them daily to make sure they are in order and that pictures, posters and products have not faded in the sun.

You

Looking polished and presentable is part of every salon role, but as the first personal representative of your salon that a client will see, it's all the more important that you look flawless.

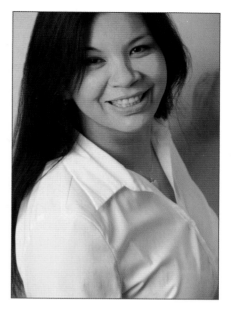

A warm welcome is essential

Greeting and communicating

Good communication is as important here as it is at every other point in your client's journey through your salon.

> Always acknowledge a client the moment they step through the door. If you are serving another client or speaking on the phone, remember that you can still take a few seconds to greet the newcomer with a warm smile and good eye contact.

> Keep all your interactions respectful, polite and friendly. Your body language should reflect a positive and friendly attitude. Never slouch or stand with your arms crossed. Stand or sit straight, with your shoulders back and your head up. Actively show you are listening by maintaining eye contact, leaning forward slightly, nodding where appropriate and summarising key points in what your client is saying.

> Adjust the way you speak and behave to accommodate each client. Use an even, clear tone of voice and make your communication appropriate to their age, social group and ability. If you receive any clients with disabilities (e.g. clients who are hearing or sight impaired, have learning disabilities or use a wheelchair), think carefully about how you can assist them respectfully.

> Find out your salon procedures on greeting people. You may have a script or a series of prompts to work to. Your salon manager may want the phone answered with the same greeting every time (e.g. 'Good morning. Electric Hairdressing. Sarah speaking. How can I help you?').

> Answer the phone with a smile – your caller will hear it in your voice.

> Quickly assess the caller's needs. They may be calling for a number of reasons, not just to make an appointment. They may have a service or price query; they may need hair or product advice; they might need directions to the salon or information about parking. Make sure you give your client your attention, listen carefully and do not interrupt. If a client or potential client walks into the salon, you should follow the same process to identify their needs quickly. Always summarise your understanding of their needs to show that you are listening and give them a chance to add further details.

> 'Read' your client (difficult over the phone, but still possible) – be sensitive to their body language, facial expression, eye contact, tone of voice and the vocabulary they are using. Frowning, fidgeting, sighing, crossed arms and tapping fingers may all be signs of anger or confusion. Ask open questions to understand how you can assist them further.

> Understand the full range of literature your salon offers so that you know which information is right for each enquiry.

> Keep everything you will need (e.g. note pad, appointment book, vouchers, receipts, pens, stapler) close to hand so that you can find them quickly and efficiently. When taking a message, write down who the message is for and who it is from, the time of the call, a contact number, the message itself and the action that is required (e.g. call back). Check your salon's policy on communicating messages. Are they placed in the stylist's column (their sequential list of clients for that day), handed to them at the workstation, posted in the staff room?

> If your salon uses email or text, make sure you check for messages regularly. Email may be a source of appointment or information requests, especially if messages are fed through from the salon's website. Deal with these requests as promptly as your workload permits.

> While each client is waiting, make them as comfortable as possible and find out what your salon's policy is on customer service in reception. Invite them to take a seat, offer them access to magazines or coffee-table books, and, if possible, offer them some refreshment from the salon menu.

> If a client makes a complaint in person, acknowledge their dissatisfaction in a respectful way. Keep calm and do not raise your voice or allow your body language to become defensive (e.g. crossing your arms). Listen without interrupting, use eye contact, nod appropriately and summarise briefly when they have finished speaking. Tell the client that you will ask the relevant staff member to speak with them and then contact that team member promptly. If the relevant team member isn't available, involve your salon manager or supervisor. There is more information on dealing with complaints in Unit G17 (Give clients a positive impression of yourself and your business).

Managing and sharing information

Reception is where most clients will first seek information about the salon and its services, where most information about clients will be collated, and where staff receive their daily schedules and greet their clients. A great deal of information is exchanged here.

> Take the time to learn everything about the services and products your salon offers. Learn what each service is and when it's appropriate, understand the time it will take to conduct the service and the price. If the service is POA (price on application)

<table>
<tr><td>Activity</td></tr>
</table>

Calculate the following:

1 How long will it take for a shine treatment, half-head highlights and a cut and blow-dry?

2 In which order should the services be scheduled?

3 How much would the total bill come to with a mid-range stylist in your salon? (Alternatively, use a price list from a local salon.)

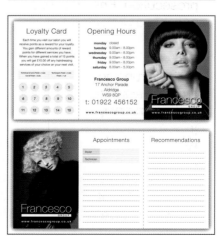

Get to know all the literature available

or price on consultation, learn the range in which the service can fall and why it's different for different people (e.g. hair length). Understand the products you retail and for whom they are appropriate.

> Think carefully about each of the professionals within your salon. Think about the prices they charge, the type of work they excel at and the type of personality they have. Then do your best to match clients who have not been recommended to a specific stylist with the one that is best suited to them. Good rapport between client and stylist will increase the probability of the client rebooking.

> Keep your reception area stocked with all the relevant information you need, such as price lists, product leaflets, new offers, newsletters and 'recommend a friend' cards.

> Keep at least two days' supply of reception stationery topped up and close to hand. Stationery might include:
    > appointment cards
    > headed paper
    > compliment slips
    > tip envelopes
    > client record cards
    > business cards
    > receipt books
    > gift vouchers and envelopes
    > client feedback questionnaires.

> Take each client's details for collation into the salon database. You need to treat the information in accordance with the Data Protection Act 1998 (see Unit G17 for a summary of the Act). Keep client information confidential. Do not leave any client record cards in open view and use your discretion when it comes to sharing client information. Only share client information with relevant staff and your supervisor or salon manager. The Data Protection Act is a matter of law and its misuse can mean prosecution. Ensure your salon database and client records are password protected and input the data with great care to ensure accuracy.

> Be a good liaison point between the client and their stylist. If the stylist is running late, politely inform the client and apologise for the inconvenience. Equally, if the client calls and lets you know they are running late, make sure you inform their stylist.

> If you have specialists on your team, such as colourists and beauticians, and you are presented with a query that you feel unqualified to answer, explain that you would like to refer the client to an expert and ask them to wait. Promptly contact the relevant member of staff. For all other enquiries that you feel unqualified to answer, involve your salon manager or supervisor.

Scheduling appointments

Salon appointment systems effectively run the business. Whether it's a book or a sophisticated computer system, it will require effective management, perfect information input and efficient booking processes and procedures.

> Your salon appointment system has a number of purposes (some only apply to computerised systems), including the following:
>> efficient use of staff time
>> scheduling staff and resources
>> monitoring and forecasting the flow of business
>> efficiently serving client needs
>> collating client data, including contact details, services purchased and products purchased
>> targeting clients for marketing purposes
>> communicating effectively with clients
>> monitoring stock sales and interacting with the stock system
>> providing clear and precise information on the day-to-day demands of the business
>> keeping financial sales data
>> monitoring promotions and commissions
>> collating reports.

> Find out your salon's abbreviations for services and people (e.g. NC – new client, NTS – new to stylist, CBD – cut and blow-dry).

> Correctly identifying each client's needs takes practice, but asking plenty of open questions (those that require an explanatory answer) will help you. A client may not know the correct name for the service or technique they want, but they will know the type of look they want.

> Learn the length of time it takes to conduct different services and in what order they should be conducted (e.g. treatment, full-head highlights, cut and blow-dry). This will ensure that clients are not kept waiting and staff are not left with spaces in their client column or appointment list that could have been put to better use.

> Learn the price for each service and the price level that each of your team members is on. If necessary, create a 'quick glance' grid of the information to help you.

> If you are using a written system, write very clearly and neatly, logging all the information in the spaces provided.

> If the client doesn't ask for a specific day or time, ask questions to help them. 'Which day of the week is best for you? Mondays are the best day to come if you don't like hustle and bustle, as later in the week it is very busy.' 'What time of day is most convenient for you?'

> Where possible, offer the client a choice of appointment times.

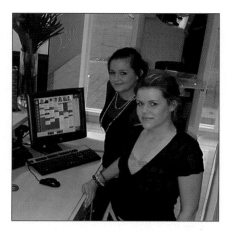

Computer-based salon appointment system

Always respond promptly to requests for appointment by phone, email or in person. If your reception is very busy, with paying and waiting clients and the phone is ringing, try to excuse yourself momentarily to pick up the phone and acknowledge the call, and either ask the caller to hold or take a number to call them back. Make sure you attend to all clients as quickly as possible.

> If the client is having colour, explain the skin test process to them and ask them to drop by at least 24 hours before their planned appointment (see Unit GH9 and Unit G7 for more information on skin testing).

> Log the date and time, the stylist, the service, the name and the full contact details of the client. Some salons find it helpful to log the fact that the client is new or is an existing client who is new to the stylist, and so on. Find out your salon's policy.

> Summarise the details of the booking for your client. If they are present, write them down on a card for them to take away for their records.

> Be sensitive to the fact that staff will need breaks and book sensibly. Overbooking, double booking, badly scheduled appointments that cause bottlenecks and wrongly booked appointments will quickly see the day descend into chaos. Staff will become frustrated and stressed and clients will have cause for complaint.

> If you are in any doubt, turn to a team member or your supervisor/salon manager for help. A client will appreciate you seeking help to meet their needs rather than ignoring the problem or failing to serve them correctly.

> If a client walks in without an appointment, do your very best to accommodate them, be understanding if they are disappointed and try to book them in as soon as possible.

> If a client arrives late, quickly assess the options. Are they still early enough to have the service without impacting on the next client or the quality of their own experience? Is there another stylist available who can help them immediately? Give the late client all the ideas and options promptly and politely. Never let them feel victimised or embarrassed because of their lateness.

> If a staff member is unable to come to work or is taken ill and leaves for the day, you should immediately set about contacting all their clients and rescheduling. This is why it is so important to get mobile, email, work and home contacts, so that clients aren't disappointed. Consider if you can offer them the same time/same day with another stylist.

Taking payment

Taking payment and handling the financial aspects of every appointment is essential to an efficient reception area and a successful salon. Wrongly calculating bills, giving the wrong change, overcharging clients, accepting counterfeit money or fraudulent

Activity

1 Create a mock column of four stylists with 45-minute appointments.

2 Schedule 22 clients, making sure that you leave your stylists room for breaks.

3 Schedule 2 sets of highlights with a cut and blow-dry, 7 blow-drys, 8 full-head tints, 4 of which include a cut and blow-dry, 3 salon treatments and 12 further cut and blow-drys.

cards will all result in a loss of funds for the business. There are many things to consider when taking payment.

Till types

Cash box

This is a lockable box, with sub-compartments for coins and a space beneath the coin tray for notes. A cash box is usually accompanied by a cash book to manually log sales.

Electronic till or cash register

An electronic till has many buttons and functions that can be programmed to represent services, commission rates and discounts and a variety of values. The till can calculate totals and change, and give running totals during the day and a total for close of business (at the end of the day). The till drawer will open once the transaction total is calculated.

Computerised till

This is part of the computerised salon management system. The keyboard and monitor often sit on the desk, while the drawer sits below it, offering extra security. This much more sophisticated system often has a touch screen and will automatically calculate bills and totals. The computerised till can produce many summaries and reports at the touch of a button (e.g. treatments sold today, revenue total for Sarah).

Payment methods

Cash

While the vast majority of payments will be electronic, cash payments will require you to keep a cash drawer or till and a float. A float is a sum of money in a variety of denominations that remains in the till to allow you to make change. The float is 'extra' to the amount transacted and should be removed at the end of the day before the cash transactions are counted. A float will include notes and coins. If the float denominations dwindle, you should alert your supervisor or salon manager, as a member of staff may need to go to the bank for more change.

Gift vouchers

Your salon will almost certainly offer gift vouchers that can be exchanged for services to the face value of the voucher. Change cannot be given, so recommend that the service chosen exceeds the value of the voucher and is topped up with another payment method. Log the voucher as redeemed in your salon's records and put the voucher in the till, along with any cash.

Traveller's cheques

Traveller's cheques are a safe way of moving money. They are the equivalent of cash and are guaranteed by the bank if lost or stolen.

Top Tip

Calculating correct payment is an essential part of reception duties. If you do not have access to an electronic or computerised system, use a calculator, pen and paper or even the application on your phone. Miscalculating either the total or the change given will upset the client and lose money for the salon.

Top Tip

Always place the money the client has given you at the edge of the till to prevent you from losing track of the change required.

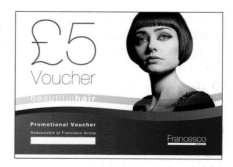

Salon gift vouchers

Check to see if your salon accepts traveller's cheques. If it does, only accept traveller's cheques that are presented in pounds sterling (GBP), as this will avoid any currency exchange problems.

Cheque

Ensure that all cheques are correctly written and signed. Find out the exact wording that should go next to 'Pay' for the salon and inform the client. Ensure that cheques bear the correct date and amount in a legible hand and that they are signed. The amount written in figures must match the amount written in words. Every cheque must be accompanied by a cheque guarantee card. There is an amount limit, usually £100, inscribed in the hologram motif. The cheque should not exceed this amount. The sort code, name and account numbers on the card should match those on the cheque, and the date the cheque will be redeemed must be within the card's validity dates. If the service total exceeds the guaranteed sum, ask the client to write cheques that are below the guaranteed sum to total the amount.

Card payments

All card payments require a chip and PIN except for Cardholder Not Present (CNP) transactions. For these, you will require the card type, the long number on the front of the card, the valid from and to dates, the name as it appears on the card and the final three-digit security code on the back of the card. You should check your salon's policy on CNP transactions. All cards will have the chip read through a PDQ (process data quickly) machine, which is an electronic terminal that connects to the bank over the internet. Your salon should also keep a manual imprinter and imprint slips to ensure you are covered in the event of a power cut or the telephone connection being lost.

Debit cards

These behave like cheques, but are debited directly from a client's current account and credited to the salon's business account. Switch, Maestro, Delta, Electron, Visa debit and Solo are all examples of the types of systems that debit cards use. The card's chip will be read through the PDQ machine and the client will need to enter their PIN (personal identification number).

Credit cards

Typically Visa or MasterCard, payment with these cards levies a charge on the salon, so make sure you get to know which ones are accepted in your salon. All card transactions now require chip and PIN, so if your client cannot remember their PIN you will not be able to make the transaction. The card has a maximum limit of credit which cannot be exceeded.

Charge cards

Cards like American Express must be settled in full monthly. Once again, use of these cards levies a charge against the salon by the card operator, so check beforehand which cards are accepted.

Activity

1 Research the different signs for the cards described here and note if each one is a charge card, credit card or debit card.

2 Find out which payment types your salon accepts.

Preventing fraud

For every payment type, including cash, there is a risk of fraud or counterfeit. Card fraud is by far the fastest growing type. To avoid fraud of all kinds you need to consider the following.

Cash

> Does the note 'feel' right? Often counterfeiters are unable to reproduce the quality of paper.
> Is there a continuous metal strip on one side that shows a shiny in-and-out weave on the other?
> Is there a hologram present that shows the denomination which matches the value of the note?
> Is there a watermark of the Queen?
> Make sure that the note is in GBP (Scottish notes are legal tender throughout the UK). Euros might be accepted by some salons, but find out your salon's policy and contact your salon manager for every euro transaction.

Cheques

Did you see the client write and sign the cheque? If not, ask them to sign another piece of plain paper and compare this signature with the one that appears on the cheque guarantee card and the one that appears on the cheque signature strip. If you do not recognise the issuing bank (e.g. Lloyds, Barclays, Santander) or the cheque feels wrong in some way, contact your supervisor or salon manager for reassurance.

Cards

Every card issuer has a 24-hour helpline for traders and a complete training pack of information. If you are in any doubt concerning either the ownership or the validity of the card, phone the number on the back of the card. Cards should meet the following criteria:

> be undamaged, with all electronic chips, magnetic strips, lettering and numerals, signature strip and hologram intact
> be within the validity dates
> be chip and PIN protected – the client should know the PIN in order to process the transaction
> carry the card member's name legibly – check the name of the card against the name of the client who has had the service (it is conceivable that they have been authorised to use a card that does not bear their name, but it's worth checking)
> all ID numbers should be present and legible – the long number across the card front, the validity dates and the security ID number at the end of the signature strip on the reverse
> the signature strip should be signed and legible
> the hologram should carry the recognised mark of the card issuer – check your salon reference material for an example.

Card authorisations

Card issuers will issue an authorisation code for every transaction. To obtain an authorisation code, you need to process the payment according to the card issuer's requirements.

Processing payments

Check that the terminal is on and in sale mode. Insert the card into the card reader, chip side up, and enter the correct amount for the total transaction. Pressing ENTER will connect you to the card company. After a few moments, a prompt will require the client to enter their PIN number. Allow the client an element of privacy to do this. The payment will either be authorised or declined. The receipt issued by the card reader will carry the relevant codes.

If the authorised amount is exceeded or the cardholder or the card are in any way suspicious, call the authorisation number to speak to the card issuer.

Retaining cards

In some cases, the card issuer may ask you to retain the card. In this instance, you must follow your salon's policy, but in all cases, place the card with all receipts in an envelope for return to the card company. Remain firm but polite and never put yourself at risk from abuse.

Code '10' authorisation calls

These calls are made in instances when you suspect the authenticity or validity of a card or the card is unsigned. Call the number of the card issuer given on the back of the card and follow the electronic prompts.

> **Activity** Name ten things that would make you suspicious about a method of payment.

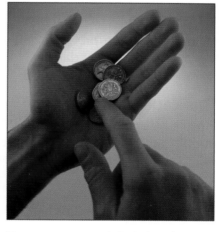

Tips are common in hairdressing

Handling tips

Tips are a recognised part of staff remuneration. A client will sometimes hand tips directly to the staff member, but more often they will leave them in the care of reception when they pay. Clients may tip just their stylist or every member of staff who has attended to them, including the apprentice. Find out your salon's policy on tips.

Receiving tips

Thank the client on the staff member's behalf.

Caring for tips

Place the tips in an envelope and clearly mark the envelope with the name of the staff member and the name of the client, then place the envelope in the till or cash drawer.

Top Tip

Tips represent a taxable part of your income and should be declared. Talk to your salon manager or supervisor about declaring tips.

Retail

Product sales don't happen at reception; they are a natural outcome of a positive hairdresser–client relationship. The client will have been educated throughout their visit on the type of care products that are appropriate to their hair type and the type of styling products they will need to care for their hair between visits. Reception plays a role in offering clients the opportunity to purchase products.

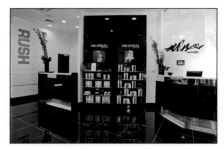

Home hair care is important to customer service

Be informed

Clients may arrive at reception with questions about price, availability and product ingredients. Know your products well and be able to define the main benefits and results they will achieve. Hold the product as you talk about it and encourage your client to smell the scent or feel the texture of the formulas.

Speak up

Do not assume that if the client isn't asking for a product they don't want it or cannot afford it. Offer every client the opportunity to purchase products. You could remind them of the products that were used on their hair that day and tell them they are a great way to keep their hair looking good between visits.

Check the product

Before packaging products and giving them to the client, examine them for any signs of damage, cracks, fading from exposure to sun, leaking or prior use.

Package well

Beautiful packaging adds value. Where available, ensure that products are placed in the correctly sized bag and nicely presented. Product manufacturers may offer their own branded bags for use.

Add to the bill

Ensure that product sales are added to the bill and the sale is logged against the correct member of staff, so that all commission is calculated correctly and passed on.

Communication when taking payment

Clear and accurate communication is important to ensuring that payment processes run smoothly. There may be instances in which you need to communicate sensitive information. Always remain polite and calm. Consider the following points.

Check for understanding

Ask your client if they are ready to pay and if they have everything they need for their visit that day.

Rebooking

Ask the client when their stylist recommended they return in order to maintain their style and offer to book a future appointment. If the client does not have their diary, offer to arrange a time at which it is convenient to call them to book the appointment.

Asking for payment

When a client 'checks out', total their bill accurately and clearly state the amount due. If your client is at all concerned or confused, offer to talk them through an itemised list of services on their bill and tell them how you arrived at the total. Ask how they will be paying (e.g. cash, credit card, cheque, debit card).

Check and recheck

Accuracy is key. Make sure that you give the correct change for cash; that cheques are correctly written and that you log the guarantee card; that PDQ amounts are correctly inputted and that the client has checked them.

Discrepancies

You will need to notify your salon manager if there are discrepancies in the till transactions at the end of any trading period. You will also need to notify your salon manager if you discover theft, fraud or illegalities. Your salon manager may involve the authorities. Be prompt in notifying the right staff member of any difficulties.

When authorisation is denied

If your client's card is rejected or they are unable to supply a guarantee card with a cheque, inform them politely and discreetly. Ask if the client would like to offer an alternative method of payment, and if you do not suspect fraud, return the card or cheque. Your client may be genuinely shocked and distressed, so be sensitive and, if necessary, call the credit card company on their behalf. Be discreet, but do not leave the reception area unattended to speak to a client.

Record logs

It is essential that you keep good records of every transaction and offer them to your clients.

Till receipts

Till receipts can be issued by your electronic till or computerised salon system. The system will log the transaction for the salon records and the client can receive a copy of the receipt.

Cash book

A cash box is usually accompanied by a cash book to manually log sales.

> **Activity** When you make a purchase in a store, note the process the cashier uses. Watch as they handle payment for other customers and see if you can spot opportunities for improvement in the following areas:
> - body language and tone
> - keeping the desk tidy
> - answering questions and providing information.

PDQ receipts

Make sure the receipt rolls on your PDQ machine do not run out. Most rolls are marked with a pink strip when they are nearing the end, so keep an eye out for it. If your receipt roll runs out and the transaction has been processed, there will be no record for your till or for your client.

Administration and marketing

There are lots of tasks that take place at the reception desk that assist in the smooth running of the salon and in helping to grow the business.

> Input all new client records and review existing ones. It's important to keep records up to date and store essential information, such as contact details, tint formulas, hair and scalp health, so that you have them to refer to at another time.

> If your salon uses text services, you may be required to set up text reminders for appointments, messages on offers and promotions, and alerts on newly available appointment times.

> Scheduling information on staff shifts and holidays must be entered into books and computer systems. You may also be asked to provide data to help your team members create the schedules.

> Any letters to clients will more than likely be sent out from reception, so you should know how to fold letters professionally and make sure they are dispatched promptly.

> Client questionnaires and research could well fall within the responsibilities of reception. Everything from asking how a client heard about the salon as they book, to inviting them to complete a questionnaire before they leave the salon, provides a rich source of information for your salon manager, to help him/her shape the business. Reception may also be responsible for follow-up service calls – a phone call to the client a few days after their visit to ask how satisfied they were with their experience and their hair.

> Current promotions will be managed at reception, as most promotions will give the client something (either money off or a gift with purchase) as they exit the salon. Learn your salon's policies on logging each response, as the information will help your salon manager to run effective marketing and promotions in the future.

> Running reports from the salon software will give your salon manager lots of business information. Each software system will offer a wide variety of reports, from 'average bill' to number of retail units sold.

> Your manual or computerised stock system will allow you to calculate stock levels and help with running stock checks – yet another task that frequently falls to reception.

Security

The reception area is a busy place that is vulnerable to crime. There are simple precautions you can take to avoid it.

> Never leave reception unattended. If you need to leave the reception area for any reason, ask an available and qualified member of staff to step in for a few moments.

> Intruders or clients with threatening behaviour should be reported immediately to your salon manager or supervisor. If you think you are at serious risk of harm and you are in a position to do so, dial 999 and ask for the police.

> Keep tills closed, cash boxes locked and secured and charity collection boxes in a visible place. Keep salon keys and any valuables either locked or shut away from public view.

> Don't keep excessive amounts of cash in the till and make regular trips to the bank. Vary the times you leave the salon with cash, to avoid theft.

> At night, before locking the salon, empty the cash drawer in the till or remove the cash box and place it in the safe. Make sure that you follow the salon's policy. Leave the till drawer open so that potential burglars can see that no cash is available.

> Leave the salon's 'night lights' on to discourage break-ins.

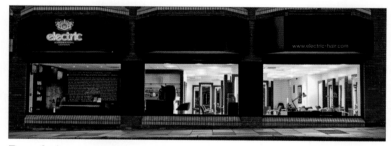

Be safe, be secure

Preparing the reception area

Below is a simple checklist to help you start your day on reception.

> Make sure the reception desk, waiting area and retail area are tidy and free of dust and dirt.

> Switch on the computer and cue the salon appointment system or set up your appointment book.

> Check email and messages sent and left overnight.

> Check that the reception desk is stocked with all the relevant literature.

> Check that you have enough clean gowns and hangers for the day.

> Switch off the telephone system's night service.

> Unlock the doors.

The law

At reception, you should act in accordance with the following laws.

Data Protection Act (1998)

(See Unit G17 for a summary of the Act.)

Sale of Goods and Services Act (1980)

This Act protects the consumer's purchasing rights. In summary, it states that:

> the goods and services must be of an acceptable quality

> the goods and services must be fit for purpose

> the goods and services must be as described in marketing literature, advertising, labelling and by staff.

Trade Description Act (1968)

The law requires that any descriptions of goods and services given by a person acting in the course of a trade or business should be accurate and not misleading. You may not:

> apply a false or misleading description to goods by written or verbal means

> supply or offer to supply goods to which a false or misleading trade description is applied.

Summary

Understanding how a salon reception is run effectively and efficiently, and contributing to its success, will benefit your entire team and salon business. The reception area provides many opportunities to enhance the overall experience, but also to deliver a great first and last impression on the customer. Never underestimate the importance of either a superb reception service or your responsibility to make it happen. From answering the phone with a smile in your voice, to opening the door for a client and thanking them as they leave, great salon reception service demands vigilance and a commitment to customer satisfaction.

G17: Give clients a positive impression of yourself and your salon

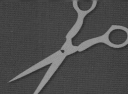

In this chapter, you will learn:

> **the key elements of great communication and how to build rapport**
> **how to provide exceptional customer service**
> **how to be proactive in responding to your customer's needs and wants.**

You will be assessed against your knowledge and ability to:

1 Meet your salon's requirements of appearance and behaviour.

2 Understand your salon's guidelines and procedures on handling customers.

3 Greet clients well, with manners and respect.

4 Assess and respond to a client's needs and expectations effectively and efficiently.

5 Keep clients informed and involved in their service, and observe their comfort levels and body language.

6 Communicate flexibly, source the right information and understand when you should ask for help and to whom you should turn.

From the moment a client calls to make an appointment, to the moment they pay and leave the salon, they are making constant assessments about your salon and about you. There may be many reasons why a client ends up in your styling chair and in your salon, which might include reputation and recommendation, or simply that it looks like 'their kind of place'. Whatever the reason, once they visit you, it will be you that makes the largest difference with regard to whether or not they will return. As a hair professional, your client is buying into 'the brand of you' – you are basically a business within a business. A good impact, great hairdressing and a positive service experience will not only encourage your client to return, it will also make them more likely to recommend you to their friends. Put effort into giving your clients an exceptional salon experience and it won't only greatly benefit you, it will benefit the reputation of the entire salon.

There are many elements to creating a positive impression of yourself and your salon. No single one will give you overall good results. You need to consider everything that influences a client's opinion and work on all of them.

Activity Look at the team members in your salon or the fellow students in your class. Select a good example of a positive salon appearance and explain why. Then select an example of someone whose appearance can be improved and explain why. Be positive when sharing feedback.

Your appearance

Looking (and smelling!) appropriate will help people to make the right judgements about you. Our industry is all about appearances, and when you are advising and helping your clients to achieve their personal best, you need to walk the talk!

> Dress appropriately for the type of salon in which you work. A youthful business will demand a trend-driven image, while a local barber's may require something more classic.

> If your salon has a uniform policy or even a clothing colour policy (e.g. everyone dresses in black and/or white), make sure you follow it.

> Your hair will be under scrutiny from your client. They will find it easier to trust your judgement if your hair looks its best. Think about the condition, maintenance and finish every day – it's what you do for your clients, so make sure you do it for yourself.

> Wear clothes that are right for the season and the work that you do. Getting hot and sweaty isn't good for you or your clients.

> Make sure shoes are comfortable and appropriate because you will be on your feet nearly the whole day.

> Ensure accessories such as scarves, long necklaces, earrings, rings and bracelets are not likely to snag on the clients' clothes or hair, or interfere with your work.

> Keep clean, use scents and deodorants, but don't overdo it! Wash and dry your hands thoroughly between clients to avoid dermatitis and skin complaints. Where appropriate, use a good hand cream or moisturiser. For more information, go to the Bad Hand Day Campaign (www.hse.gov.uk/hairdressing).

> Keep your hands and nails well manicured. Your hands will often be the focus for a client as you touch your client constantly. Protect your skin, using moisturisers, gloves and barrier creams to avoid dry skin, dermatitis and infections.

> Use teeth cleaning, mouthwashes, mints or breath fresheners to maintain good oral hygiene. You are in close contact with your client and strong or bad breath odours will offend.

> Don't smoke, or if you do, try to leave enough time before greeting your client to wash your hands and clean your teeth or freshen your breath. Cigarette smoke lingers on your clothes, hands, breath and in your hair, and it's definitely not a scent that you want your clients to associate with their salon experience.

> Your posture is important for health reasons, because good posture will prevent strain and injury from the sustained movement and standing required by hairdressing. Posture will also communicate a lot about you to your client. Good posture will illustrate pride, energy and confidence, while slouching and dragging your feet will make you look less than the professional you are.

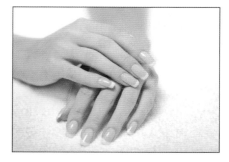

Your clients will appreciate well-kept hands

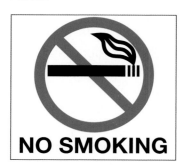

Make sure your clients don't suffer from your smoking habit

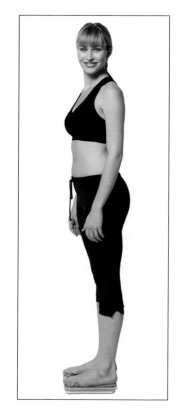

Good posture is healthy and looks good too

Case study
It's not all hair

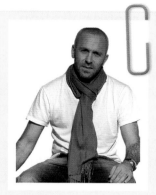

Edward Hemmings is Director of Alan d, the largest private provider of work-based NVQ education in the London area. The academy guides the NVQ careers of hundreds of trainees each year.

'We surprise our trainees by telling them that the actual cut, colour and finish in hairdressing will be a relatively small part of their job. Making a client feel special and important is really what we do. Focusing on a great attitude and a service-oriented mindset will empower you to give a little more than a client really expects and they will remember you for it. A hairdresser with a great technical standard who leaves a bad impression on the client won't be rewarded with that client's loyalty and business. We train our NVQ learners to the standard that would be expected in a salon charging £100 because we know that once this benchmark has been achieved then it's easy for a young professional to give a great first impression. We train them to put the client, not their hair, at the centre of the service. Doing that will mean that the focus is on delivering the experience rather than the cut, colour or finish.'

Edward Hemmings, Education Director, Alan d Academy

Your communication

Great communication enables great hairdressing and great customer service. Your ability to listen, ask good questions, share information and ideas, negotiate, reassure and understand correctly will lie at the centre of your development as a professional. Every client who comes to you will have a unique set of needs and desires. By listening and obviously taking clear steps to meet those needs and desires, you will create an overwhelmingly positive impression.

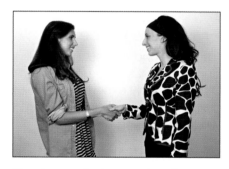

Greet your clients warmly, with genuine feeling

Greet well

When you greet each client, walk towards them with a natural, welcoming smile and seek out eye contact. Use open, relaxed body language (i.e. with your arms loosely at your sides, palms turned slightly forward). If appropriate, shake hands or briefly rest your hand on their upper arm to establish natural physical contact.

Name game

Call your client by their name and introduce yourself. Remember their name and use it again through the service. Never refer to the client as 'my client' or 'my lady/gentleman'.

The consultation

The consultation is one of the most important interactions you will have with your client. This is the point at which you will quickly build rapport and establish your credentials as a trustworthy professional. Unit G7 examines the consultation in depth, with many suggestions for positive body language and open questions (i.e. questions that require explanatory answers).

Do not rush the consultation. Take your time and let the client share all the information and concerns they might have about their hair and their visit. Use visual tools, such as colour swatches and magazines, to help you both achieve a common understanding. Maintain eye contact and, when appropriate, sit beside your client to discuss their visit. Look carefully at their clothes and accessories, ask questions about their lifestyle and the way they currently care for their hair. Examine their face, body shape and colouring to help you to offer them ideas. Thoroughly examine the health of their hair and scalp.

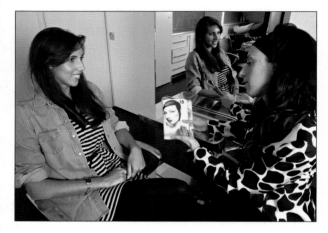

A great consultation starts with great communication

At the end of the consultation, always summarise and check your understanding. Be sensitive to the fact that your client may feel nervous about any dramatic changes. A thoughtful consultation is a powerful way to make your client feel valued and respected.

Frame the process

It's useful and reassuring to talk your client through what will happen during their visit. The client journey in your salon may be different to that previously experienced. Tell the client about the different areas of the salon they will visit and introduce them by name to the staff who will be attending to them.

Pay attention

Communication is a two-way process, so pay attention to your client's body language as well as the words they speak. Be sensitive to tone and choice of words, and look at their eyes and face so that you can interpret their expressions. If you see your client fidgeting, crossing their arms and/or legs, looking uncomfortable, tugging at their hair or ears or avoiding eye contact, then it's likely that they are unhappy about some aspect of their treatment or service. Asking a simple open question, such as 'How are you feeling now?' will help to draw out the source of the problem so that you can address it. Never ignore these signs! An ignored problem will only get worse.

Speak well

The language you use and your tone of voice can help to make a positive impression. Your salon may have guidelines on how you refer to clients, team members and services, so take the time to find out what these are (e.g. some salons refer to clients as 'guests'). Adjust your communication to suit your client. Keep slang and buzz words to a minimum, unless your client uses them first. Ensure that you never swear, and always use words that are appropriate to your client's age and social network. Use adjectives (descriptive words), but also make sure that you are clear on key points, such as length, texture and shade. There are lots of terms in common usage, such as layered, graduated and feathered, which may have a completely different meaning for the client than they do for you. Ensure that your client shares your view of these techniques and use pictures where necessary. Use a clear tone of voice at a comfortable pitch. Feel free to communicate energy and enthusiasm. Mumbling and very quiet voices will make the client feel that you lack confidence, while a high-pitched tone will feel nervous or aggressive.

Your expertise

Demonstrate your skills

Having good skills isn't enough in itself to provide great hairdressing service. You need to be able to demonstrate that skill clearly, share knowledge and information, be open and honest at all times and work effectively as part of a salon team. Your client will feel more relaxed in your care and trust your judgement with confidence if you can achieve these things.

Prepare yourself

Familiarise yourself with your clients before they arrive. At least take a list of their names and, if they are not a new client, get to know the types of services and products they have purchased in your salon on previous visits.

Prepare your client

> Help your client out of their coat and hang it up.
> Help your client into a clean and neatly pressed gown and fasten the ties or Velcro to protect their clothes.
> If your client is wearing a polo neck or high collar, offer to show them to a changing room or toilet to allow them to remove it and put on the gown.
> If the salon has locker storage and the client has bags, offer to store them in a secure place during their visit.
> For colour clients, use a dark or colour-resistant tinting gown, carefully place a towel around their neck and shoulders, and secure the towel at the front with a plastic hair claw. If you notice any stains on a client's clothes before you gown them, tactfully point them out to the client. You do not want to be held responsible afterwards for staining clothes with tint or product.
> Seat your client in the consultation area.
> Loosen the hair with the fingers and then brush or comb through,

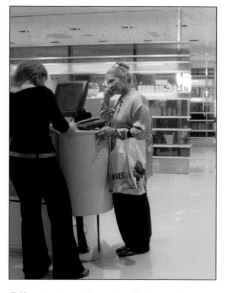

Offer to store the client's bags in a secure place

using the right tool for their hair length and texture. Be careful to remove tangles without tugging or pulling on the client's scalp. If necessary, hold the hair with one hand, above the tangle, to prevent tension.

> Conduct a full and thorough consultation.

> Introduce your client to other team members who will be attending to them during their appointment, and guide your client to the shampoo or tinting area.

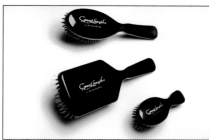

Protect your client and their clothes

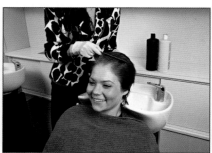

Check your client is comfortable

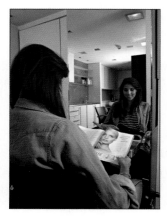

Offer your client magazines

Know your equipment

Use your combs, brushes and scissors appropriately to create the look that you have agreed on with the client. (For more information about tool choice, go to Unit GH12, where you will find a comprehensive list of tools and their uses.)

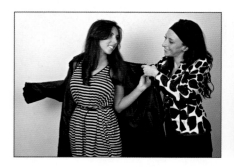
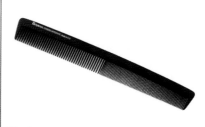
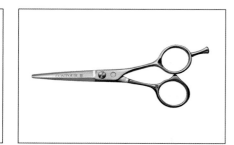

Salon equipment

Know your services

Talking knowledgeably about the range of services your salon offers will not only show you to be a well-rounded professional, but may also get a client interested in purchasing more. Colour services, treatments, extensions, nail services, hair up and beauty may all be included in your salon's service menu. Be clear and honest about pricing; never add a price-bearing service to a client's bill without their full knowledge and consent. Keep a price list or service menu close to hand, so that you can quickly check on the range, description and price of every service.

Share your knowledge

It's a great idea to tell clients what you are doing. Tell them why the shape and colour selected suits them. Tell them what the techniques used will do for them. Tell them how the care and styling products recommended to them will help them achieve the look at home, and tell them when they need to return to keep their hair looking its best. Sometimes clients express a desire for shapes, textures or colours that will not suit them. Use your knowledge to tell them tactfully why there are better choices available. Be sensitive, as they may have set their heart on their hair looking just like their favourite celebrity's.

Answer questions

If a client asks you a question, you are lucky. They are handing you a golden opportunity to meet their needs and show yourself as an expert. Answer their queries and requests promptly and respectfully, and if you don't have the information to hand, excuse yourself and ask a colleague.

Involve others

Your client will appreciate it more if you involve a colleague on any subject than if you try to deal with situations that are outside your area of expertise. If your salon has dedicated colourists, trichologists, extensions experts or beauticians, and your client has a need or request in their area, make sure you involve them promptly. Introduce your colleague to the client by name and give them space and time to discuss the issue.

Your conduct

A lot about the way clients perceive their visit will be connected to your demeanour and the atmosphere in the salon. Take the trouble to find out your salon guidelines on conduct and behaviour, and ask what processes and procedures are in place to guide you.

Be attentive

Concern yourself with your client's comfort. Check that they are sitting comfortably. (See Unit G20 for more information.) Ask if your client would like some refreshment and, if available, bring them a refreshment menu. Ask if your client would like any magazines to read and, if so, what type. Make sure that magazines are current and in good condition.

Remember, remember

Try hard to remember details about your client and their lives (e.g. if they have children, what kind of work they do, major events in their

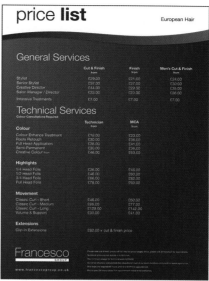

Talk knowledgably about the services you offer

lives). Your client will feel valued as an individual and know that you take an interest in them as such.

Excuse me!

Do not answer your mobile, talk over the client or take your attention away from them for any reason other than absolute necessity. If you must interrupt their service, excuse yourself respectfully and tell them how long you will be.

Say what?

Always be polite and respectful, even if your client isn't. Learn to read your client's body language and conversation, and make a judgement about whether they want to chat or whether they want to sit in peace and quietly enjoy their service. This takes practice, and learning when not to speak is a very useful skill. Do not chat with your colleagues around your workstation unless it is a conversation in which your client is involved.

Team talk

A good atmosphere is one of the reasons that is often quoted by clients in their choice of salon. How you and your colleagues communicate between you will contribute greatly to the salon atmosphere. If you are as respectful, kind, warm and helpful to one another as you should be to your clients, you will create a positive impression.

Appropriate behaviour

Do not engage in or allow to go unchecked behaviour that is inappropriate or sexual in nature, whether this is directed to a team member or a client. Report any behaviour you have witnessed or experienced to your supervisor or salon manager. Only touch your clients in ways that are relevant to the service you are providing, and do not either initiate or get drawn into discussions that might be deemed inappropriate. Do not gossip about other clients or your teammates – your client will feel that you are untrustworthy and may well be gossiping about them too.

Handling difficult client interactions

If your client is unhappy or upset about any aspect of their service, either while they are in the salon or once they have returned home, you need to ensure that you do everything you can to turn a negative situation into a positive outcome for your client, yourself and your salon.

> Read the signs by watching your client's body language and facial expressions. If they frown, look sad, fidget, sigh, raise their shoulders or keep their arms/legs crossed, there is every chance they are unhappy about something. Don't ignore it – ask!

> Take prompt action and, if possible, take your client to a quiet area or room within the salon.

> If your client complains, listen calmly and patiently. Do not

interrupt, and pay attention to the information they are giving you. When the client has told you how they feel, take the heat out of the situation by saying, 'Thank you for giving us the chance to solve this.'

> Use active listening, open body language and open questions to get to the bottom of the situation. If required, involve your supervisor or salon manager.

> Use empathetic language, such as 'I can understand how that would be disappointing for you.' Be careful not to become defensive, and if you feel the client is attacking you personally, then politely bring the focus back to the problem.

> Decide on which course of action you will take. If the client's hair is damaged, agree a time-related plan of care to rehabilitate it. If the client's clothes or jewellery are damaged, take them in for cleaning or repair. If a financial settlement or 'money back' situation is required, follow your salon's policy accordingly. Whatever the agreed steps are for achieving client satisfaction, make sure that they are agreed and recorded between everyone concerned.

> If you feel uncomfortable with the way a client is treating you, either verbally or physically, involve your supervisor or salon manager. You are not required to tolerate abuse.

> If your client insists on pressing for compensation, your salon manager should notify their insurers about the claim.

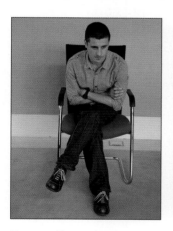 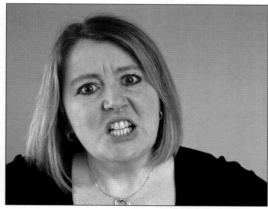

Be sensitive to body language and expression

Your long-term commitment

People naturally like to feel involved and cared for as part of a 'community', and having a vision for your client's long-term style management will help them feel that way.

> Never treat a client as if the current appointment is the only time you will ever see them.

> Record all the details of the services your client has had in the salon, plus any other relevant information, on a client record

card or in your salon database. Act in accordance with the Data Protection Act and give your client the opportunity to receive information by email or text from your salon.

> Tell your client when they need to return to the salon to keep their style looking its best. Either offer to book an appointment for them or encourage them to do so at reception. Your salon may offer a service where, if the client does not have their diary with them, the receptionist will call them at an arranged time to make a booking.

> Find out your salon's policy on 'between appointment services', such as complimentary fringe trims and styling advice, and share these with your client.

> Talk to your client about the products you have used, tell them why you have used them and show them how to care for and style their hair at home.

> Give your client any information that might be interesting or relevant, such as a current price list, current newsletter, salon offers, product samples or information about products and hair care.

> Invite feedback by either offering your client any feedback forms that are available or asking them how they felt about their service and how it might be improved. Always give the client a comfortable amount of time to respond and thank them for any feedback, which you should receive respectfully.

> Hairdressing salon businesses predominantly grow on word-of-mouth recommendations. Assuming your client is clearly happy with their service, don't be afraid to give your client your card and ask them to recommend you to their friends. Your salon may even have a card or marketing offer related to 'recommend a friend' to help you make your request comfortably.

> **Activity** For each client you see in the next week, think about their next appointment or next few appointments and the way you would progress their look. Share your ideas with them to communicate your long-term commitment.

Contribute improvement ideas

Industry standards and client expectations are constantly changing, and your salon will need to keep developing their policies and approaches to remain competitive. As a member of the team, you have an obligation to help them achieve this goal.

> If you spot opportunities to improve the experience for your customers, share them with your supervisor or salon manager.

> Think of things from your client's perspective, experience new services such as treatments for yourself and consider how you can maximise the experience for your client.

> Take the opportunity in team meetings to open discussions about service improvements, as your team members will have valuable experience too.

Your obligation under law

There are some areas of law that will govern the way in which you treat your clients. These include the following.

Data Protection Act (1998)

> Personal data shall be processed fairly and lawfully.

> Personal data shall be obtained only for one or more specified and lawful purposes, and shall not be further processed in any manner incompatible with that purpose or those purposes.

> Personal data shall be adequate, relevant and not excessive in relation to the purpose or purposes for which they are processed.

> Personal data shall be accurate and, where necessary, kept up to date.

> Personal data processed for any purpose or purposes shall not be kept for longer than is necessary for that purpose or those purposes.

> Personal data shall be processed in accordance with the rights of data subjects under this Act.

> The holder of the data can be prosecuted for misuse.

> Personal data shall not be transferred to a country or territory outside the European Economic Area unless that country or territory ensures an adequate level of protection for the rights and freedoms of data subjects in relation to the processing of personal data.

> The individual retains the right to access all information held about them.

For more information you can see the Act in detail at the Information Commissioner's Office online (www.ico.gov.uk).

Equal opportunities and the law

The Equal Opportunities Commission has defined a number of Acts that protect the rights of the individual against discrimination. You are obliged to offer equal opportunities to all clients and be offered equal opportunities by your employer. The main Acts include the following.

Disability Discrimination Act (DDA) (1995)

This Act outlaws discrimination based on disability in the areas of employment, education, access to goods, facilities and services, and in relation to land and property.

This Act also requires public bodies to promote equal opportunities for all individuals, regardless of ability, and it addresses the issue of equal access to public transportation by setting minimum standards for ease of use by all passengers.

Sex Discrimination Act (SDA) (1975)

This Act outlaws discrimination on grounds of sex, marital status or gender reassignment.

> Direct discrimination occurs when a person is treated less favourably because of his/her sex than a person of the other sex would be treated in the same circumstances.

> Indirect discrimination occurs when rules or circumstances are applied equally but clearly to the detriment of one of the sexes.

> There is victimisation as a result of an individual bringing a discrimination claim against their employer. Victimisation is outlawed under the SDA. Victimisation occurs if an individual is treated less favourably than someone who has not brought a discrimination claim.

Employment Equality (Age) Regulations (2006)

These regulations protect people against discrimination on grounds of age, and prohibits less favourable treatment of a person because of their age. This can include people of any age who are discriminated against, harassed or victimised.

Summary

Great customer service starts with you. You are a customer too and you know exactly the kind of service that delights you, so apply some of that good experience to your own role as a service provider. Clearly thinking through every aspect of your client's journey through the salon will help you to structure the way in which you give a positive impression of yourself and your salon. Help your clients to buy into 'the brand of you' by greeting them warmly, delivering a personalised service in a professional manner and giving them every opportunity to see you as an expert. Keeping clients is much easier than finding new ones, so you will invest your effort wisely in making every client feel special, every time they visit you.

Case study

Apprenticeships: in-salon learning

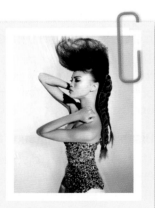

'When looking for a salon to serve an apprenticeship, look for one you admire, award-winning salons or 'the' salon in your area. Generally successful salons have good training.'

'Look for ones who have a good balance of services and that is up to date with the latest hairdressing innovations, techniques and trends. Make sure you will be trained in all aspects of hairdressing – women, men, colour, perming, Afro and dressing. Also a salon where training is a priority, do they have more than one training night a week, do they have educators come to the salon or give you the chance to go on training courses?'

'Be careful though because, as there is no one standard hairdressing apprenticeship, you need to make sure they train to NVQ standards. This may be done in the salon or by attending a college once a week. Also think about your daily trip to work, how far it is and how much it will cost. Spending hours travelling can be expensive, tiring and demoralising. With a good apprenticeship you could be on the salon floor within two and a half to three years, so do your research and take your time.'

My apprenticeship:

'I went for an interview in a well-known salon in the West End and spent all day there. I turned up in a suit and tie; I must have been the smartest apprentice ever!

I followed the boss round, watching and chatting to everybody, I really enjoyed it. But at the end of the day, he said, "You'll never make it as a hairdresser, you're too chatty and too tall, you'll have back problems." He just walked away – no 'thank you for coming', no niceties. It knocked my confidence. It was one of the worst things someone could say to a 16-year-old. I'd known I wanted to be a hairdresser since I was five and this was just the sort of busy West End salon I aspired to – I was mortified.'

'It took me a week to pull myself together and I decided to keep trying. I got a job in a salon and worked under Paul Edmonds, who was just the best teacher and mentor. After seven months, Paul decided to move to Neville Daniels' salon, and I went with him. I found myself one of 18 trainees so there was lots of competition, plus I had to restart my apprenticeship, but it paid off. The training was great and after only two months at Neville Daniel I became head junior. Two years later, I qualified and went onto the shop floor.'

'I learnt so much from my apprenticeship and I would always go and assist anybody and everybody. Charles Martin, who worked in the salon, did the Queen's hair at the time and I even went to Buckingham Palace to assist!'

'A good apprenticeship will give you a great foundation for your career as mine did, so take time to find the best salon you can. Expect competition though, places in good salons are sought after, so you'll have to try extra hard to get the job and keep it. And remember, it's not just about training; it's also about experience. Take every opportunity you can to assist both in and out of the salon and watch and learn all the time.'

'My apprenticeship has led me to an MBE, a top London salon and work that's in demand all around the world. Where will yours lead you...?'

Errol Douglas MBE, Errol Douglas Salon, Knightsbridge, London

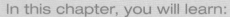

> In this chapter, you will learn:
>
> **>** **how to identify and deal with the main risks that you come into contact with in your workplace**
>
> **>** **how to take appropriate responsibility**
>
> **>** **how to give or source the correct help in connection with the health, safety and general well-being of everyone in the salon.**
>
> You will be assessed against your knowledge and ability to:
>
> **1** Understand your salon's health and safety policies and your obligations under law.
>
> **2** Identify and understand all workplace instructions connected with safety equipment and protective clothing.
>
> **3** Protect your client, yourself and your colleagues from harm or the potential of harm.
>
> **4** Identify and tackle hazards and risks in the salon.
>
> **5** Identify the people to whom you should turn in the event of an illness, injury, accident or emergency.
>
> **6** Document and report correctly any incidents.

Hard, polished floors, large surface mirrors, running water, harmful chemicals, electrical appliances, heavy boxes and the sharpest scissors and blades all add up to the hairdressing salon being a potentially harmful environment. Knowing good health and safety practice and your roles and responsibilities within it is absolutely vital to becoming a good hairdresser – it's not only a matter of common sense and good teamwork, it's a matter of law! The laws, guidelines and policies that apply to you are there to protect you, your team and your clients. You must show that you understand and acknowledge health and safety laws. You must adhere to them and take responsibility for potential problems you see.

Case study
Safety as service

Edward Hemmings is Director of Alan d, the largest private provider of work-based NVQ education in the London area. The academy guides the NVQ careers of hundreds of trainees each year.

'Health and safety is a fundamental part of what we do. In a busy salon you are surrounded by any number of potential hazards that we need to be aware of. The potential for lawsuits, injury and

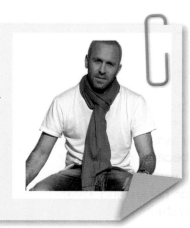

worse can be minimized by good practice. We drill it into our NVQ learners very early on so that it becomes a natural part of offering a service, rather than a chore or simply something else that they must think about. Gowning a client, protecting a client and making sure that they are comfortable are not just health and safety issues but good service. Equally, protecting yourself and taking responsibility for the equipment you use and the environment in which you work will avoid everything from unnecessary upset to a career cut short. Learning and repeating best practice in health and safety will make it a habitual part of every hairdresser's day-to-day job and that can only be a great thing.'

Edward Hemmings, Education Director, Alan d Academy

Health and Safety at Work Act (1974)

Also referred to as HASAW or HSW, the Health and Safety at Work Act is the most important piece of legislation covering health and safety relevant to your working environment and all the people operating within it. The law is subject to review, but you can find the latest version on the Health and Safety Executive website (www.hse. gov.uk). At the time of writing (2010) the law can be summarised as follows:

> Your employer has a legal obligation and responsibility to protect the health, safety and welfare of everyone in the salon or those affected by its services. They are obliged by law to appoint a 'competent person' to be their health and safety representative and offer a single point of contact.

> Employees have a duty of care and a responsibility to themselves, their peers, their clients and the salon owner to uphold health and safety law and take reasonable measures to protect them from risks and hazards.

Note: For businesses with more than five employees, the employer is obliged to conduct a risk assessment survey, to record the results and to have a written health and safety policy that is well communicated to all employees.

Hazard and risk – what's the difference?

A hazard is something that has the potential to be harmful. A risk is something that has a probability of becoming harmful. For example, an electrical styling tool with a long cable that coils to the floor is a hazard; an electrical styling tool with a long cable trailing across an area where people walk is a risk. While the cable coiled to the floor it was potentially harmful; once people were likely to trip on it, it became probable that it would cause harm.

If you spot a hazard, either deal with it directly or notify your manager or health and safety officer and, where there is one present, the first-aid officer. If you spot a risk, act quickly to minimise or remove

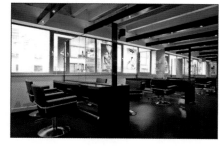

The salon space has many hazards and risks

it and/or notify one or all of the key staff immediately. If you are in any doubt as to what course of action to take, or if you are unsure whether something represents a threat, notify key staff immediately.

Identifying, assessing and handling risk

You share responsibility with all your colleagues for contributing to a safe and healthy workplace. Make sure you know the following:

> your salon's health and safety policy
> where to find first-aid supplies and either how to use them or who your first-aid officer is
> the correct people to contact for hazards, risks and emergencies
> the hazardous aspects of your role and how to handle them
> the location of the safety equipment, such as fire extinguishers and alarm switches, and how to use them
> the location of electricity master switches and how to turn off the main flow of water to the salon.

Your responsibility to the well-being of your workplace and health and safety is best summarised in three steps:

> identify
> assess
> address.

Become aware of the areas in which your salon environment might prove harmful to team members and clients. Remember that a hazard has the potential to cause harm, so assess the situation carefully. Observe and think about the likelihood of someone being hurt. Address the situation directly or involve a relevant member of staff. In health and safety law, addressing a situation is termed 'control' and requires that you bring any hazard or risk down to an acceptable and manageable level. In accidents and emergencies, this whole process may take moments, but in all cases it is you who will make the difference. Common hazards and risks are outlined in the table opposite.

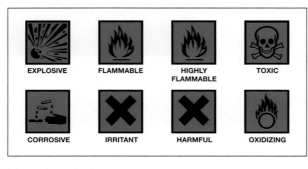

Hazard symbols

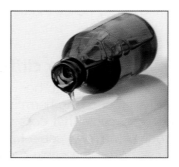

Chemical spills need urgent attention

Identify	Assess	Address
Bottles of product that may contain chemicals that could be harmful	If the bottles are labelled and stored correctly, with lids secure, then risk is minimal. If the bottles have missing labels, are spilled or are left open or in the wrong place, the risk may be high.	Clear up chemical and product spills, taking adequate and appropriate precautions. Always read the manufacturer's instructions. Dispose of products correctly, according to policy and COSHH (Control of Substances Hazardous to Health) regulations. Replace lids and store products in the correct place.
Heavy boxes	Incorrect lifting may cause injury.	Identify where the box must be moved to and where it can be stored safely. Lift by bending your knees to prevent injury, and seek help where appropriate.
Chemicals	Chemicals and food must be kept in separate areas to avoid contamination. Chemicals might give off toxic fumes and should be handled in a correctly ventilated room. Protective clothing will be required.	Store chemicals correctly. Remove food from the vicinity. Wear protective gloves and/or aprons. Handle in a ventilated room. Always read the manufacturer's instructions and dispose of chemicals in accordance with COSHH (Control of Substances Hazardous to Health) regulations.
Blocked passageway, stairs, fire exit or doorway	Obstructions create a risk of tripping, stumbling and falling and may restrict evacuation in an emergency. There is a significant risk of injury.	Clear thoroughfares, storing or disposing of items appropriately.
Electrical styling appliances and salon equipment	Misused, faulty and incorrectly stored or maintained appliances can cause injury or death.	Keep electrical appliances away from water. Check cords and plugs for fraying and damage. Switch off and allow to cool after use. Store away when not in use. Make sure that appliances are checked under health and safety laws. Never use electrical appliances with damp or wet hands.
Long cords on appliances	Cords that trail to the floor offer a small tripping risk; cords that trail across thoroughfares are a significant risk.	Coil cords and store appliances appropriately.
Spills or slippery floors	Spilled water, product on the floor and even hair cuttings can make the floor slippery and cause falls and injury. Make sure you assess whether the spill itself is harmful before you deal with it.	Clean up spills appropriately and dispose of them. Sweep up hair clippings and clean slippery floors. Where appropriate, put out warning and safety signs.

Identify	Assess	Address
Worn or damaged floors, doors, mirrors, chairs, etc.	There is a risk of injury from poorly maintained salons and broken items such as chairs and mirrors.	Alert your salon manager or health and safety officer so that the situation can be addressed. If necessary, cordon off the area to prevent access by team members and clients.
Blown light bulbs	Lack of light can make it difficult to see safely, especially in important areas such as stairwells and fire exits. Broken light bulbs can cause injury.	Remove and dispose of light bulbs safely. Replace with the appropriate wattage and connector. Use safe equipment, such as step ladders, to reach the bulb. Alert your salon manager or health and safety officer.
Cupboards, shelves and drawers	Open cupboards and drawers can cause injury. Badly stacked shelves may cause harm.	Keep cupboards and drawers closed, and use stepladders to reach shelves when taking things down. Do not put heavy items at a high level.
Hot water	Wrongly calibrated thermostats can cause scalds and burns with very hot water.	Always check the temperature of your water before directing the flow onto clients or team members. Check the temperature by passing the flow quickly over your hand. If the water is dangerously hot, alert your salon manager or health and safety officer.
Scissors, razors and blades	Exposed blades left unattended represent a risk of cutting and injury.	Close scissors and store in a holster or box. Remove blades and dispose of in a 'sharps' box, which in turn can be disposed of through the salon's local authority. Carry blades in their correct storage container. Never walk around or run holding scissors.
Cups, saucers, glasses and plates	Chipped or cracked cups, saucers and glasses could cut and cause injury.	Dispose of any imperfect china and glassware immediately. Wrap these items carefully in newspaper or paper towels and place in the regular bins.

Common hazards and risks

This list of hazards does not describe all the hazards and risks you might face on a daily basis; that relies on your common sense and your ability to spot and assess problems, both real and potential, in all situations. To conduct a risk assessment you must:

> identify the hazard
> decide who might be harmed by it and how they might be injured

> decide how to address the hazard or risk and take action
> record your findings and actions in the relevant documentation (e.g. accident book)
> review with your manager or health and safety officer all your findings, and, if necessary, update your health and safety documentation, policies or procedures.

Note: If you notice any contradictions or differences between your salon's health and safety policies and the manufacturer's instructions supplied with products and appliances, you should bring it to the attention of your salon manager or health and safety officer immediately.

Accidents, illness and emergencies

Whether it's an accident, illness or an emergency, it needs urgent attention. Make sure you are informed and prepared, so that you are ready to act quickly.

Reports and records

After any event, complete the relevant report to be included in your salon records. You might include the following information.

> Your name and role and the name(s) and role(s) of the person/ people involved.
> The date, location and area where the incident occurred.
> A description of the incident, what happened and the actions taken.
> The outcomes (e.g. admitted to hospital, sent home).
> Your signature.

Fire

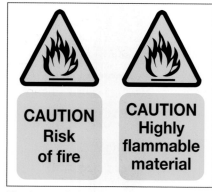

Fire hazard signs

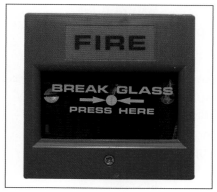

Central fire alarm

Salon fires can have a number of origins and flammable sources. How you treat the fire will depend on what type of fire it is. Fires spread quickly, with devastating effect, so if you are in any doubt, call the emergency services and ask for the Fire Service. Fires have different classes and require different extinguishers.

Classes of fire

> Class A: involving solid material such as paper, wood, hair (yes, it's very flammable).

> Class B: involving liquids and chemicals that are combustible, including grease oil, hydrogen peroxide (which can ignite combustible material on contact).

> Class C: involving electrical equipment, such as appliances including hairdryers and irons, wiring, lights, circuit breakers and sockets.

> Class D: involving combustible metals, such as magnesium, titanium, potassium and sodium, which are unlikely to be present in the salon.

Types of fire extinguisher

The type of fire dictates the type of extinguisher you would use.

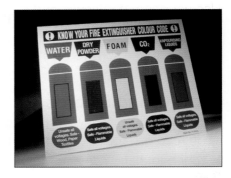

> Water extinguishers: bright red and full of about 2 gallons of air-pressurised water. These are only appropriate for Class A fires.

> Dry powder extinguishers: red with a blue panel and filled with sodium bicarbonate or potassium bicarbonate. These are appropriate for Class B and C fires.

> Carbon dioxide (CO_2) extinguishers: red with a black panel and filled with a pressurised, non-flammable gas. Carbon dioxide is most effective on Class B fires.

> Foam extinguishers: red with a cream panel and filled with a foaming water mixture. It has limited effectiveness on Class A fires, so should only be used on very small incidents and is most commonly used for Class B fires.

Fire extinguishers

Note: Class D fires require special powder extinguishers that are rarely provided in a salon environment. Using a Class A extinguisher on a Class B fire will actually make the fire bigger, and using a Class A extinguisher on a Class C fire can cause you to be electrocuted, so you need to get to know the equipment.

Other tools used to fight fires

> Fire blanket: ideal for smothering small, confined fires, such as on stove tops or in waste-paper baskets. They can also be used for protection during evacuation of a burning building.

> Fire bucket: contains sand or water. Sand is useful to smother small fires, and to confine or mop up spills of chemicals and liquids. Water is only safe to tackle Class A fires.

> Fire escapes: should be clearly marked and clear of all obstructions. There should be a clearly identified route of escape and a procedure in place to evacuate the building – these should be detailed on a map and a sign. The map should clearly show the safe assembly point to gather at when you have left the building. This will help to identify quickly anyone potentially trapped inside. If your salon or building has a fire certificate, then

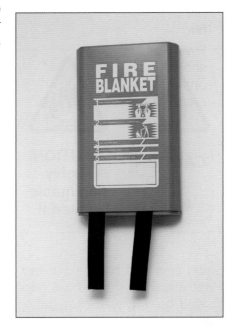

Fire blanket

there will also be emergency lighting powered by an independent power supply to light your means of escape.

> Fire alarm: the building you work in may be fitted with a central fire alarm. Make sure you are aware of how to raise the alarm in the event of a fire.

Note: All firefighting equipment should be checked regularly by a qualified fire officer and stored correctly. Fire extinguishers are not doorstops! For further tips and advice on dealing with fire risks and avoiding harm, visit the government website Fire Kills (http://firekills. direct.gov.uk).

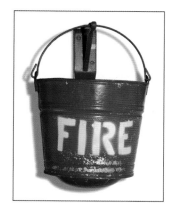

Fire bucket

What to do about fire

Use your common sense and do your best to prevent fire.

> Don't smoke inside the building.
> Dispose of cigarettes safely.
> Be careful with lighted candles.
> Switch off equipment at the wall when not in use.
> Empty bins frequently and dispose of contents outside the building.
> Store flammable materials according to the manufacturer's instructions.

If you spot a fire

> Identify quickly the source of the flames.
> Assess whether the flames are controllable and raise the alarm.
> If you are alone, dial 999 and ask for the Fire Service. Alternatively, if someone is with you, ensure that they do so.
> Address the fire with the correct firefighting tool. If the fire does not immediately come under control or begins to spread, you should evacuate.
> Even if you have been successful in putting out the fire, you should evacuate the building and meet at the assembly point until your health and safety representative readmits you to the premises. Smoke and toxic fumes may result from fire and remain in the atmosphere after the fire is extinguished.

Note: Some sources of fire give off toxic fumes as they burn, and all smoke is damaging to the lungs. Do not attempt to enter a burning room or tackle a fire you know to be toxic.

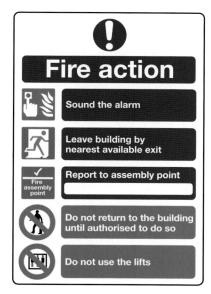

Evacuation sign

Activity

1 Describe a Class A fire.
2 What sort of extinguisher is used on a Class A fire?
3 What type of fire safety device would you use to protect yourself as you leave a burning building?
4 Name three potential sources of flammable material in a salon.

First aid

It is common for salons to have a first-aider, or someone trained in first aid, as well as the mandatory first-aid kit, as salons are obliged by health and safety law to provide adequate provision of assistance. You can find out more about first aid in leaflets available from the Health and Safety Executive (www.hse.gov.uk) or through training courses and information from St John Ambulance (www.sja.org.uk). In every instance where help is required after an accident, illness or emergency, make sure that you notify the correct personnel. If you are in any doubt as to your ability to provide adequate care, dial 999 and ask for an ambulance.

First-aid kit – what's in it?

Every salon should have a first-aid kit and all staff should know where it is. A well-stocked kit might contain the following.

> A leaflet giving general guidance on first aid, like the ones available from the Health and Safety Executive.

> Twenty individually wrapped sterile plasters of assorted sizes and preferably hypoallergenic.

> Two sterile eye pads.

> Four individually wrapped triangular bandages, preferably sterile.

> Six safety pins.

> Two large, individually wrapped, sterile, unmedicated wound dressings.

> Six medium-sized, individually wrapped, sterile, unmedicated wound dressings.

> A pair of disposable latex-free gloves.

> Eye wash phials for cleansing eyes and wounds.

> Sterile wipes.

> Burn dressings.

> Microporous tape.

> Small scissors for cutting dressings and bandages.

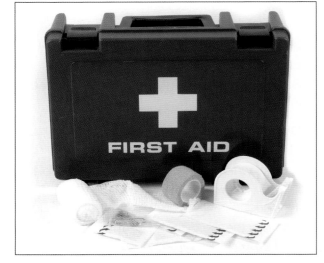

First-aid kit

From a client fainting, to a flooded kitchen, to the colleague who has cut themselves – all these incidents require you to take proactive action. The table shows some of the most common occurrences you may be called on to tackle in your career.

The potential challenges you may encounter at your salon and the actions that should be taken are outlined in the table opposite.

Note: Always record incidents in the correct documentation.

> **Activity** Make a risk assessment of your salon. List all the things in each area which are a hazard, describe how they might become a risk and what controls you would put in place to reduce the probability of anyone coming to harm.

Accident, illness or emergency	How you should act (in all instances, send for help)
Unconscious person	Check there are no visible signs of injury. Check that there is no obstruction in the mouth or throat and tip the head gently backwards to open the airway. Check that the person is breathing. Stay with them until medical help arrives.
Unconscious person not breathing	If there are no obstructions in the mouth or throat and the head is tilted back, but there are still no signs of breathing, perform artificial respiration if you are qualified to do so.
Minor cuts	Put on protective gloves and apply a sterile dressing to the wound, pressing firmly until the flow of blood abates. If necessary, apply a second dressing on top, but do not remove the first dressing and expose the wound again.
Serious cuts	Check that there are no objects embedded in the wound. Put on protective gloves and, using a clean towel or cloth, apply pressure to the wound, where possible raising the wound above the level of the heart. If there is an embedded object, press either side of the object, not directly on it.
Shock	People can experience shock even after minor injuries. If their breathing is shallow, their pulse is fast and they are pale and clammy, keep them warm, lay them down and raise their feet above the level of their heart. Loosen any restrictive clothing.
Anaphylactic shock	Allergic reactions can be life-threatening. If you notice someone with a swollen face, mouth or tongue and blotchy skin, breathing difficulties and a rapid pulse, and you suspect an allergic reaction, dial 999 immediately. Some allergy sufferers carry a pre-loaded adrenalin syringe, which you can help them to administer or inject them with if you are trained to do so.
Chemical burns	Despite obvious skin damage, redness, swelling or blistering, chemical burns can also cause coughing, dizziness and shortness of breath. Remove the casualty from the location where the burn occurred and remove any contaminated clothing. If you know which chemical is involved, check the manufacturer's instructions. Using large volumes of cool, clean water, wash the burn for at least 20 minutes. Cover it with sterile dressings or a clean cloth and seek medical attention.
Burns	If the burn is large, dial 999 immediately. If not, cool the skin by running the injury under cool water for at least ten minutes. Cover the burn with a lint-free, sterile dressing or kitchen cling film and seek medical help.
Electrocution	You need to break the connection between the electricity and the person as soon as possible. Switch off the electricity at the mains if it is safe to do so. If you cannot turn off the electricity, stand on non-conductive material, such as thick paper, and push the victim away from the electricity source with something non-conductive, like a wooden broom. Then dial 999 and ask for an ambulance. Where necessary and possible, administer first aid.
Eye injuries	If chemicals have splashed into the eye, flush the eye for at least 15 minutes, with the eye as wide open as possible. Do not cover the eye, and seek medical assistance as soon as possible. If there has been a blow to the eye, lightly apply a cold compress and seek help. If there are cuts or objects in the eye (e.g. glass), do not wash out or try to remove them. Cover the eye with a rigid shield, such as the bottom half of a paper cup, and seek medical help immediately.

Accident, illness or emergency	How you should act (in all instances, send for help)
Broken bones	If you suspect a casualty has a broken bone, try to keep them as still as possible and support the break with rolled-up blankets or clothes. If they cannot be moved, dial 999 and ask for an ambulance. Broken bone victims often experience shock, so look out for the signs. If the skin is also punctured, gently hold a clean, sterile dressing to the wound.
Sprains or strains	A sprain typically occurs at a joint and a strain along a limb or body part. In all instances, rest the injury, apply cold compresses, support the injury with a bandage or soft padding and, where possible, elevate it above the level of the heart.
Back or neck injuries	If you suspect a neck or back injury, it is essential that the casualty does not move. Cover the casualty in a blanket. Kneel behind the person's head and hold either side gently but firmly with both hands. Support their head, neck and shoulders with rolled up towels or clothes and wait for help to arrive.
Fire	As detailed above (page 38), the way you treat a fire relies on the source of the flames. Ensure that you are familiar with policies and firefighting equipment in your salon.
Flood	For floods and damage caused by broken pipes, alert your health and safety officer, turn off the electricity at the mains with dry hands, and turn off the water at the mains.
Gas leak	If you smell gas or suspect a leak, alert your health and safety officer, open all the windows and doors, and turn off the gas supply to the salon. Evacuate the salon without using a mobile or landline phone, and without smoking or switching on any lights. Alert the gas supplier from another location.
Intruder	If you are threatened by the presence of someone behaving strangely or inappropriately, immediately alert your salon manager, who will decide whether to involve the authorities.
Bomb threat or suspicious package	If you receive a bomb threat or find a suspicious package left in the salon, alert your salon manager immediately.

Potential challenges

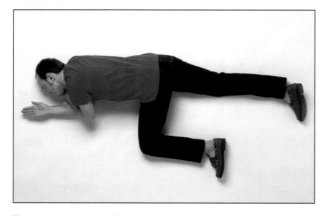

The recovery position

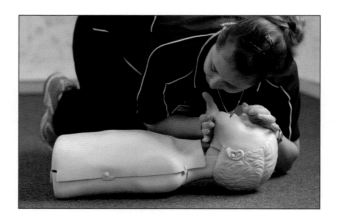

Practising CPR (artificial respiration)

Keeping a clean salon

The cleanliness of your salon communicates a lot to your clients. A spotless, well-kept salon will give the impression of a team that takes pride in its work and believes in offering great customer service and high standards – and that's even before the client has finished their appointment.

A clean, well-kept and orderly workspace is also safer than one that isn't, and it helps you to uphold your health and safety responsibilities. Without doubt, salons are hard to keep clean – product, hair cuttings, water, refreshments, high footfall all make mess – but with constant and vigilant care, you can and should play your part in creating a clean and safe salon environment to be proud of. The warm, damp atmosphere caused by all those dryers and so much running water combine with the high volume of people in the salon space to represent a perfect breeding ground for germs and infection. Think carefully about the appropriateness of the cleaning methods and how thorough you are in carrying them out.

Styling chairs

Hair can get trapped in the seat and underneath the base. Use a dryer to blow cuttings away from the chair so that they can be swept up. If any hair remains or there is product or tint on the chair, wipe it away, making sure that you are wearing the proper protective clothing/gloves. Regularly wipe down the chairs completely, using disinfectant or antibacterial cleaning materials. Report any damaged chairs to the salon manager, as cracks and tears can be a breeding ground for germs.

Floors

Sweep up hair cuttings immediately and dispose of them. Mop up and clean spills as soon as they happen, making sure you put out the correct safety signs and wear protective clothing where required. Mop the floor whenever needed and at the end of every day, taking care with textured surfaces which can trap germs. If it is snowing or raining outside, your floor in reception is likely to become wet and slippery. Put out appropriate safety signs and mop as required. Be thorough, clean in corners, behind doors, at the base of backwashes and freestanding workstations, and so on.

Reception

Reception areas have counters and seating that have lots of traffic. Keep the area tidy, picking up and organising any magazines or books, clearing away any used crockery and disposing of any rubbish left behind by clients. Wipe down reception counters and coffee tables every day, using disinfectant or antibacterial cleaning material. If the surfaces are polished, make sure you leave them smear-free.

Retail areas

Keep shelves clean, remove any bottles that have been tampered with and report any poorly maintained shelving that may fall and cause injury.

Workstations and mirrors

Keep mirrors spotless, as they are a key tool in cutting hair; dirty mirrors reflect very badly on the salon. Polish at the beginning or end of every day and check regularly through the day. The workstation may have shelves, product cubbies, appliance holsters and back mirrors, which all need to be wiped down and/or polished regularly.

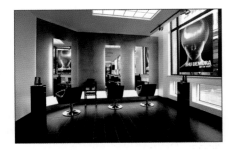
Workstation

Windows and glass doors

Glass doors and windows can quickly become dingy and covered in hand and finger prints. Your salon may employ a professional window cleaner, but keep your eye out for smears and dirt and attend to these as needed. Glass can be hard to see when it is very clean, so make sure that where relevant the glass carries a sticker or image to make it easily seen. Door handles need wiping down regularly, with disinfectant or antibacterial cleaning materials.

Shampoo area

Wipe down the sink and surrounding area after every use and clean with the correct cleaning material at the end of the day. Restock any backwash products, refill towel stores and wipe down the backwash chairs with disinfectant or antibacterial cleaning materials.

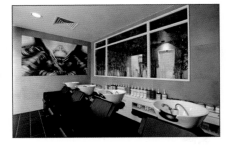
Backwash area

Toilets and changing rooms

The toilets, sinks and mirrors should be cleaned at the end of every day, and checked regularly throughout the working day to restock toilet paper and towels and to clean if required. Any changing rooms should be checked on regularly throughout the day. Don't forget to sweep and mop changing rooms too and keep any mirrors spotless.

Kitchens, dispensaries and prep areas

Keep kitchen surfaces clean at all times. Put dirty crockery, glasses and utensils in the dishwasher. If your salon is not equipped with a dishwasher, carefully hand-wash all cups, saucers, plates, glasses and cutlery in warm, soapy water. Wear gloves to protect your skin and carefully clean each item, paying particular attention to the rims of cups and glasses. Either leave your items to air-dry and polish with a clean, dry cloth, or dry thoroughly and store. Never use a dirty sink, sponge or drying cloth to clean your items. Always begin with a clean work area. Keep perishable food and liquids in the fridge. Clean out coffee machines, fridges, kettles and microwaves

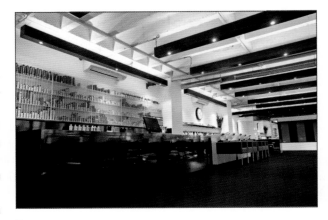
Dispensary

regularly, according to the manufacturer's instructions. In dispensaries, store all materials appropriately, dispose of used tint tubes and bottles, clean tint bowels and brushes. Make sure you wear protective gloves and clothing where necessary. In all areas, make sure that cupboard doors are kept closed.

Bins and waste disposal

General salon waste should be placed in a lined bin with a lid. Empty the bin when it is full and at the end of every day, and replace the bin liner. Regularly clean bins inside and out with warm water and disinfectant or antibacterial cleaning materials. Dispose of chemicals and tints in accordance with the manufacturer's instructions and in line with COSHH (Control of Substances Hazardous to Health) regulations. Some chemicals can erode pipes and contaminate water supplies and should not be disposed of in the sink. Where necessary, wear protective clothing.

Blades and sharps

Your salon will have a 'sharps box' for the disposal of blades and needles. These should not be put into the general waste. Your salon manager will contact the local authority to arrange collection when the box is full.

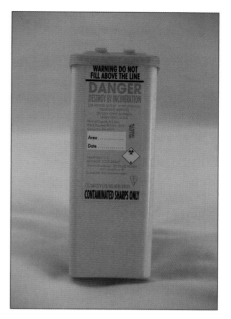

Sharps box

Activity Create a timed work plan that schedules cleaning and spot checks for the salon throughout the day. Repeat tasks as often as you feel is necessary.

For example:

Time	Salon area	Task
9am	Reception	Check and polish glass doors, door handles, retail shelves
9.15am	Toilet	Check toilet paper, wipe down sink, check floor

Keeping equipment clean and safe

Clean and well-maintained equipment will prevent injury and the spread of infection, as well as presenting a good impression of you and your salon. Methods of cleaning equipment include the following.

Sterilisers

Steam sterilisers (autoclaves) kill bacteria at high heat and can be used on metal and non-heat-sensitive equipment. Allow the autoclave to cool to a safe temperature before opening. Other heat sterilisers include dry-heat cabinets.

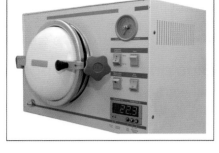

Steam steriliser

Disinfectants

Immersing tools, including plastics such as combs and brushes, in an industry-grade disinfectant (such as Barbicide) will successfully kill organisms. Change the disinfectant frequently to ensure it retains its effectiveness. Some sterilising fluids can be corrosive, so check the manufacturer's instructions.

UV radiation

Placing equipment in a light cabinet with UV radiation will kill the organisms exposed. You must not expose yourself to the light and you may need to turn the equipment.

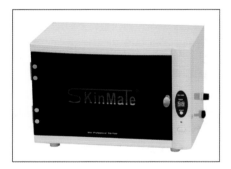

Light cabinet

Sanitisation

A good wash and spray with hot water and antibacterial soap will help to kill some bacteria, but does not qualify as sterilisation.

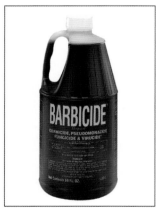

Barbicide

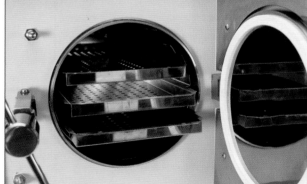

Autoclave

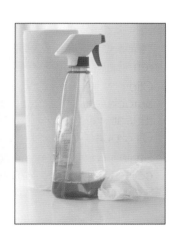

Cleaning solution

Equipment should be cleaned as follows:

> Neck brushes – make sure you wash your neck brush regularly in warm water with a detergent, and spray it with an antibacterial spray. Leave to dry naturally.

> Scissors – regular sterilisation in an autoclave or industry-standard solution such as Barbicide is recommended. Get your scissors

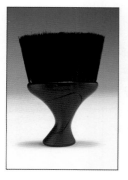

Neck brush

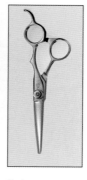

Scissors

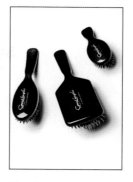

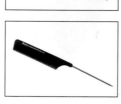

Combs

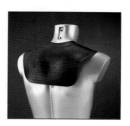

Brushes

Cutting collar

professionally sharpened approximately every six months and keep them oiled.

> Combs – place in an industry-standard sterilising solution such as Barbicide for at least ten minutes to remove all germs.

> Brushes – use your comb and/or tail comb to comb the hair out of the bristles or pins of your brush. For resistant hair, use the tail of the comb to pick it out. Wash in soapy water, then treat with an industry-standard disinfectant. Do this regularly.

> Cutting collars – wash in hot, soapy water and immerse in industry-standard disinfectant solution for at least ten minutes.

> Brushes and tint bowls – wash away all signs of tint, chemicals and product, according to the manufacturer's instructions.

> Equipment trolleys – remove the trays and clean with disinfectant or antibacterial cleaning materials, and wipe down the trolley carcass with the same solution. Allow to dry naturally.

> Tint aprons – wipe tint aprons after use with a warm cloth to remove all chemicals and splashes.

> Clippers – if possible, remove clipper blades and place them in an autoclave or industry-standard disinfectant solution. Make sure that all hair is removed first, and replace and realign worn blades. Oil clipper heads as necessary.

> Styling irons – make sure the styler is turned off, unplugged and cool. Wipe casings, plates and rods clean with disinfectant wipes,

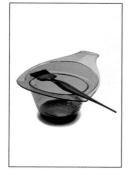

Tint brush and bowl

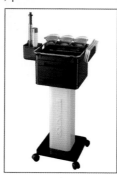

Equipment trolley

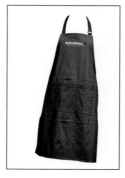

Tint apron

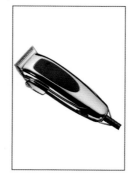

Clippers

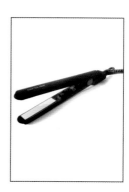

Styling irons

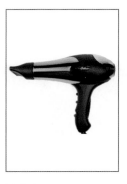

Hairdryer

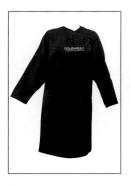

Gown

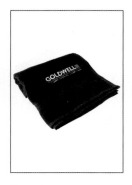

Towel

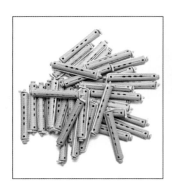

Rollers

ensuring that you remove any product residue. Allow to dry completely before using again.

> Hairdryers – before you clean your dryer, make sure it is turned off, unplugged and cool. Professional dryers have replaceable filters. To clean the intake grill, brush lightly with a nail brush to loosen hair and fluff, then vacuum the surface. To clean the casing and flex, wipe the surface with antibacterial wipes and allow to dry completely before using again. Wash detachable diffusers and nozzles in warm, soapy water and allow to dry naturally.

> Gowns – hairdressing gowns should be freshly laundered for each client. Hair cuttings should be removed from Velcro fastenings with a fine tooth comb or vacuum. You may wish to keep gowns for tinting separate to those for cutting, as tint can stain.

> Towels – your salon may have a towel-cleaning service or a laundry room. Use clean towels for every client and then place them in the towel bins provided for washing. You may wish to keep towels for tinting separate to those for cutting as tint can stain.

> Grips and section clips – regularly wash in hot, soapy water, and immerse in industry-standard disinfectant solution for at least ten minutes.

> Rollers and rods – regularly wash in hot, soapy water and make sure you remove all trace of chemicals. Immerse in industry-standard disinfectant solution for at least ten minutes.

> Computer screens and keyboards – use specially purchased antiseptic wipes and sprays on your keyboard and screen to kill germs.

> Phones – wipe phones, handsets and keyboards with antiseptic wipes.

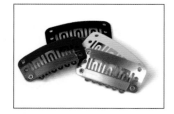

Grips and section grips

Preparing your work area

It's really important that you spend a few minutes each day, and before receiving each client, gathering the things you need to hand. Placing items within easy reach and getting products and equipment in an unhurried manner will guard against hazards and possible accidents for both yourself and your clients. You should follow the steps set out below.

Inform yourself

Check your list of clients, or the list of the stylist you are assisting, and try to think ahead. Gather together client records for each person you will be seeing, so that you can familiarise yourself with them and the typical services they enjoy. For all client records, act in accordance with the Data Protection Act (1998).

Be product-prepared

Ensure your workstation has the right range of styling products, serums, and so on, close by. Make sure you know the key benefits of each product and the results you should achieve.

Get tooled up

Ensure you have cutting collar, neck brush, back mirror, tissues and electrical styling tools to hand at your workstation. Check your kit roll for your scissors, combs, brushes, section clips, and so on.

See to the equipment trolley

Prepare a trolley with a good range of pre-cut and folded foils, a range of rods and curlers, pins and grips, disposable neck capes, disposable gloves, tint removal wipes, cotton wool and anything else you might need. Do not pre-mix tint or lay out bowls.

At the backwash

Before you start, check that the backwash sizes of all types of cleanser and conditioner have a good quantity of product. Make sure that towel tidies are stocked and pick up towels before each shampoo.

At reception

Check that there are clean gowns in the gowning area so that there is no delay or problems with gowning your client.

Protecting your client and yourself

Sound

A buzzing salon with appropriate music makes a great place to work and spend your salon appointment, but if the music is persistently loud it can irritate conditions such as tinnitus (ringing in the ears) and affect mood. Keep volume at an acceptable level.

Eyes

When you are using spray products, make sure that you spray away from your own eyes and use one hand gently to shield the eyes of your client. Be very careful with tint and bleach and don't overload the brush, to avoid splashes and splatters.

Water

Check the water temperature before putting it to your client's scalp by quickly passing your hand beneath the flow of water. Ask if the water temperature suits them.

Disability

Salons are obliged to do everything feasible to accommodate disabled clients and offer them the same freedoms and services as everyone else. People who use a wheelchair, are mobility impaired, hearing impaired, visually impaired or have learning difficulties may all need extra assistance in the salon. Check your salon's policies and use your common sense to keep these vulnerable clients safe and well.

Shampoo area

Use a cushioned neck support at the backwash to relieve pressure on your client's neck. During the consultation, always ask if they have any back or neck concerns that they would like to tell you about. If possible, and if your client would like it, raise the foot of the chair to bring their body more in line with the backwash. Do not cause the head to jerk or the neck to twist during the backwash service.

Comfort

Ensure your client is seated comfortably at the workstation. Where available, point out the foot rests on the chair and encourage them to use them. They will be sitting still for some time, so you must make sure that their position won't place them under physical stress. Move the seat to the correct height using the hydraulic pump, so that you can begin the service comfortably.

Accessories

Remove any rings, bangles, bracelets, pendants, necklaces, scarves or earrings that might interfere with the service you are offering. Long hair can also be a hazard, so tie it back where necessary.

Infections, conditions and diseases

Airborne germs

Be careful around clients who have symptoms of cold or flu. Keep tissues close by so that they can 'Catch it, Bin it, Kill it'. When you are removing hair cuttings from a client's neck or face, *never* blow on them, always use the neck brush.

Blood-borne diseases

HIV is the virus that causes AIDS and it can be caught through the transmission of blood from one person to another. HIV stands for human immunodeficiency virus, and AIDS stands for acquired immune deficiency syndrome. Hepatitis B and hepatitis C (HBV and HCV) are carried in the blood and can cause serious liver disease.

If you become aware or suspect that either yourself or your client is a carrier for any blood-borne diseases, and you or your client has any cuts, grazes or sores, make sure that you wear protective gloves and take every necessary precaution. If your scissors or equipment get any blood on them, wash and sterilise them immediately. *Never* let blood get into your mouth or eyes.

Dermatitis

According the Health and Safety Executive (HSE), up to 70 per cent of hair professionals will suffer some sort of work-related skin damage at some point during their career. Dermatitis is the most prevalent and can bring careers to a full stop. This skin problem causes the skin to redden, swell, itch, crack and dry out, and can be a site for secondary infection. Dermatitis is caused by either an allergic reaction to chemicals and products or contact with them. The HSE runs a Bad Hand Day campaign to raise awareness and recommends five steps to keep dermatitis at bay.

> Step 1: Wear disposable, non-latex gloves when rinsing, shampooing, colouring, bleaching, and so on.
> Step 2: Dry your hands thoroughly with a soft cotton or paper towel.
> Step 3: Moisturise after washing your hands, as well as at the start and end of each day. It's easy to miss fingertips, finger webs and wrists.
> Step 4: Change gloves between clients. Make sure you don't contaminate your hands when you take the gloves off.
> Step 5: Check skin regularly for early signs of dermatitis.

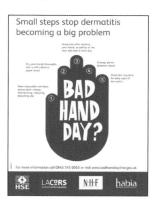

Wear gloves to protect against damage and disease

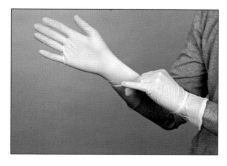

Bad Hand Day is dedicated to educating professionals

Protection

Always gown your clients to protect their clothes. Make sure that you wear appropriate gloves and aprons when handling chemicals. Non-latex gloves are recommended for wet work.

Conduct

Inappropriate and unwelcome behaviour should be avoided. If you experience or witness any such behaviour, make it known to your supervisor or salon manager. Take care only to touch clients in a professional manner and as required in the course of your job.

Your health

Hairdressing is a physically demanding career! You will be in the best shape to do your job if you take good care of yourself. So consider the following points.

Clothing and shoes

Dress appropriately for the physical demands of your job. Wear comfortable shoes that offer good support.

Posture

When working, think about your posture and how you use your body, in order to avoid strains and repetitive strain injury.

Exercise

Take regular gentle exercise. Even if your job is physically demanding, it will help to relieve stress and build stamina.

Water

Stay hydrated! Salon environments, with hot air, humidity, air conditioning, artificial lights and constant activity, can dehydrate you. Dehydration can give you headaches and affect your concentration. Drink at least 2 litres of water every day.

Smoking

Try to give up! Smoking is bad for your health, and even after a spray of breath freshener you will almost certainly bring smoking odours back into the salon and to your clients. Go to www.smokefree.nhs. uk for advice on quitting.

Cleanliness

Shower or bath and put on clean clothes every day. Use a good quality deodorant and wash your hands with antibacterial soap after every client and before and after eating. Check yourself daily for hair splinters (tiny shards of cut hair). They can lodge themselves in the skin almost anywhere, but are typically found around the nails, waistband, between the fingers (and toes if you are wearing sandals) and in the creases of your joints. Hair splinters can cause discomfort and become a site for infection; they can also get into your eyes, so take care. Simple personal hygiene can avoid lots of potential health problems, from eye infections to stomach upsets.

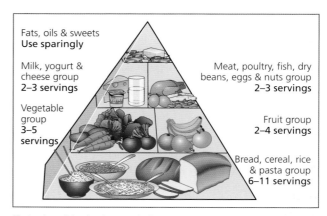

Eat a healthy balanced diet

Diet

Eat at least five portions of fresh fruit or vegetables every day and maintain a healthy balanced diet. The right nutrition will help you stay healthy, maintain energy levels and fight off illness. Avoid excess alcohol and *never* drink during working hours.

Activity

1 Find out your body mass index and whether it falls within healthy parameters (see www. nhs.uk/Livewell).

2 Find out the safe number of units of alcohol that an adult can consume per week.

3 Find out the amount of hours of weekly exercise recommended by the health authorities.

4 Think about ways in which you could improve your diet.

Environmental awareness

Your salon is obliged to work with the health and safety regulations to operate environmentally friendly working practices. Such regulations include the Control of Substances Hazardous to Health Regulations (COSHH) (2002) and the Waste Electrical and Electronic Equipment (WEEE) directive. These regulations mean you must:

> dispose of chemicals and hazardous waste appropriately and safely (COSHH), without allowing them to damage or pollute the environment

> find a suitable way to recycle broken or unwanted electrical appliances (WEEE) – your salon manager can contact the manufacturer or the local authorities for advice.

There are other ways in which you could thoughtfully help the environment, including the following:

> switching off lights in unused rooms where it is safe to do so

> using towels and placing them in the laundry bins only when necessary, to reduce the environmental cost of cleaning them

> ensuring that taps are switched off completely after use to reduce waste water

> working smart to eliminate waste products being left in tubes and disposed of.

Health and safety law

The following are the key regulations that apply to you. It is your responsibility to be proactive in upholding the Health and Safety at Work Act (1974) described at the beginning of this unit. You are not required to remember the detail of each regulation, but it's worth familiarising yourself with them. The information, tips and advice in this unit, combined with your own common sense and experience, will give you a great structure.

Management of Health and Safety at Work Regulations (1999)

This confirms the ways in which employers are obliged to uphold health and safety law and dictates that they must:

> conduct a workplace risk assessment

> make arrangements for implementing the health and safety measures identified by the risk assessment

> appoint competent people (often themselves or company colleagues) to help

> implement the arrangements

> set up emergency procedures

> provide clear information and training to employees

> work together with other employers sharing the same workplace.

Data Protection Act (1998) (see also Unit G4)

All companies and organisations that hold any personal details about living people must register with the Information Commissioner.

> Data should be held safely and securely.

> Data should be fairly and lawfully processed for a defined and limited purpose.

> Data should be appropriate in content, depth and volume.

> Data should be kept in an accurate and timely manner.

> The keeping of data does not interfere with personal rights.

Workplace (Health, Safety and Welfare) Regulations (1992)

These regulations describe aspects of the salon/working environment and include the following:

> workplace and equipment maintenance

> ventilation and temperature control

> lighting

> cleanliness and the removal of waste

> space allocation and room to work

> workstation and seating fit for purpose

> free and safe circulation of people and traffic in designated 'routes'

> rules for transparent doors, dividers, windows, and so on

> provision of adequate sanitary and washing materials

> provision of a water supply that is clean and safe to drink

> facilities to rest and eat meals

> facilities to change

> changing and storage facilities for clothing.

Electricity at Work Regulations (1989)

These regulations refer to the maintenance and handling of electrical equipment and states that:

> safety is the responsibility of the employer

> the employer is responsible for maintenance of fixed and portable appliances, which must be regularly inspected

> all electrical test certificates are in place and carry the following information: date of inspection, date of purchase or disposal, the contractor's details

> the employer must maintain an itemised list of equipment, along with serial numbers.

Portable Appliance Testing (PAT)

This is a recognised method of upholding the Electricity at Work Regulations and is:

> recommended annually
> carries a date, number and signature of the tester
> made in addition to regular visual inspections by staff
> recorded in a log.

Control of Substances Hazardous to Health Regulations (COSHH) (2002)

COSHH is the law that requires employers to control substances hazardous to health such as tints and peroxide. An employer must:

> assess the health hazards
> decide how to prevent harm to health
> provide control measures and make sure they are used
> provide information, instruction and training for employees
> plan for emergencies.

A substance is deemed hazardous if it can cause harm when it is ingested, inhaled, absorbed through the skin, injected or introduced through a wound.

Waste Electrical and Electronic Equipment (WEEE) Regulations (introduced 2007)

These regulations are actually part of environmental rather than health and safety law, but they apply readily to salon businesses. WEEE states that:

> all businesses that use electrical and electronic equipment (EEE) must comply
> for all non-household WEEE, either the producer (manufacturer) or end user (you or your salon) is responsible for the disposal of the products
> if your employer gives your WEEE to someone else, they must ensure that it is taken to a suitable facility to be treated and recycled
> proof must be obtained and kept to show that your WEEE was given to a waste management business and was treated and disposed of in an environmentally sound way.

Personal Protective Equipment (PPE) at Work Regulations (1992)

Employers have basic duties concerning the provision and use of personal protective equipment (PPE) at work. The regulations require that:

> PPE is properly assessed before use to ensure it is suitable
> PPE is maintained and stored properly

> employees are provided with instructions on how to use PPE safely

> employees use PPE correctly.

Hazards requiring PPE include many things commonplace in salons, such as chemicals, electrical equipment, heated appliances and sharp tools.

Note: PPE is provided by law for free and as an employee you cannot be charged for necessary protective equipment.

Manual Handling Operations Regulations (1992)

Any activity that requires you to lift, support or move a load with your body is manual handling, and employers are required to carry out a risk assessment of work processes that involve lifting. There are guidelines available on acceptable weights. Employers must assess the following:

> risk of injury

> the ways in which a load is moved manually

> the strains the load will place on the bearer

> the way the working environment will limit or support the operation

> the worker's individual capabilities

> ways to minimise risk.

Reporting of Injuries, Diseases and Dangerous Occurrences Regulations (RIDDOR) (1995)

This regulation places a legal obligation on the employer or manager to report work-related deaths, major injuries or injuries resulting in more than three days away from work, plus near misses and dangerous diseases. There is an extensive list of reportable incidents, which include:

> fractures

> permanent or temporary loss of sight

> loss of fingers or toes

> illness as a result of toxic exposure

> electric shock

> skin diseases, including dermatitis

> infections such as hepatitis or anthrax.

Summary

Health and safety is a very relevant and integral part of your role as an employee, a professional and a team member. Knowing how to spot, assess and address a hazard or risk will help to avoid concerns before they become problems. Your great health and safety conduct can have a very real impact on the productivity and profitability of your salon. Knowing even rudimentary first aid will make you more confident and competent to deal with everyday and out-of-the-ordinary occurrences. Health and safety rules and policies aren't there to make extra work or stop you enjoying your job; they make a difference on every level. They illustrate standards and a caring environment to staff and clients; they support best practice in avoiding illness, accidents and harm; and they even help to protect the environment.

Activity What law applies in the following instances?

1 Someone in your salon receives an electric shock.
2 Someone in your salon slips and breaks a wrist.
3 Your professional dryer breaks down and must be replaced.
4 You are mixing tint.
5 The salon heating breaks down.
6 You are taking client information.

Describe and explain your choice in each case.

Section 2

With the client

This is where hairdressing happens! Every client is different, with different needs, desires, challenges and expectations. The skills in this section will give you the power to transform not only your client's looks, but the way they feel too, and that's career gold dust! As a people business, hairdressing thrives on great communication and that's just where this section starts, with the client consultation. The perfect consultation gets you off to a flying start because you learn a lot about your client, share a lot about your skill and lay the foundation for a long-term client–hairdresser relationship. The practical modules guide you through the essential skills needed to deliver good hairdressing for both women and men. Don't forget that mastering these skills will give you the confidence to explore your own creative ideas, so practice truly does make perfect.

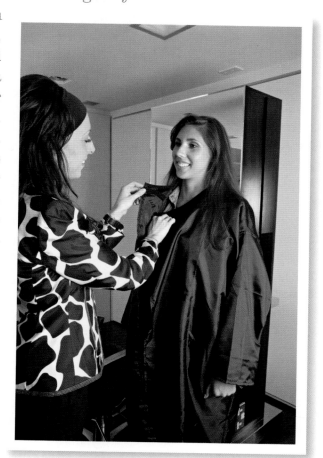

In this chapter, you will learn:

> **the essential skill of successful client consultations**
> **how to fully understand your client's needs**
> **to assess the condition of the hair and scalp**
> **how to make appropriate suggestions.**

You will be assessed against your knowledge and ability to:

1 Understand and remember your salon's and your own legal responsibilities towards your client.

2 Share information about the services your salon offers and the prices.

3 Successfully identify your client's needs and wants and make appropriate and suitable suggestions.

4 Communicate appropriately in an open, honest and respectful way that meets client expectations and salon policy.

5 Use positive verbal and non-verbal communication and be sensitive to your client's communication.

6 Use all the tools available to communicate successfully.

7 Judge when to involve other staff and professionals and know who to contact.

8 Understand the main structures and functions of the skin, scalp and hair.

9 Confidently identify, diagnose and recommend a course of action for common diseases, conditions and complaints of the hair and scalp.

10 Check your client's understanding of the situation and secure their agreement to the service.

11 Create and maintain accurate client records and treat them in accordance with the law.

Case study

Consultation success

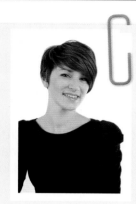

Anya Dellicompagni is Director of Hairdressing of the Francesco Group, a 31-strong salon group with three academies in the Midlands, which serve a large number of work-based NVQ learners.

'I teach all of our staff and students that the consultation is the single most important starting point for the salon service. As hair professionals, it's our opportunity to spend time uncovering the detail of our clients' wants and needs and understanding them and their hair.'

'We teach a simple but very effective consultation structure that focuses first on the past, then the present and lastly the future. The past examines real detail with the client – how they feel their hair has and hasn't worked, the concerns they have, the styling problems, etc. The present takes a snapshot of where they are today, their lifestyle demands, what they are able to change, the amount of time they can invest in their style, the health and condition of their hair and scalp. The future allows us to discuss how we might progress their look, what life events are coming up, how they plan to maintain their look.'

'As trainees learn and in the early months, we recommend the use of a consultation form to help keep them on track. Most frequently, learners just don't spend long enough or go into enough detail to get all the information they need so a structured form really helps. It can also be tough to master all the science and theory such as hair and skin structure, head shape and growth patterns, but as an experienced professional I spend time with staff until they are confident because it's so important. The condition, texture and structure of hair along with its growth patterns dictate how it behaves. Add hair behaviour to the head shape and these things will dramatically affect the way you cut and colour and the style that can be achieved. A good consultation will deliver good results and let a client know that they have been listened to – that builds trust and confidence and the start of a great relationship.'

Anya Dellicompagni, Francesco Group

The perfect consultation

Clients value being listened to, but they also value your professional opinion, so become confident about sharing your ideas and building on the information you get from your perfect client consultations.

Why is it done?

The consultation is your first real interaction with your client and is an excellent way to source information and build trust. It's your opportunity to assess and then constantly reassess your client's needs *and* their wants, along with the essentials like health. It's also your opportunity to reinforce your strengths and skills, and educate your client about the services and products your salon offers.

What should I do?

As with all great skills, practice makes perfect. A list of bullet points or even a basic script can help you in the beginning. Use consultations to achieve the following.

Get eye-to-eye

Conducting your entire consultation 'through the mirror' puts unnecessary barriers between you and your client. Where appropriate, sit beside the client and look them in the eye.

Manage expectations

Talk your client through the 'client journey' and explain the purpose of the consultation, who they might meet, where they will go and what will happen while they are visiting your salon. Talk broadly about all the services your salon offers, to show that all their needs can be met.

Discover likes and dislikes

Talk about the 'no-go' areas in every client's needs (e.g. they don't want to show their ears) and discover the things they love too.

Assess your client

Look at their clothes, shoes and accessories. What is your client's personal style? Are they classic, current season, funky? Do they have an outgoing or introverted nature?

Examine your client's physical attributes

Face shape, body shape, eye colour, skin tone, natural hair shade, hairlines and growth patterns all have an impact on the choices you make. What physical challenges do they have? Do they use a wheelchair? Do they wear a hearing aid or use spectacles?

Talk about their lifestyle

What a client does for a living and how they spend their leisure and family time all contribute to the requirements they will have for their style.

Discover their level of commitment

Short hair and some coloured hair requires more maintenance than long, natural layers, so talk about how frequently the client should return to the salon and the potential upkeep costs of different looks. This is also an early way to introduce the idea of booking their next appointment before leaving the salon (e.g. 'With a short look, you would need to return to the salon every six to eight weeks to keep it looking its best').

Do a health check

Assess the type and condition of the hair and the health of the scalp. Keep a sharp lookout for any challenges, problems or diseases, all of which may affect your choice of style, service or the final result.

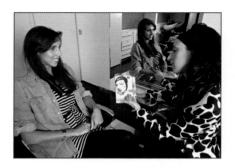

A comprehensive consultation is the first step towards a great client relationship

Ask about neck or back problems, to make sure that these issues are handled well at the backwash and styling area. Ask about any history of allergic or adverse reactions to any product or service, and carry out a skin test or strand test if necessary.

Look at what's gone before

Which services has your client had in your salon or other salons before? Is there evidence of existing colour, perm or chemical straighteners on the hair? Does the client use any products that might prove incompatible with salon treatments and services? The tests you conduct on the hair should also provide you with good information.

Get the right people involved

Your peers and colleagues might be in a better position to advise your client in more depth, so, where necessary, involve a colour expert or even recommend doctors or trichologists. Never be embarrassed to ask – you are doing the right thing for your client.

Brainstorm ideas

The consultation is your opportunity to showcase your creativity, *share* ideas and work *with* your client to plan a way forward for their hair.

Price the job

Some services, such as colour, hair-up and extensions, are priced on consultation. Your salon will have an hourly rate that they like to achieve from every professional hour purchased. Knowing this figure and the time required for the work involved will help you to give the client a clear expectation of what they might pay. If you are in any doubt, talk to your manager or supervisor, as under-pricing a job will not build long-term business or help your salon's bottom line. For example:

> Apply half-head extensions for length = 3 hours for two staff
> One professional salon hour = £45
> Number of hours = 6
> Price for the service = £270 plus the cost of materials.

Summarise

Let your client know the results of their consultation and hair/scalp diagnosis, and check your understanding of their needs and no-go areas; talk about the plans for their current visit and the type of care and conditioning products they will need to maintain healthy hair. Don't be afraid to talk about longer-term plans for their style – this shows that you have vision and a commitment to the client beyond their current visit.

Record the outcomes

Capturing information about hair type, condition, scalp health, face shape, product usage, product recommendations, colour and style ideas will help both you and your client. Make certain that you keep *all client records* confidential, in accordance with the Data Protection Act (1998), and respect your client's right to privacy. You have a legal and moral obligation to your client. If you do not adhere to your obligations, it may result in a legal or civil action against you or your salon.

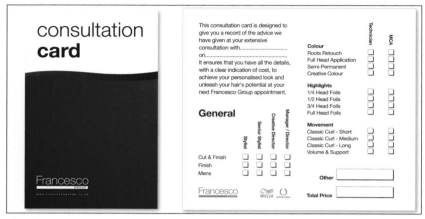

Keeping excellent client records is essential

Legally speaking

As well as the Data Protection Act (1998), you are bound by the Trades Descriptions Act (1968 and 1972) and the Sale of Goods and Services Act (1980) (see Unit G4), to honestly represent any product or service in communicating with the client, so make certain you know what each item in your service menu represents and how to describe it well. The Prices Act (1974) is also in force to ensure that prices are displayed to the client so that they are clear about the costs involved. Your salon is likely to charge differently for varying services and levels of staff experience, so make sure you know how much is charged and why. For prices on consultation, discuss the final price with the client and write it down for the record. Make sure the client understands that services such as conditioning treatments at the backwash will bear a cost.

Remember to do a thorough consultation *every* time and *never* rush.

> Your client may have completely different needs from one visit to another, or their circumstances may have changed, so don't assume that you know what they want.

> A thorough consultation helps you discuss new ideas and keep your client's look fresh.

> A rushed consultation will have a big negative impact on the way a client feels about their experience.

Consultation tools

There are lots of useful tools you can use for perfect client consultations.

Magazines

Use celebrities, models and good examples of shade/shape and texture to develop a mutual understanding. Your client may have a completely different understanding of the terms 'layered' or 'trim' than you do.

Shade charts and swatches

Colour manufacturers provide comprehensive shade charts and pre-treated hair swatches to help you to communicate colour.

Consultation cards

Keep a written record of the points you have covered with your client (or potential client) and store the details safely.

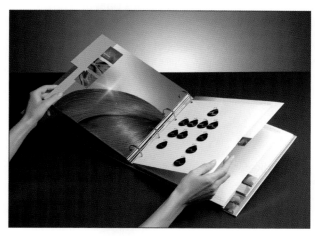

Use visual tools to talk about colour

Your brain!

As a trained professional, you are the best person to advise your client, so take time to really think carefully about them and share your ideas effectively.

Communicating for success

Questions, questions

How effectively you communicate will have an enormous impact on how successful you are as a hair professional. Your client will learn a lot about you and your salon's capabilities/services from their consultation; giving them a positive impression and lots of information will help grow your column and your salon's revenue. In your client consultations, seek to ask mostly open questions – open questions are those that require a more complex or longer response, while closed questions are those that can be answered with a simple yes/no or single-word response. Open questions draw out more information and give even shy clients more opportunity to share their thoughts. Useful questions are shown in the table overleaf.

Activity

1 Role-play with your friends, family and fellow students by working through a consultation as if you were in a salon. Tell them your ideas for their hair, assess their hair and scalp and, above all, take time to *listen* to their needs.

2 If you are not working in a salon already, visit professional salons and either observe consultations from established hairdressers or ask for a complimentary consultation for yourself.

3 Practise asking and hearing open questions in regular conversation. Remember that open questions tend to begin with 'what', 'why' and 'how' and require a more complex response.

Question	Purpose
How do you feel about your hair right now? What do you like about your hair?	Find out what's working and what's not, and discover those all-important 'no-go' areas (e.g. I want to keep my ears covered!).
What styling tools do you use regularly at home? How long do you spend on your hair each day?	Uncover their current time commitment to their style.
Tell me about your typical day. What you do for a living? What you do to keep fit?	Reveal the demands their lifestyle might place on their overall look.
Which celebrity hair do you really admire at the moment and would love to achieve for yourself?	Gives you and your client a clear and common understanding of the look they would love.
What kind of products do you use on your hair?	Allows you to explore condition, volume and styling.
How did you rate your last haircut?	Ensures you understand *this* client's past and helps you to understand their likes and dislikes.
Describe for me… Tell me more about… What are your thoughts on…? In what way…?	Use these phrases to draw out more information on any subject you are discussing with your client.

Using open questions

Vocabulary and tone

> When talking to a client, ensure that you never swear and make sure you use words that are appropriate to your client's age and social network.

> Keep slang and buzz words to a minimum, unless your client uses them first.

> Use adjectives (descriptive words), but also make sure that you are clear on key points such as length, texture and shade.

> Use a clear tone of voice at a comfortable pitch. Feel free to communicate energy and enthusiasm. Mumbling and very quiet voices will make the client feel you lack confidence, while a high-pitched tone will feel nervous or aggressive.

Body language

The spoken word represents only a tiny part of our communication. *How* we communicate has a much greater impact than *what* we communicate. So consider your body language in all your interactions. Other people read our body language, which includes tone of voice, gestures, facial expressions, your posture, eye contact and the distance between you and the person you are communicating with.

Why is it important?

> Body language has a big impact on the way your client will feel about you and their experience.

> Being aware of positive and negative body language helps you to read your clients and how comfortable or happy they are.

❯ Good body language helps you to diffuse and avoid potentially difficult situations (e.g. sensing when a client is unhappy).

Body language types

Eye contact

Refusing to meet another person eye to eye is a sign that one party is uncomfortable, lacks confidence or feels in some way embarrassed. Looking away while you speak makes the other person feel dismissed or unimportant. Locking eyes with someone feels hostile or intrusive. Maintain comfortable eye-to-eye contact at all times.

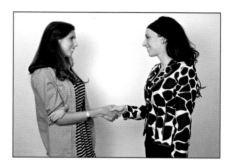

Maintain good eye contact

Facial expression

Smiling is the easiest way to welcome a client and the best way to judge a great end result. Be natural! A genuine smile will usually involve the whole face, including the eyes. Narrowing of the eyes, pursing of the lips and biting of the lower lip can communicate anger or nervousness.

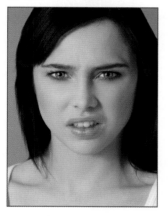
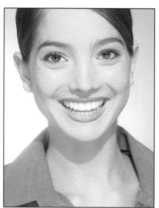

Be aware of facial expressions and what they mean

Arms and hands

Crossed arms and clenched fists can communicate defensiveness or anger, while upturned, open palms and raised shoulders can imply a lack of personal responsibility or knowledge about a situation. Relaxed arms and hands or purposeful movements will communicate confidence and comfort.

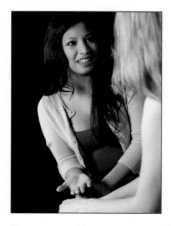
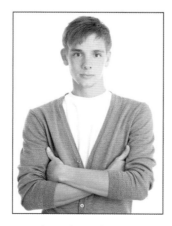

Be aware of how you are using your hands and arms

Posture

Hunched shoulders, looking down or hugging yourself are signs of insecurity and discomfort. Standing balanced on both feet, with shoulders and hips aligned, communicates confidence and attentiveness.

Closeness

Standing too close to someone can make them feel intimidated, or make you appear aggressive or even a little creepy! A gap of around 60 cm, or 'arm's length', is a comfortable distance from which to interact.

Physical contact

Be respectful. Hairdressing requires close physical contact, but when not actually conducting a service, think carefully about how and why you are touching your client. Resting a gentle loose hand on a shoulder or arm can be reassuring and warm. Touching someone with a firm open palm can be perceived as aggressive.

Gestures

'Talking with your hands' is very useful in hairdressing to help you describe shape and movement. Very fast and wide gestures make the listener feel that you are nervous or angry. Keep your gestures smooth, assured and close to your body.

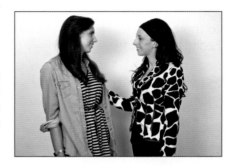

Use touch reassuringly

Active listening

Clients value being listened to; it makes them feel that you are responding to their unique needs and treating them as an individual. Above all, it helps them to choose you over the competition. The key principles of active listening include the following.

Leaning in

A subtle inclination of the head and body towards the client will help them feel that you are listening only to them.

Eye contact

Look at your client's lips and face as they speak.

Concentrate

Don't answer the phone, speak to a colleague or start doing something else while your client is speaking, unless it's a safety issue. Give them your undivided attention.

Head movement and expression

Nod or shake your head, smile or frown slightly where appropriate. Reflect the feelings that your client is exhibiting or expressing.

> **Activity** Next time you watch your favourite programme, switch your TV to mute. Consider what the expressions, postures and gestures of the people on screen are communicating, and really study their body language.

Don't interrupt

Allow the client to finish everything they are saying. Don't finish their sentences for them or assume you know what they are about to say.

Ask clarifying questions

Ask questions that invite your client to expand on points they have covered.

Summarise

'So what I'm hearing…', 'So my understanding is…' Repeating back to the client the key points of their communication will be undeniable proof that you have been paying attention.

Activity Take notice of the way in which you are listened to: by family and friends, in the bank, at the doctor's. Note the behaviours and how they make you feel.

Suitability

The style you create should maximise your client's positive attributes and suit their head shape and face shape. The human form isn't truly symmetrical, so you will have to think carefully through your cut to compensate for everything, including pronounced occipital bones, varying ear heights and different brow shapes. Make careful judgements about features such as a weak jaw, sticking-out ears or a large nose, and try to assess whether these are issues for the client.

Face shape, head shape, body shape

Face shape

Face shape can be divided into five categories: square, oval, long, round and heart-shaped.

> Square shape is best suited to softer, rounded styles that mask a heavy jawline. Longer styles and side-swept fringes also help to give the face a softer geometry.

> Oval shape is the ideal and this client can carry off any style. Make sure you take into account all the other factors, such as condition and lifestyle, before you get carried away!

> Long shape needs width and texture to balance the face. Avoid height, as this will add length. Solid fringes work well, as they shorten the face, but avoid centre partings.

> Round shape requires height, not width, so keep the side

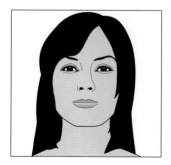

Square face

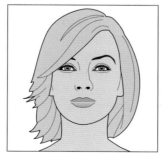

Oval face

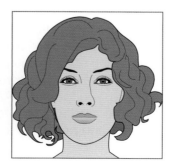

Long face

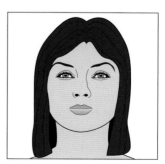

Round face

sections close to the head and avoid jaw-length styles. Longer lengths with fullness below the jaw work well.

> Heart shape loves textured, chin-length styles, but keep the perimeters soft as this shape can have a sharp chin. Height and side-swept, wispy fringes are good; avoid blunt fringes, as this can make the shape look harsh.

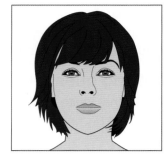

Heart-shaped face

Head shape

The basic structure of the skull will affect your choice, especially in profile. Knowing the bones of the skull is important to following technical step-by-steps. The sides of the skull are formed by the parietal and temporal bones. The back and nape are formed by the occipital bones, and the forehead by the frontal bones. Take heed of cheekbones and eye sockets (orbital bones) too, as these may well affect the overall look.

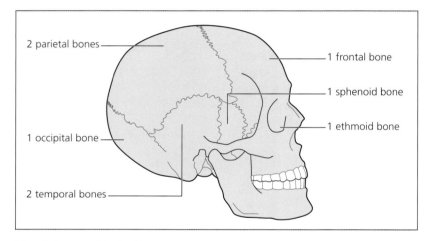

Head shape with skull bones

Body shape

Take a good look at your client's overall body shape. Consider the length and width of the neck, the width of the body and the overall outline. A great style will work with the whole person!

Age and lifestyle

Age

Make the style you create for your client age-appropriate, but also specific to their personality. Young people may prefer classic styles, while the young at heart may want something more fashionable. Observing your client's street clothes, accessories and general demeanour will help you to make a judgement. As a rule, keep it practical for kids, softer for mature clients, sharp for professionals, easy-to-manage for young parents and quirky for teenagers.

Lifestyle

Your consultation will reveal plenty about how your client spends their time. If they are active and do lots of sport, or have little time on their hands, go for manageable styles. Regular swimming and exposure to chlorine will impact colour and should affect your choice of shades and tones. If they are fashion-conscious, you can select something that requires styling time and maintenance. Ask plenty of open questions to help you.

Activity

1 In day-to-day life, try to identify the face shape and body shape of the people you meet and assess whether their hairstyle is maximising their features. Think how you would do it differently.

2 Complete the grid below.

Face shape	Best suited to...
Square	
Oval	
Long	
Round	
Heart	

Skin tone and eye colour

Your colour consultation should include plenty of tools such as swatches and charts, but you should also get to know the general rules when it comes to colour suitability, and look carefully at your client's natural skin tone and eye colour. Skin tones generally fall into warm and cool.

Warm tones

These are represented by an underlying apricot tone in the skin. Warmer colour palettes work in harmony with warm skin tones, so it's important to choose the right tone and shade depth of any colour to compliment the skin. For example, a brunette might be a warm oak or leather; a blonde might be a sand or warm gold. Most dark skin has a warm tone.

Cool tones

The undertone of cool skin is a rosy red or pinkish hue. For cooler skin tones, work with cherry reds, champagne blondes and sienna browns, as these will enhance and compliment cooler skin shades.

Eye colour

A great colour choice can make eye colour really 'pop', and make a big difference to your client's overall appearance. Generally, dark hair works well with dark eyes, and extremes of tones (e.g. light blonde,

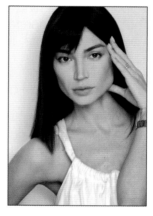

Warm skin tone

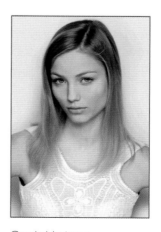

Cool skin tone

deep black) work well with blue eyes. Always defer to the skin tone when making a colour choice.

Assessing skin, scalp and hair

Never forget that you are a professional specialist in your field, so make it your business to know the key facts about hair and skin, and the typical challenges and diseases you might see over your career. These facts will give you the confidence and the knowledge to help your clients, and to understand the way in which these things will affect the style, services and products you choose. Preserving or enhancing the condition of your client's hair and scalp must be your constant goal. You also have a duty of care to protect yourself and other clients against infection, so you must be able to spot potentially contagious skin, scalp and hair problems efficiently, and be able to deal with the situation tactfully.

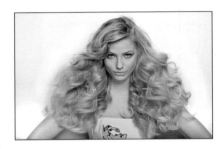

Dark eyes

Skin

Skin is our largest and most resilient organ, constantly renewing and replenishing itself and protecting us against disease and infection. It's also covered in hair! Getting to know the structure and functions of skin will help you to understand the part it plays in the way our complexion and our hair looks, feels and behaves.

Blue eyes

What is it?

Skin is a complex organ made up of three main layers.

The epidermis or outer layer

This is the layer that we see and touch and which comes into direct contact with our environment. The epidermis alone has five layers of cells:

> horny layer (stratum corneum) – the layer that we shed
> clear layer (stratum lucidum) – with no melanin (colour), but lots of keratin (the protein that makes hair)
> granular layer (stratum granulosum) – the tissue that separates the two layers above from the soft ones below
> mixed layer (stratum spinosum) – contains melanin and active keratin growth cells called prickle cells
> germinating layer (stratum germinativum) – most active growth cells.

The dermis or middle layer

This is the thickest layer and has lots of jobs to do. The dermis is where the hair follicle is formed and contains blood vessels, lymph vessels, sweat and sebaceous glands, nerve endings and the connective tissues collagen and elastin. The dermis nourishes the epidermis and gives us the ability to interact with our world through our senses, including pain, touch and temperature.

The subcutaneous layer or base layer

This is made up of fat and collagen. It acts as an insulator and buffer against injury.

What does it do?

Apart from growing hair, our skin has key functions, including the following.

Protection

It shields our organs from damage and infection.

Information

The skin is profoundly sensitive and provides us with constant feedback about heat, pain and pleasure!

Storage and secretion

The skin stores essential water, fat and vitamins required for body function, while excreting sweat (mostly water and salt) and oil to moisturise and lubricate the skin.

Temperature

The muscle at the base of the hair (erectile pilli) and the sweat glands team up to keep us cool or warm.

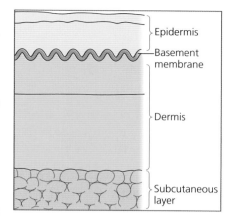

Structure of the skin

What structures are important to me?

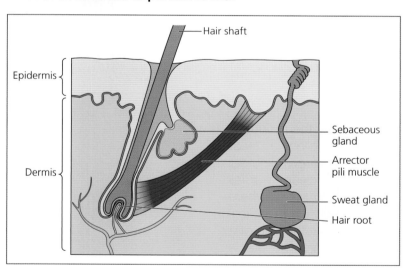

Hair follicle and muscle

The hair follicle and hair muscle

At the bottom of tube-like gaps in the dermis and epidermis are nerves and blood vessels called papillae. The papillae are surrounded by a matrix, which creates cells with melanocytes (colour) to form the hair bulb. The base continues to generate cells, which push others up and forms hair fibre at the surface of the skin. There is a muscle attached to the outer hair shaft which constricts, causing the hair to point up and the skin to bunch, creating 'goose flesh'.

The sweat gland

This lays in the dermis, alongside the follicle, and produces sweat (mostly water and salts) in response to heat or stress. Sweat glands help to keep the body cool.

The sebaceous gland

This secretes sebum into the hair follicle to retain a protective and waterproof layer on the skin and scalp, as well as keeping the skin supple and healthy. The oil secreted is called sebum and its chemical properties give our skin an antibacterial barrier.

Skin allergy test

What's it for?

Before you apply any chemicals to your client's hair that will come into contact with the scalp, you *must* carry out a skin allergy test (sometimes called a patch test). It is your responsibility to follow the manufacturer's instructions for skin tests precisely. While there is no law to enforce skin testing, it is your legal obligation under health and safety law to protect your clients from harm. If no test is conducted and your client has an allergic reaction, you expose yourself and your salon to the risk of prosecution. A properly conducted *and recorded* test will protect the interests of you, your client and your salon.

What is it?

A contact skin test is conducted prior to a full chemical service, in order to assess the client's potential reaction to the chemicals that the tint or perm contains. Make sure you test the actual product at the intended concentration to ensure a true result.

How is it done?

You should always follow the instructions provided by the product's manufacturer. However, in general terms, test your client at least 48 hours prior to the planned service – it only takes a few minutes. Prepare a small amount of the exact product and clean a small area either behind the ear, on the inside of the elbow or anywhere else on the body that is unobtrusive. Clean the area with medical alcohol, apply the tint with cotton wool in an area about the size of a large coin, and leave it to dry naturally. If, after 48 hours, the skin is unchanged and there is no redness, itching or raised areas, you may proceed with the service.

How do I position it with the client?

> Use every opportunity to educate your client – tell every client during every consultation that you skin-test for colour.

> Emphasise that the skin test is for their protection, safety and health.

> Offer every client a skin test, regardless of whether they are having colour or not. Record the formula and concentration you use.

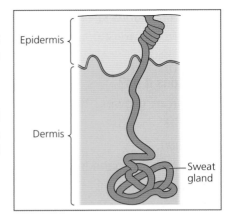

Sweat gland

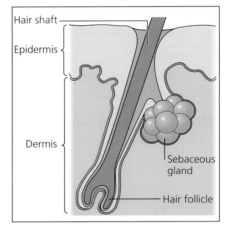

Sebaceous gland

> Where possible, ask your clients to sign their skin test results to confirm that they are not experiencing symptoms of allergy.

Hair

Hair is your fabric, and understanding every tiny weft and weave will help you cut some gorgeous designs for your clients. The biology and structure of hair affects its behaviour, and it's important to conduct a range of tests to truly understand the fabric that you are working with for your individual client. The tests described in this section will give you lots of information about the type of styles, colours and textures that are possible. The results will also help you to explain to your client why, for example, a full-head tint or short fringe are inadvisable.

What's hair made of?

> Carbon, hydrogen, nitrogen, oxygen and sulphur are nature's ingredients for long chains of amino acids that are called polypeptides or proteins.

> The most prevalent protein in hair is called keratin and it's this that allows hair to be stretched, styled, curled, and so on.

> Keratins form long coils that are bonded together with links called disulphide bonds (or bridges), made of salt, hydrogen and sulphur.

> Salt and hydrogen bonds are relatively weak and easily broken. Sulphur bonds, more commonly known as disulphide bridges, are stronger, but can be altered chemically.

> Keratin in its natural state is called alpha keratin. Keratin that has been styled and had its shape changed is called beta keratin.

> The shape of hair is temporarily changed through setting and styling by breaking the salt and hydrogen bonds.

> Once moisture is reabsorbed into the hair shaft or it becomes wet, keratin will relax back to its former shape.

What's its structure?

The hair is made up of three distinct structures: cuticle, cortex and medulla.

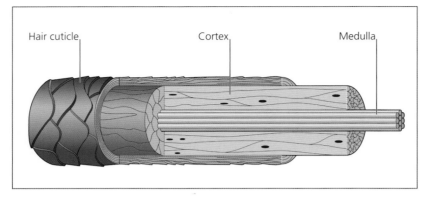

The structure of a single hair

Cuticle

The cuticle is the outer layer. It's transparent and made up of scales that overlay one another, sealing in moisture. In healthy, untreated hair, the scales lie flat and all point towards the end of the hair. Dry, damaged or chemically treated hair will have missing or elevated cuticles and absorb more moisture. In chemical processes the cuticles are raised intentionally, to allow colour and chemical to reach the inner cortex and change the hair.

Cortex

The cortex is made up of intertwined fibres of protein and gives the hair its strength, elasticity and colour. Chemical tints and perms must reach the cortex in order to work effectively.

Medulla

The medulla is the very centre of every hair and has a honeycomb appearance. It's only present in coarse, thick hair.

Hair grows in three stages: anagen, catagen and telogen.

Anagen

Anagen is the active growth phase. Hair grows at about 12 mm a month, although many factors, such as age, ethnicity and health, can affect the rate of growth. This phase can last from months to years, and at any time approximately 85 per cent of the hair is in this phase.

Catagen

The catagen or transitional phase lasts about two weeks, during which time the hair is no longer growing and the follicle shrinks, causing the papillae to break away beneath and enter a rest period.

Telogen

The Telogen phase lasts for five to six weeks, and eventually the papillae begins to generate a new hair bulb. The new hair that forms will push out any unshed hair as it grows.

How does the structure affect the way it looks and behaves?

> Hair follicles are formed mostly at an angle in the dermis, which is why hair grows in a defined direction. A successful style works with the direction in which the hair grows.

> Thickness of the hair is defined as: very fine, fine, medium or coarse.

> There are three main human hair groups: Caucasian, Black and Eastern Asian. Caucasian hair tends to be very fine to medium, and straight or slightly wavy. Black hair is very tightly curled. Eastern Asian hair is very coarse, thick and straight.

> Straight hair tends to be symmetrical in cross section, wavy hair mostly oval, and curly hair quite flat.

> Hair absorbs water from the atmosphere and washing (hygroscopic). The tiny gaps in the hair allow moisture in, so the more gaps caused by damage, the more water will be taken on, making it harder to style and hold a styled shape. Curly hair naturally has more gaps, making it more sensitive to humidity and meaning it takes longer to dry.

> Hot air causes the hair to swell, which raises the cuticle. Raised cuticles let in moisture, environmental damage and cause the hair to look dull and lifeless.

> The cortex holds the hair's natural pigment (melanin). Black and brown shades contain eumelanin. Red and blonde shades contain pheomelanin. UV and environmental damage can drain or bleach the natural and chemical pigment from the cortex.

> The cortex stores moisture. Overuse of heated styling appliances and damaging hair tools can cause voids in the cuticle or the moisture inside to evaporate. Dry hair becomes brittle and inelastic.

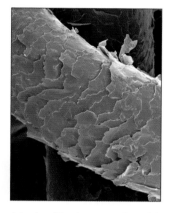

A hair with damaged cuticle

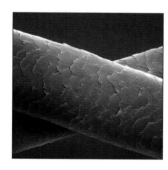

A hair in good condition with cuticle closed

What do I need to know about good condition?

> Hair is in good condition when the cuticle is lying flat, and a healthy cortex makes it strong and elastic.

> The flat cuticle, fed by good inner moisture levels, will cause the hair to shine.

> The flat cuticle means that the hair is easy to comb.

> Good moisture levels and healthy proteins in the cortex will make it strong and supple.

What do I need to know about bad condition?

> Hair is in bad condition when the cuticle is raised, damaged or missing, and when the cortex is swollen or damaged. If you see this kind of damage, carry out porosity and elasticity tests.

> When the inner cortex (or ends) dry out or suffer trauma, it can become split or frayed.

> When the cuticle is raised, hair does not reflect light and looks dull.

> **Activity** Define the following:
> 1 The main functions of the skin.
> 2 The main growth stages of the hair.
> 3 The key attributes of hair in bad condition.

> When the cuticle is raised, it locks together with other strands, much like a zip, causing knots and tangles.
> When the hair has been subjected to too many chemicals, it becomes bloated or eroded, making it porous and weak.
> Overuse of mechanical and heat-styling tools will cause the hair to dry out, making it porous, dull and brittle.
> Damaged hair absorbs and holds moisture, which means it takes longer to style and loses shape more readily.

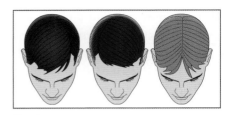

Partings can vary

What are the main growth patterns in hair?

If you do not clearly identify the natural growth patterns in your client's hair, you will struggle to get the look right. Cut the hair, working *with* the natural growth patterns and hairlines.

Natural partings

These can be anywhere and may not run in a straight line from front hairline to crown.

Hairlines

Square hairlines, high hairlines, low hairlines, receding hairlines, low

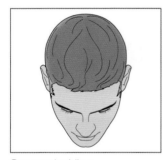

Square hairline

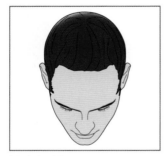

High hairline

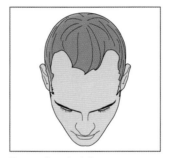

Receding hairline

nape hair will all have an impact on the type of style you cut. Your client may feel embarrassed, so be sensitive.

Cowlick

This is hair that grows back or up at the hairline and can make cutting a fringe difficult. Leave plenty of length and internal layers (weight) in the fringe section to encourage the hair to lay flat.

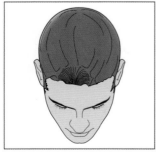

Cowlick

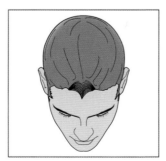

Widow's peak

Widow's peak

This is where the hair forms a 'V' shape at the front hairline. It can cause the hair to fall into a parting on short fringes.

Double crown

The hair grows in a circular direction at the crown, and some people have two areas of circular growth on the head. If the hair is cut too short, it will stick up.

Nape whorl

Strong hair growth that can be in any direction and forms a distinct whorl or curve in the direction of the hair. Nape whorls normally occur

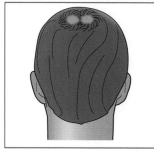

Double crown

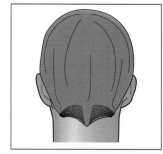

Nape whorl

at the centre back hairline or anywhere along the back of the head and will make short, graduated shapes very difficult.

Hair tests

The tests described in the table will help you decide which services and products are most appropriate for your client.

What is it?	When do I do it?	How do I do it?
Incompatibility testing 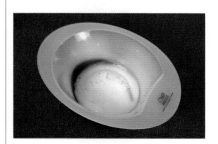 This tests how your client's hair will react to a particular product, to make sure there will be no adverse reactions.	You only need carry out this test if you have become aware of the fact that hair has been home-coloured using a product containing 'metallic salts' (products such as Grecian 2000) or if you feel the hair may contain some product or coating that may react to hair colour.	Cut a small lock of hair and secure the strands using tape, place it into a glass bowl containing a small amount of hydrogen peroxide and alkaline perm lotion. The hair should remain in the solution for approximately 30 minutes. If the hair does not contain any metallic salts, nothing will happen. If the solution bubbles, fizzes, begins to give off heat or the hair changes colour or begins to dissolve, perming lotions or hair colour products containing hydrogen peroxide should not be used on the hair.

What is it?	When do I do it?	How do I do it?
Porosity testing 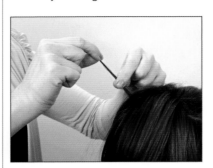 If the cuticle is damaged, hair is more porous, which will affect how the pigment is absorbed. Porous, brittle and dry hair will be damaged further and may break, and can cause patchy or poor colour results.	You must assess the condition of every client's hair prior to any chemical process, testing to make sure that hair is in adequate condition to withstand the proposed chemical process.	If the hair feels rough and coarse when you rub strands with the ends of your fingers, it is porous. Porous hair remains heavy and saturated even after towel drying.
Elasticity testing 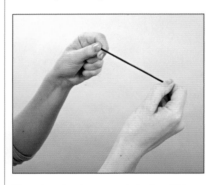 If cortex is damaged, hair will have poor elasticity. This indicates the overall strength and suppleness of the hair. Hair that breaks easily, remains stretched or is weak will return poor colour and styling results, and may be damaged further.	You must assess the condition of every client's hair prior to any chemical process, testing to make sure that hair is in adequate condition to withstand the proposed chemical process. Hair that has been previously bleached or coloured is likely to show weakness.	Hold a few strands of hair between the fingers of both hands, at the root and further along the shaft too. Apply pressure and tug lightly on the hair. If the hair breaks but does not stretch, the cortex is damaged. If it stretches but does not return to its original length, the elasticity is compromised.

What is it?	When do I do it?	How do I do it?
Strand testing 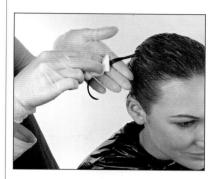 This is to assess what the colour result will be.	This test helps you to judge the colour result first hand, and should be done towards the end of the manufacturer's recommended development times.	Open a foil or lift a section of tinted hair and rub away the excess tint with gloved fingers or the back of a tint comb. Visually assess the hair to see if the process has optimised.
Test cutting 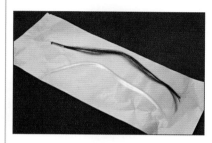 This allows you to see first hand how hair will react to chemicals before applying them to the client. It is the same as a strand test, but is not conducted while the hair is attached to the client.	Conduct this test when you are in any doubt about how hair will react to any colour, perm, bleach, etc.	Cut a tiny section of hair from the nape. Lay the section on a foil and apply the chemical. Check the development time and the results.

What is it?	When do I do it?	How do I do it?
Pre-perm curl test Different hair textures will require different rod sizes, development times, etc. This test gives you the right choices for your client.	Create a test curl before any perm is done.	Take one or two sections and wind on to rods. Choose the underneath sections of hair. Apply the lotion and process accordingly. Assess the results. Adjust rod size, etc., as required.
Development curl test Check the development of your perm during processing to assess progress.	Neutralising will set the wave, so make sure you are confident you have achieved just the right level of curl or wave beforehand.	Carefully unwind a rod and push the hair back on itself to assess how well the curl has developed. When the optimum curl is achieved, you can begin neutralising.

Hair tests

Activity When and why would you conduct the following tests?

1 Porosity.

2 Compatibility.

3 Test cutting.

Record the results!

Everything you have learned about your client and their skin, scalp and hair is important information. Record the results of your consultation and tests clearly in the salon database. Refer to history and reassess your client each time they visit. Using the information you have will help you to create successful styles for your client, recommend the right products and services and help them feel treated as an individual – which all adds up to a happy client! Make sure that you respect the data protection laws and your client's right to privacy (see Unit G20 for more information).

Diseases, problems, conditions

Parasites, fungi, viral and bacterial infections, along with inherited or topical problems, can all cause challenges for the hair and scalp. Trichologists are professionals who specialise in the study of the function, structure and diseases of the hair and scalp. It's sufficient for you to be a generalist, but make sure you are a good one! There are many diseases that must be reported by the employer or salon manager under the Reporting of Injuries, Diseases and Dangerous Occurrences Regulations (RIDDOR) (1995) (see Unit G20 for more information). Refer to the Health and Safety Executive website for a full list of reportable diseases (www.hse.gov.uk/RIDDOR).

Look out for the following diseases, problems and conditions.

Contagious and infectious

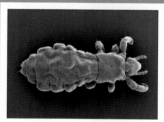 Head lice (pediculosis capitis) Contagious	Most often seen in school-age children, head lice are parasitic, grey/brown insects that grow to about 2.5 mm. The insect clings to the hair, biting the scalp, causing irritation and itching, and feeding on the host's blood. It then lays eggs (nits) that are firmly attached to the hair shaft close to the scalp. The egg hatches after approximately seven days. Head lice cannot jump, hop or fly. Head-to-head contact is required. As soon as you part the hair, especially near the hairline, you will see adult lice, black/brown eggs or white empty egg casings.	Treatments are available in the form of lotions or shampoos from chemists and alternative health stores. Normal cleaning/ washing of equipment, towels and gowns after contact with head lice is all that's required.
 Scabies (Sarcoptes scabiei) Contagious	Scabies is caused by a mite that burrows beneath the skin and lays eggs. Extreme itching and a rash are caused as a result of an allergic reaction to the mite. The rash may develop anywhere on the body. The burrows or initial site of infestation are usually on the hands. Extreme scratching can cause a secondary infection. Scabies are transferred by skin-to-skin contact.	Scabies is treated with insecticide cream and the client should be referred to a doctor.

Contagious and infectious

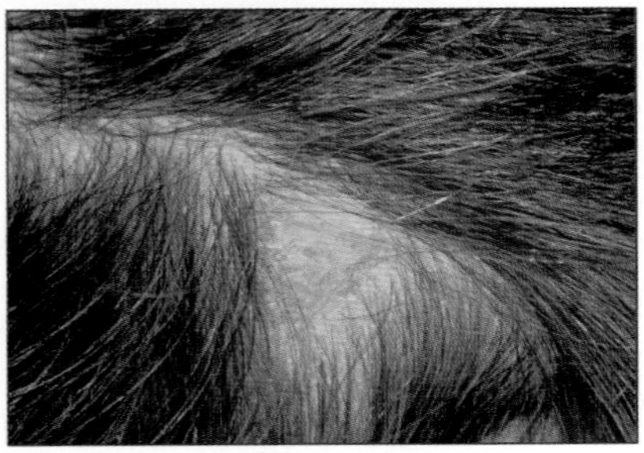

Ringworm (tinea capitis)

Fungal/contagious

This is most common in children and leaves a small area of hair loss enclosed by a red, slightly raised ring. There may also be some flaking and scaling.

Treatment is in the form of prescription antifungal creams. Refer your client to a doctor.

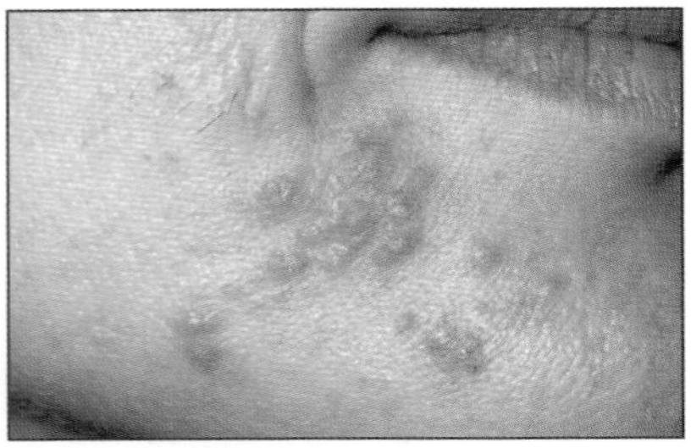

Cold sore (herpes simplex)

Viral/contagious

Herpes infection can lay dormant in the body, but flairs up to form a burning, itching inflammation that will first blister, then crust. Most commonly found on the face. Cold sores are transmitted by skin-to-skin contact.

Topical cream is available over the counter, but refer your client to a doctor if they are experiencing recurrent infections.

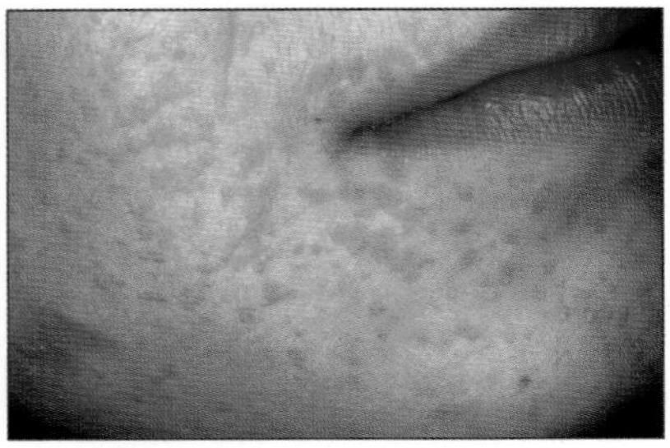

Warts

Viral/contagious

More common in children, warts are caused by the human papilloma virus that flares up to form an overgrowth of skin. Growths are usually a slightly different colour to the healthy skin.

Over the counter, topical remedies are available. Referring your client to a doctor is recommended.

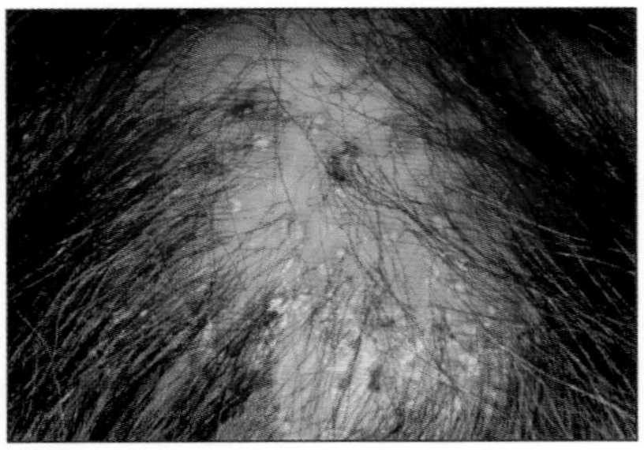

Folliculitis

Bacterial/viral
Contagious and non-infectious types

Any infection or inflammation of the hair follicle can be a form of folliculitis. Non-infectious folliculitis appears when bacteria have entered an area of damage caused by irritation such as shaving. It presents as red swelling and pustules.

Refer your client to a doctor. Treatment depends on cause.

Contagious and infectious

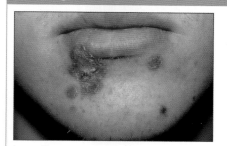

Impetigo

Bacterial/contagious

Redness, burning and itching is followed by spots that cluster and become blisters that eventually have a yellow crust. This infection spreads quickly from skin-to-skin contact.

Refer your client to a doctor. Treatment is usually an antibiotic cream.

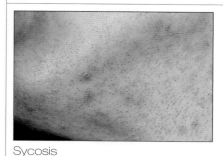

Sycosis

Bacterial/contagious

Typically found in the beard, neck and hairline. This bacterial infection of the follicle can result in permanent destruction. An inflamed follicle with burning and irritation are the main symptoms.

Refer your client to a doctor.

Non-infectious or non-communicable

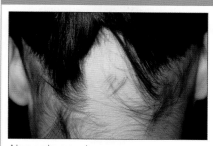

Alopecia areata

Non-infectious

The most common form of alopecia is usually seen in circular patches of baldness about the size of a ten pence piece. They can cluster and join and usually start above the ear. When hair regrows, initially it can be paler than the rest of the hair or even grey. Causes can be varied, but stress is generally recognised as the main catalyst.

Referral to a trichologist is recommended.

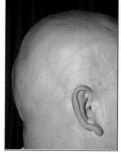

Alopecia totalis

Non-infectious

Total scalp hair loss can be as a result of extended alopecia areata.

Referral to a trichologist is recommended.

Non-infectious or non-communicable

 Scarring alopecia (cicatricial) Non-infectious	This spontaneous inflammation permanently destroys and damages the follicles, causing scarring and baldness. Causes are usually associated with illness.	Referral to a trichologist is recommended.
 Alopecia universalis Non-infectious	Total hair loss over the entire body.	Referral to a trichologist is recommended.
 Male pattern baldness (androgenic alopecia) Inherited	Most men will experience some inherited baldness by the time they are in their sixties. Typically affects the front hairline and crown and is caused by a change in the way follicles react to hormones. Follicles begin to shrink, the hair weakens and eventually it stops growing.	Treatment includes wigs and scalp surgery, and medications are available on private prescription that report some success in restoring growth or delaying loss.
 Thinning and hair loss (telogen effluvium) Symptomatic	General thinning of hair can be the result of medication, bad diet, sudden weight loss, childbirth, cancer treatment or environmental factors such as stress or sun. Examine the scalp carefully and ask the client tactful questions.	Dietary supplements/ diet change. Referral to a trichologist.

Non-infectious or non-communicable

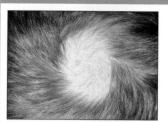 Traction alopecia Mechanical	Overuse of styling tools, plaiting, brushing or tightly securing hair can pull the hair free of the follicle before that stage of the growth cycle has been reached. Usually seen around the crown and hairline. Look out for clusters of fine regrowth.	Once the tension is consistently released, the hair will grow back.
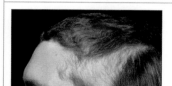 Trichotillomania or compulsive hair pulling Habitual	Obsessive hair twirling, tugging, sucking and ripping is a compulsive disorder that leaves alopecia-like bald spots and missing sections of hair.	Cognitive behaviour therapy and hypnosis are two potential sources of treatment, but refer your client to a medical professional for help.
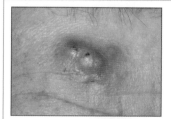 Boils and abscesses (furunculosis) Non-infectious	An ingrowing hair or blocked pore can become infected, painful and inflamed, with a pus-filled centre. Often there will be localised heat and the client may experience chills or fever.	Refer your client to a doctor.
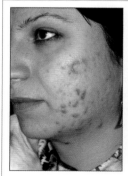 Acne Bacterial/non-infectious	Typically affecting the face, neck, shoulders and upper arms. Acne causes a range of skin and hair follicle problems, from pus-filled spots and raised bumps to deep lesions and scarring. The cause is overactive sebaceous glands and can lead to secondary infections.	There is a wide range of treatments that work together to improve the condition. Refer your client to a doctor or skin specialist.

Non-infectious or non-communicable

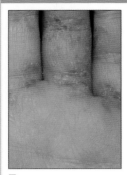 Eczema Atopic/non-infectious	Symptoms can range from mild redness to severe splitting of the skin with weeping. Eczema is itchy, uncomfortable and can scar. Atopic eczema starts after someone with a familial tendency is subjected to a trigger such as soap and detergents.	Refer your client to a doctor.
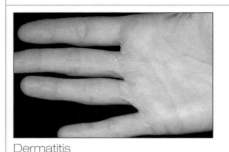 Dermatitis Non-infectious	Dry, itchy and uncomfortable red skin, most often seen on the hands as a result of contact with or an allergy to an irritant, such as detergents or cosmetics.	Use of gloves and barrier creams to prevent contact will help, but refer your client to a doctor too.
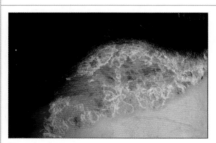 Psoriasis Non-infectious	Thick, reddened, inflamed and flaking skin patches, sometimes large, and usually seen on the scalp and joints. Causes are varied and the condition can be chronic.	Refer your client to a doctor.
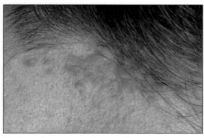 Seborrhoea and cradle cap (seborrhoeic dermatitis) Non-infectious	Excessive secretion of sebum from the sebaceous glands of the scalp causes hair to become lank and can cause an inflammation of the scalp (even in adults) that is commonly called cradle cap. The build-up of sebum and dead skin cells can develop into a fungal infection.	Recommend specialist cleansing and scalp treatments.

Non-infectious or non-communicable

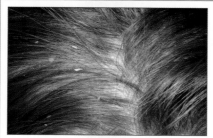

Dandruff (pityriasis capitis)

Non-infectious

Dry flakes and scales fall from the scalp, causing irritation and itchiness. Causes can be varied, including harsh cleansers, excessive heat styling and dry environments.

Recommend specialist cleansing and scalp treatments.

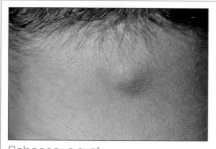

Sebaceous cyst

Non-infectious

Cysts form as a result of the skin cells multiplying and forming 'pools' of keratin cells beneath the skin. They are benign and can be left or removed under medical care.

Refer your client to a doctor.

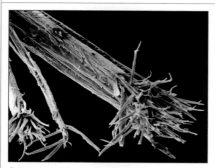

Split ends (trichoptilosis)

Mechanical/environmental

The hair looks frayed and shattered at the ends, as a result of poor maintenance, bad condition, harsh chemicals or overuse of styling tools.

The best solution is simply to cut the split ends off, but restorative treatments and conditioners can help.

Beaded hair (monilethrix)

Inherited

Caused by a keratin mutation. The hair has regular nodes along the shaft and is very weak and fragile. The hair breaks easily and often never grows to any great length.

There is no treatment. The hair is too weak to sustain chemical or mechanical processes.

Non-infectious or non-communicable

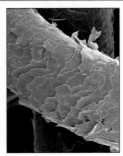 Cuticle damage (fragilitas crinium) Mechanical/environmental	The hair is brittle and can be torn and damaged at any point along the shaft. There are often voids in the cuticle layer. Hair is unmanageable and dull. Cuticle damage is often chemical, mechanical or the result of poor maintenance.	The best solution is simply to cut the hair off, but restorative treatments and conditioners can help. Damaged hair should be rehabilitated before being subjected to chemical treatments.
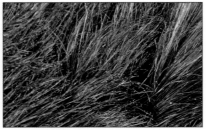 Trichorrhexis nodosa Mechanical/environmental/inherited	Characterised by a nodular hair shaft, this disorder is a result of cuticle damage and a swollen inner cortex. It can be experienced from birth, but is most often the result of chemical or mechanical damage.	Treatment can include fortifying products and a style that requires less mechanical styling. Avoid chemical treatments until the hair is restored to health.
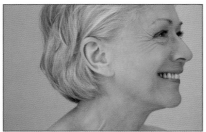 Grey hair (canities) Inherited/acquired	Grey hair is always connected with the absence of melanin or natural pigment. Albinos have white/grey hair from birth and some people grey early. Stress, fear or long-term illness can affect melanin production and bring on greying.	Tints can mask grey.

Communicating about problems

Often you will be the first person to spot a client's problem or be in a position where you will have to uncover personal details in order to make a correct diagnosis. Think carefully about how you communicate.

> Be discreet and put yourself in your client's position.

> Where possible or appropriate, reposition your client away from others before starting the discussion.

> Ask open and honest questions, such as: 'How would you describe your health at the moment?' 'What changes have you noticed in your hair and scalp recently?' 'Tell me more about the hair products and styling tools you use.'

> Frame your findings to help prepare your client. For example, 'I've completed a full assessment of your hair and scalp and I'd like to tell you more about my findings.'

> Reassure your client that, as their professional, you are ready and willing to help.

> Make sure you have a solution or a referral ready.

> Your client may get upset or even angry with you if they had no prior knowledge of the problem. Be patient and understanding. Do not reflect these negative feelings or use defensive body language. Use phrases such as: 'I understand this is a shock for you.' 'I accept this is difficult.'

Activity

1 Identify the possible diseases or problems for the symptoms described in the table below.

Symptom	Problem
A small area of hair loss enclosed by a red, slightly raised ring.	
Redness, burning and itching is followed by spots that cluster and become blisters that eventually have a yellow crust.	
Dry flakes and scales fall from the scalp, causing irritation and itchiness.	
The hair has regular nodes along the shaft and is very weak and fragile.	
Small black/brown eggs (nits) that are firmly attached to the hair shaft close to the scalp.	

2 Identify which of the following problems are contagious.

Problem	Contagious (yes/no)
Impetigo	
Psoriasis	
Alopecia	
Split ends	
Head lice	
Folliculitis	
Scabies	
Warts	
Dandruff	
Acne	

Record the results!

As before, everything you have learned about your client and their skin, scalp and hair is important information, so record the results of your consultation and tests clearly in the salon database for future reference. Make sure that you respect the data protection laws and your client's right to privacy.

Summary

The consultation will lay the foundation of your ongoing relationship with your client and demands that you know your hair science and principles well. Take the time to build that knowledge, because it will give you a firm basis for your future career. You will learn how to assess your client's hair and scalp with confidence; how to make good judgements about the style, shapes and colours that will suit them well; and how to source lots of information to tailor the look you create to their individual needs. Most importantly, your client will learn that they have found a hair professional they can trust and who listens to them.

GH8: Shampoo, condition and treat the hair and scalp

In this chapter, you will learn to:

> **understand the products, tools and terms used when providing shampoo and conditioning services**
> **shampoo, condition and treat clients' hair and scalp**
> **provide aftercare and advice.**

You will be assessed against your knowledge and ability to:

1. Understand your salon's processes and procedures with regard to promoting products and services.

2. Understand your legal and health and safety responsibilities when carrying out these services.

3. Understand your personal obligations to other team members and know when and from whom you should seek advice and assistance.

4. Maintain effective and safe methods of working, and shampoo and treat hair and scalps in a commercially viable timeframe.

5. Communicate effectively with clients, using positive listening skills, body language and verbal communication.

6. Consult with clients, diagnose hair and scalp conditions and consider other key factors when deciding on shampoo and conditioning services.

7. Carry out a variety of shampoo, conditioning and treatment services.

8. Know the shampoo area and understand the specific tools, techniques and products required in shampooing and conditioning.

9. Recognise adverse results and deal with them effectively.

10. Provide aftercare and product advice.

Introduction

Why do we shampoo hair?

Hair is shampooed to remove dirt, grease and product build-up, to make the hair both clean and easier to work with.

Why do we condition hair?

Conditioner is used to improve the look, health and manageability of hair.

What are treatments?

Treatments are specific formulas used to repair hair damage and treat various hair and scalp conditions.

What does this chapter cover?

This chapter covers Unit GH8, showing you how to provide quality shampoo, conditioning and treatment services that meet the needs of today's clients.

The art of the shampoo

As a trainee hairdresser, the first interactive client service you will probably be called on to provide is the shampoo. This does not mean it's unimportant and only to be given to those with little or no experience. Not at all – a good shampoo is an integral part of the service the salon provides. A good shampoo forms the base of all salon work and, more than anything, it is a crucial element of the client's enjoyment of the salon visit.

The shampoo is your chance to show your skill as a technician and your expert product knowledge. It is also your chance to earn tips; a skilful shampoo technician will get requests and more tips!

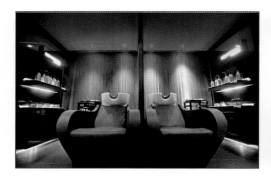 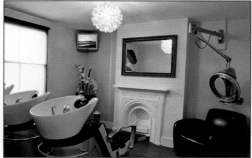

The shampoo area

While shampoo areas will vary in shape, size and location, they will fundamentally consist of the same features: basins, reclining chairs, towel and product dispensers and waste receptacles. Hair is most commonly shampooed from behind (backwash), but there are some salons that use a 'sidewash' system. The basin itself may be adjustable, as may the height and recline angle of the chair. Many salons use integral, all-in-one shampoo units that have various manual or motorised positional adjustments. The shampoo area may be on a raised platform or in a sectioned-off area of the salon. Dim lights and soft music are often used in shampoo areas to aid relaxation.

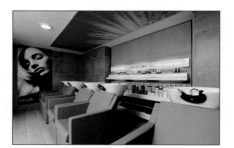

Knowing your shampoo area

In order to deliver a quality shampoo and to ensure the health and safety of you and your clients, it's important to know your shampoo area well.

Before you can start providing shampoo services, you need to learn:
> how to operate the shampoo chair and basin to position clients comfortably and correctly
> how to operate and control the water temperature and pressure
> how to use and apply the shampoo and conditioning products
> how to replenish stocks of towels, products, and so on
> what is required to maintain a clean and safe working environment.

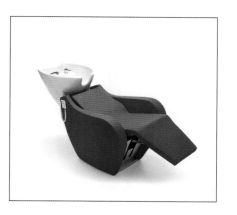
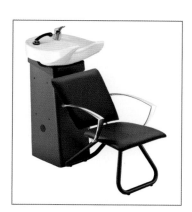
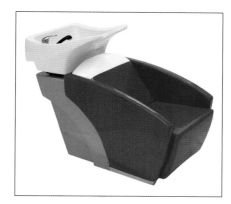

Top Tip

Practise positioning yourself and your colleagues at the shampoo basin; learn how to adjust the position for shorter and taller people.

Shampoo, conditioning and treatment products

There are countless products on the market, for both professional and home use, each with its own specific function or feature. Some salons will use a single manufacturer's full range of shampoos and conditioners at the backwash, while others will mix products from various ranges to enable them to cater to all their clients' needs. This means that it is important that you take time to learn the names, functions and quantities of the products used in your salon and any new ones that are introduced.

Confusing names...

You will soon notice that product manufacturers often use different terms and names for shampoo and conditioning products. Sometimes it can be difficult to judge if these are words that actually relate to the product's function or the result it produces, or if they are terms thought up by marketing departments.

Shampoos are sometimes referred to as:
> cleansers
> baths
> scrubs
> washes
> emulsions.

Conditioners and treatments are sometimes referred to as:

> creams
> milks
> rinses
> repairers
> reconstructors
> rejuvenators.

Therefore, it is vitally important that you know the primary use and function of your salon's products.

Shampoo

What is it?

A shampoo is a detergent-based liquid that is used to remove dirt, grease and product build-up from the hair and scalp.

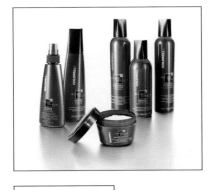

Are all shampoos the same?

While the basic principle is the same, there are many different shampoo formulas created for specific hair types, colours and scalp and hair conditions.

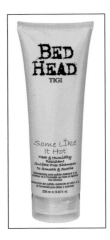

Heat and humidity resistance shampoo

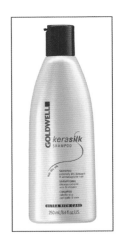

Shampoo for dry, damaged hair

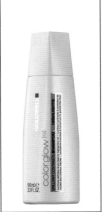

Shampoo for highlighted hair

The detergent molecules in shampoo are attracted to both grease and water and work in the exact same way as washing-up liquid. Detergent molecules have two ends: one is attracted to water and one is attracted to grease. When you wash a client's hair, the detergent in the shampoo combines with water on the wet hair and is able to spread throughout the hair and scalp. As these molecules are also attracted to grease, when they come in contact with it the other end becomes stuck to this as well. This means they are stuck to both the grease and the water. When you rinse, the detergents run off the hair with the water, taking the grease and dirt with them. (This is why the dirt stays in the bowl with the water when you wash up.)

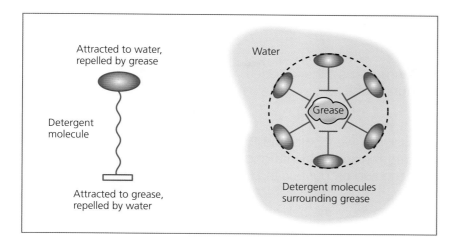

While the basic principle is the same, different concentrations of detergents and additives help the shampoo to do different things:

> Shampoos for dry hair will have a light/weaker detergent.
> Shampoos for greasy hair will have a stronger or more concentrated detergent.
> Shampoos for scalp conditions like dandruff and psoriasis will contain certain medications to alleviate or soothe symptoms.
> Shampoos for pre-colouring or pre-perming will contain few additives and will balance the hair's pH and/or porosity to aid the even processing of the hair.

Product build-up

One of the major jobs a shampoo has to do is remove product build-up. Product build-up is when the continual and long-term use of a product results in a residue being left on the hair. This residue can cause the hair to begin to look lank, greasy and heavy. It can also affect and dry the scalp, as well as 'blocking' and interfering with chemical services such as colours and perms.

Salons will have between four and eight shampoos, so take time to learn the correct use for those in your salon.

Note: If shampoo or conditioner gets splashed in your or your client's eyes, rinse immediately with cold water and check the manufacturer's advice on the product for any further procedures. You may also need to enter this in the accident book.

Top Tip

You don't need to use the same product for both shampoos. You may decide to use a combination of two shampoos for the best result. For example, you might select a shampoo for greasy hair for the first wash if the hair is particularly dirty, and a medicated shampoo for the second wash if the client has an itchy scalp.

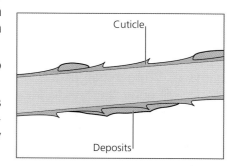

Hair conditioners and treatments

What are they?

Hair conditioners and treatments are oil-, lanolin- or synthetic-based products used to improve the feel and texture of the hair.

Why are they used?

Conditioners are used to make the hair easier to work with and to improve its sheen, while treatments will also replace nutrients and repair damage. The distinction between these two products can be a bit blurred.

Fundamentally, a conditioner works on the outside of the hair shaft, helping to close and smooth the cuticle, and coating the exterior with various fatty oils and lanolin to improve the texture and condition of the hair.

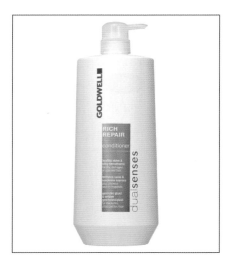

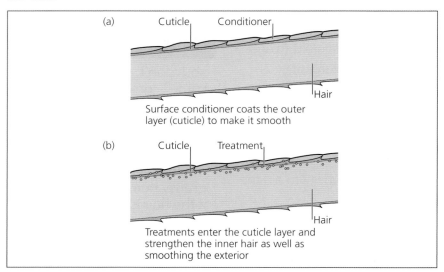

(a) Surface conditioner coats the outer layer (cuticle) to make it smooth;
(b) Treatments enter the cuticle layer and strengthen the inner hair as well as smoothing the exterior

A treatment, on the other hand, is designed to treat the hair by replacing lost moisture, amino acids and nutrients, and by repairing damage. While most of the repair will be only temporary, treatments will enter the hair to improve the elasticity and strength, as well as smoothing and improving the cuticle. If the cuticle is raised, it will cause the hair to tangle. Conditioning makes the hair more manageable and makes it look healthier.

Using hair conditioners and treatments

For best results, heat is often used with treatments. Moist heat from a steamer, or created by placing a plastic cap on the head, will help swell the hair and gently open the cuticle slightly, enabling the treatment to penetrate into the hair. Also, cooling the hair before rinsing will help to seal the product inside.

Some manufacturers have developed special treatments and

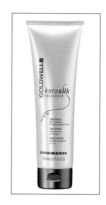

conditioners designed to be used following the use of a specific hair colour, perm or other technical service. These often have particular ingredients that either counteract a particular damaging property of the colour or perming product, or are designed to enhance or help to fix the result. You should always follow the specific manufacturer's recommendations for each technical product you use.

As with shampoos, conditioners and treatments contain various ingredients, all designed for particular functions. While using the wrong conditioner or treatment won't damage the hair, it can affect how the hair looks and feels, especially after styling. Using the wrong product can result in the hair looking lank and dull and feeling greasy.

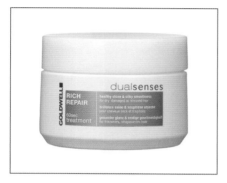
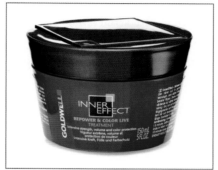
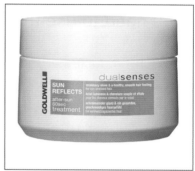

Scalp treatments

What are they?

Scalp treatments are products that are applied directly to the scalp as part of the shampoo service.

What do they do?

They treat certain medical scalp conditions and improve scalp health.

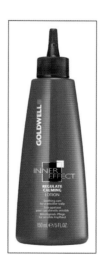

There is an increasing number of professional scalp-treating products available to salons; these are designed to deal with a number of conditions and to promote the well-being of the scalp. While some are design to treat specific scalp conditions, like dandruff or psoriasis, others are used to counter scalp dryness and sensitivity, or to stimulate and promote general good scalp health. Many scalp treatments are applied post-shampoo and left on.

Pre-treatments (pre-technical service treatments)

What are they?

Pre-treatments are products designed to be used prior to a technical service like a perm or a colour.

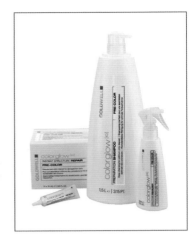

What do they do?

They prepare the hair to make sure it is in the best possible state to undergo the chemical service, protecting it against unnecessary damage and aiding a successful result.

Do you need to use them before all technical work?

No. There are products that do require use of a particular pre-treatment, but with others it is recommended as and when required.

How do I know when to use one?

During your technical and product training, you will learn what pre-treatments your salon uses and the products that require them. Always read the product's usage directions and ask your salon's educator if you need advice.

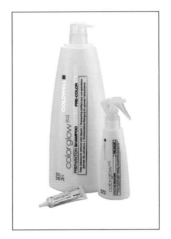

As older hair or damaged hair is more porous than virgin hair, pre-treatment products work by evening out the porosity, so that the perm lotion or colour is absorbed evenly. As dryer hair will tend to process quicker, this helps to protect dryer hair from further damage while the virgin hair processes.

Note: Products may react differently when used in combination with others, so it's important to learn about all the shampoo and conditioning products your salon uses. If in doubt, ask a colleague for advice or contact the manufacturer.

Diagnosis

The shampoo is usually the first time that chemicals and products are used on the client, so it's important to take a careful look at the hair, scalp and skin around the hairline. It's also important to check the client's record card and to ask if they are allergic to any specific substances, or if they have any conditions that may cause a reaction with the hair products you will use. You should also ask if there is anything they have been doing that may have affected their hair that you should know about.

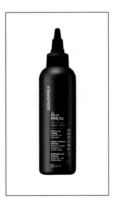

It's important to know how the shampoo and conditioning products in your salon should be used and the results that they produce. Using the wrong product could result in the hair not being properly cleaned, or a residue being left on the hair that can make the hair greasy and difficult to style. It can also interfere with other planned treatments or chemical services.

Always make sure you know how to use the products, the application amounts and processing instructions. If in doubt, always ask a senior member of the team.

Note: Busy stylists may easily miss subtle hair, scalp and skin conditions during the consultation, so always be vigilant. If you see anything that doesn't seem right with the products you've been asked to use, quietly speak to the stylist and explain why you are concerned. Never be embarrassed to check.

As well as considering what service the client will be having, you need to take a good look at the client's hair, scalp, face and skin around the hairline.

Hair – what you're looking for

> Level and amount of oil or grease – will the hair require one shampoo or two?
> Level and amount of product and product build-up
> Texture of the hair: coarse, frizzy, flyaway, and so on
> Condition of the hair:
>> Chemical damage – caused by perming, colouring or other chemical service
>> Heat damage – caused by hot stylers and straighteners
>> Environmental damage – caused by the sun or swimming, and so on
> Look at the hair in sections – roots, mid-lengths and ends – and diagnose individually; only the ends might need conditioner
> The thickness and volume of the hair
> Head lice and their eggs.

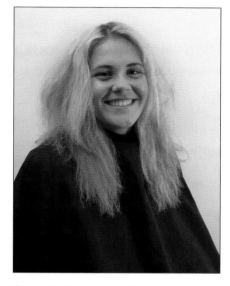

Chemically damaged hair

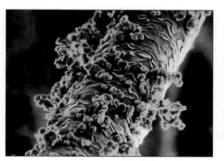

Heat-damaged hair

Product build-up

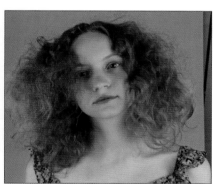

Environmentally damaged hair

Scalp – what you're looking for

> Signs of dryness, flaky skin
> Amount of oil
> Product build-up
> Signs of dandruff, psoriasis, eczema or other skin conditions
> Bumps, bruises, cuts, scratches or abrasions.

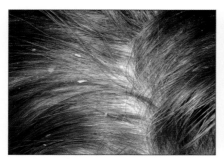

Dry scalp

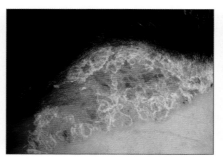

Psoriasis

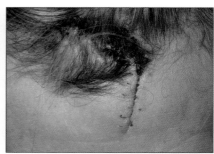

Scar

Skin – what you're looking for

> Skin disorders and infections
> Bumps, cuts, scratches or abrasions, including new scars – cosmetic surgery scars are often hidden behind the ears
> Piercings, new tattoos and jewellery.

Note: Always ask if the client has any cuts or bruises you should know about, but you must check as well as asking – the client may have forgotten they bumped their head or not think a cut or a new scar is important. Pressing on a bruise will be painful and reopening a cut or catching a new scar could be quite serious.

Also, if you discover a skin disorder, irritation or something in the hair that you are not sure about, ask for help and advice from a senior technician. Don't ever be too embarrassed to ask.

Preparation for shampoo and conditioning services

Each salon will have its own method of client preparation for shampooing that will include:

> gowning to protect the client and their clothes
> analysing the hair and scalp to make the correct product selection
> rules and guidance on your own protection and working methods.

These methods may be different from what you have learned in college or at another salon, so make sure you are up to speed with your salon's products and practices.

You need to ensure that you are prepared, with the necessary tools to hand and protective items such as aprons and gloves. You also need to prepare the client.

The client

> The client should be correctly protected, with clean gown and towels. (For clients with a low hairline at the nape, use cling film or a plastic cape tucked into the collar as additional protection.)
> A correct diagnosis should have been made and the appropriate

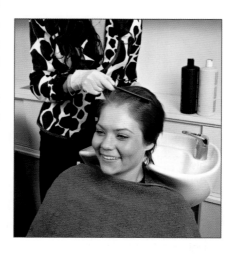

products selected for both the client's hair and scalp type, and for the further services the client will receive.

> You should check the scalp for cuts and bruises and enquire about product allergies.

> Any earrings should be removed and other jewellery should be safely out of the way.

> The client should be positioned correctly and comfortably and should be are relaxed.

> The client's hair should be brushed through and free of tangles, pins and clips, and so on.

You

> Check that the shampoo basin and chair are clean before taking the client over the shampooing area.

> Ensure that your hands are clean.

> Wear gloves to protect your hands and an apron to protect your clothes.

> Make sure that none of your jewellery will get in the way while you are working.

> Have all the necessary towels, products and clean tools to hand in order to complete the entire process.

> Make sure that any tools or equipment you use are safe and fit for purpose.

> Keep your working area as tidy as possible while carrying out your work.

> Ensure that you know how to work safely, with the correct posture, and that you are wearing clothes and shoes suitable for the service you are carrying out.

Care of your hands

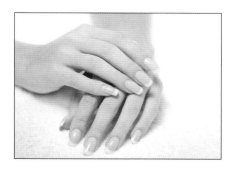

One of the major reasons hairdressers give up hairdressing is contact dermatitis (see page 51), caused in a large part by carrying out wet services like shampooing.

Taking care of your hands is *your responsibility*! Yes, your salon owner or manager has a duty of care to initiate safe working practices and to provide you with all the protective equipment you need, but it's up to you to follow the procedures and to use the equipment. In fact, you have a legal responsibility to do so. But more than that, not looking after your hands could ruin a great career.

Take care of your hands by:

> always drying them properly

> always wearing gloves when you can

> never carrying out chemical services without gloves

> using gloves when cleaning and using cleaning products

> using a barrier cream to protect your hands while working

> always using a good quality hand cream (even you guys!), especially when you finish work and at bedtime

> wearing gloves in the winter.

Note: You must advise your manager or salon owner if your hands become sore or show signs of contact dermatitis. Cease wet service work immediately and seek medical advice as soon as possible. Never ignore it!

Glove use when shampooing

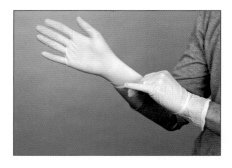

The current recommendations by the Health and Safety Executive and industry trade bodies is that non-latex, non-powdered, nitrile or vinyl gloves should be used for all wet salon services, including shampooing. Being a very tactile service, however, many hairdressers dislike shampooing with gloves, noting that it makes it hard to judge water temperature and that they can pull on the hair, making it uncomfortable for the client.

The recommendation is designed to protect you from dermatitis and skin damage, and as your salon manager has a legal obligation to protect you from injury while at work, they should take it into account when deciding salon policies. At the same time, you also have an obligation to follow salon rules and not do anything that could injure yourself or others.

More importantly, regardless of your salon's policy, they are *your* hands and it is *your* career. You do not want to put your career at risk by not taking good care of your hands in the early years.

> If your salon policy states that you 'must' wear gloves while shampooing, you must do so. Failure to do so may result in disciplinary action, but equally importantly, it would negate any claim for damages or loss of earnings if it resulted in skin injury and inability to work.

> If your salon policy 'advises' or 'recommends' glove use while shampooing, the onus is more on you. You have to take responsibility for looking after your hands and deciding on whether or not you wear gloves. If your salon has provided gloves and advised you that you should wear them, but you don't and you develop skin injury, you will find it very difficult to claim for damages or loss of earnings.

> If your salon has 'no policy' on glove use while shampooing, you still have a responsibility and duty to protect your skin. You must advise your manager if you would like to wear gloves while shampooing, or if your hands start to become affected by wet services. While your manager has a duty of care to ensure your well-being, failure to request protective gloves or to advise your manager of any problem may affect your ability to claim and the level of compensation you receive.

It would be against the law for a salon to insist that you don't wear gloves while shampooing.

Activity If the product selection is made for you by a stylist, always ask why the selection was made, either at the time or later if it's not convenient at the time of service. If you continually do this, it won't take you long to learn all the features and benefits of your salon's products.

The shampoo is the best part!

For many clients, the luxury of having someone else wash their hair is a real treat and the best part of the salon visit experience, so don't forget to make sure that the client feels at ease, so they can relax and enjoy the experience.

There are a few things you can find out that will help you to make it the best possible experience for the client:

> Would they prefer you not to talk during the shampoo?
> Do they prefer the water to be on the hot or cool side?
> Would putting their feet up on a stool make them more comfortable?
> Do they prefer a firm or gentle shampoo?
> Would they like cotton wool to stop water going in their ears?

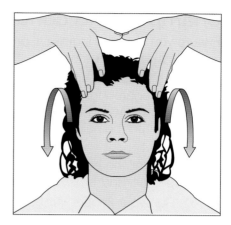
Effleurage

Shampoo techniques

All shampooing techniques are carried out using the tips of the fingers.

Effleurage

This is moving the fingers in one firm but smooth, large circular action from the front to the back of the head, covering the entire scalp. The fingers should be straight and open slightly.

Petrissage

This is moving the fingers in small, massaging, circular motions, working around the head. The hands should be 'crabbed', with the fingers open and bent.

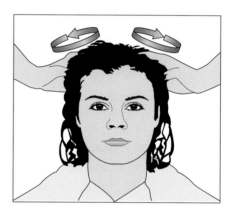
Petrissage

Scalp massage

This is massaging the head and scalp to relax the client and make the shampoo more enjoyable. It can also help to increase blood flow and stimulate the sebaceous glands. There are various techniques that use a combination of slow massaging movements and pressure.

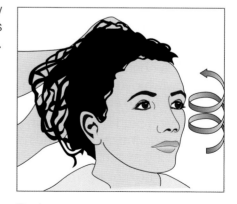
Scalp massage

Shampoo and conditioning step by step

Ensure you read the individual product's preparation, application and rinsing instructions before you start.

1 Make sure both you and the client are correctly protected and prepared for the shampoo. The client should be seated comfortably and correctly at the basin, and you should have examined the hair and scalp and have the selected products to hand.

2 Ensure all the hair is in the basin, taking special notice of the nape hair, and brush through.

> Run your fingers through the hair to see if there are any pins, grips, and so on.

> Using a cushioned paddle or grooming brush, starting at the front and with the ends of the hair, brush through to the roots, making sure all the hair is brushed backwards, away from the face.

> Brush the hair from the nape upwards, towards the crown.

> Finally, for long hair, brush through the mid-lengths and ends until it is tangle-free.

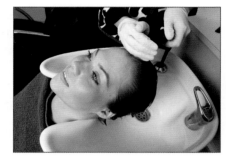

(a)

3 Turn on the water and check the temperature. (If you are wearing gloves, remember the water may be hotter than it feels to you.) Run a small amount of water on the client's head and ask if the temperature is okay.

4 Beginning at the front, shield the face with your hand while wetting down the hair (a). Ensure all the hair is completely wet.

5 Pour or pump the selected shampoo into your hand (b), taking care not to take too much (you can always add more if needed).

6 Spread the shampoo evenly across your two hands and apply to the head, spreading the shampoo evenly over the entire head.

7 Beginning at the front, begin to shampoo the hair using petrissage (c). Check that the pressure you are using is okay for the client.

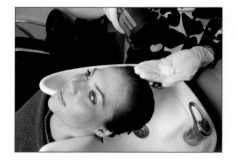

(b)

8 While continuing to shampoo the hair in this fashion, begin to slowly move your hands down the sides of the hairline to the ears. Make sure you wash all the hair in front of the ears.

9 Moving slightly back down the head, start to move back towards the centre of the head. Make sure your hands are working symmetrically on either side of the head.

10 Continue moving from the centre to the hairline as you work back down the head, until the entire head has been covered. (You may need to lift and support the client's head with one hand while you work on the nape area.)

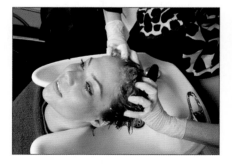

(c)

11 Once complete, use effleurage to shampoo and massage the scalp from front to back, in steady, firm, large circular motions.

12 For long hair, gently massage the shampoo through the mid-lengths to the ends (you may need to split the hair into sections if it is thick). Do not 'scrub' the hair together, as this will roughen the cuticle and tangle the hair.

13 Begin rinsing at the front, ensuring that you check the temperature before starting. Again, shielding the face with your hand, rinse the hair from front to back, pushing the water back and through the hair.

14 When rinsing the sides, tilt the client's head slightly over and use your free hand to 'cup' around the hairline to stop the water running down the client's face.

15 At the nape, if you need to, lift the head slightly and, again, cup your hand to the hairline to stop water running down the client's neck (d).

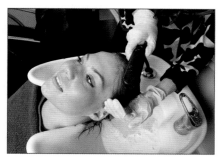

(d)

16 When the hair is well rinsed, repeat the process.

17 Once the second shampoo has been completed, turn off the water and squeeze the excess water out of the hair (e). (If the hair is in very poor condition or is very thick, you may need to give it a light towel-dry.)

18 Pour or pump the selected conditioner into your hand, making sure you don't take too much. Spread it evenly between your hands and apply to the mid-lengths and ends of the hair. Avoid putting conditioner onto the roots unless it's needed.

19 If the hair is long or thick, use your fingers to divide the hair into sections so that all the hair is covered. If you need to, apply more conditioner, but take care not to apply too much, as this may make the hair limp and greasy.

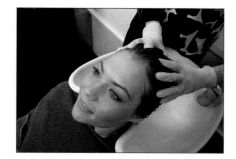

(e)

20 Using a large, wide-toothed comb, comb the hair from the mid-lengths to the ends, avoiding the roots.

21 Once complete, you may need to leave the conditioner on for one or two minutes, depending on the hair.

22 Rinse as before, again checking the temperature, and continue rinsing until the water runs clear from all areas of the head.

23 Once finished, squeeze out the excess moisture before placing a towel around the front hairline. Wrap the hair in the towel (f) before getting the client to sit up.

24 Check the towel and gown for wetness before taking the client over to the workstation.

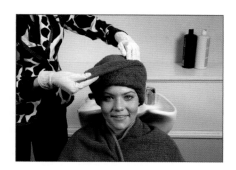

(f)

25   Comb through the hair with a large-toothed comb.

> Squeeze the hair in the towel and remove the towel.

> Beginning at the ends of the hair, begin combing up towards the roots. Take care not to scrape the scalp, as it will be soft following the shampoo. (If the hair is thick, you may need to take sections.)

> Work up the head until you reach the crown.

> Then begin at the front hairline, combing all the hair back and off the face.

> Finally, use the original towel, again squeezing the ends to remove any drips.

26   Return to the shampoo area, clean or sterilise your comb, tidy up any mess, return shampoos and conditioners to their correct place, and ensure the basin is clean and ready for the next client.

Note: Warm water and shampooing softens the scalp and makes it more sensitive. The heat can also have the effect of swelling the hair, causing the cuticle to open. Take care immediately after shampooing not to be too aggressive with the hair or the scalp, or to use strong products until the hair and scalp have had a chance to cool and settle.

Scalp treatment application step by step

Scalp treatments may be applied at the basin, but applying at a styling station will enable you to carry out the process more efficiently and will be more professional.

Ensure you read the individual product's preparation, application, processing and rinsing instructions before you start. Note that there may be a need for sensitivity or incompatibility testing before treatment.

1 Make sure both you and the client are correctly protected and prepared.

2 If pre-shampooing is required, towel-dry the hair and seat the client in a styling position.

3 Pour or pump the treatment into a bowl, making sure you don't take too much (you can always add more if you run out), or use the applicator or application process recommended.

4 Section the hair into four quarters from the crown (a), and secure with section clips if needed.

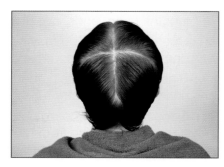

(a)

5 Use a tint brush to apply the treatment to the scalp along the partings (b). Check that the client is comfortable and the scalp is not reacting to the treatment.

6 Beginning at the crown, take a 2–3 cm section, diagonally across the top of one of the back sections, and apply the treatment to the parting.

7 Take a further section across the section, following the same line, and repeat.

8 Continue working this way until you reach the nape. Then begin working on the second back section in the same way.

9 Once complete, begin work on the top sections, again taking diagonal sections across the main section (c). Work from the crown forward, applying the treatment to the scalp.

10 Avoid applying too much treatment near the hairline, as it may run onto the skin.

11 Once all four quarters are complete, clip up the hair, cover the head with a plastic cap and place under an accelerator or dryer if required. You may also need to place a strip of cotton wool around the hairline if the product is particularly runny.

12 If using heat, set the correct time and check that the client is comfortable.

13 Set a timer for the processing time.

14 If rinsing is required, you may need to use cooler water, so carefully check the temperature with the client. Rinse thoroughly and avoid massaging or rubbing the scalp too much.

15 Carry out any subsequent shampooing or conditioning according to the instructions.

16 Put back any unused product in the original container. Only return product that has not been in contact with the hair or scalp.

17 Once finished, squeeze out the excess moisture before placing a towel around the front hairline. Wrap the hair in the towel before getting the client to sit up.

18 Check the towel and gown for wetness before taking the client over to the workstation.

19 Comb through with a wide-toothed comb.

20 Return to the shampoo area, clean up any mess, wash up your tools and ensure the basin is clean and ready for the next client.

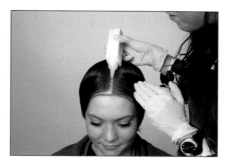

(b)

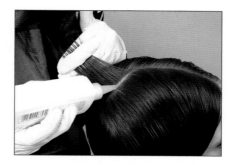

(c)

Conditioning treatment application step by step

Conditioning treatments may be applied at the basin, but applying them at a styling station will enable you to carry out the process more efficiently and will be more professional.

Ensure that you read the individual product's preparation, application processing and rinsing instructions before you start.

1 Make sure that both you and the client are correctly protected and prepared.

2 After shampooing, towel-dry the hair and seat the client in a styling position.

3 Pour or pump the treatment into a bowl, making sure you don't take too much (you can always add more if you run out).

4 Section the hair into four quarters from the crown (a) and secure with section clips.

5 Beginning at the nape, take a 2–3 cm section from one of the back panels and clip away the remaining hair.

6 Use a tint brush to apply the treatment to the mid-lengths and ends only (unless the roots also require treating – (b), (c)).

7 Using your hands, work the product down the hair shaft (d), making sure that the ends are adequately covered.

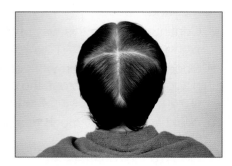

(a)

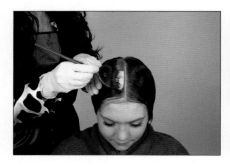

(b)

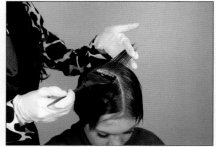

(c)

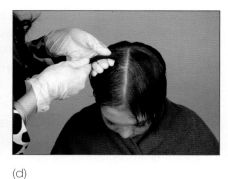

(d)

8 Use a large, wide-toothed comb to comb the section through thoroughly (e).

9 Once complete, repeat the process, taking sections up the head until you reach the top.

10 Use a section clip to clip up the treated section before repeating the process on the three remaining quarters.

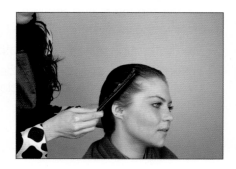

(e)

11 Once all four quarters are complete, combine the sections (if possible) and secure with one clip.

12 Place a plastic cap over the head and place under an accelerator or dryer if required. You may also need to place a strip of cotton wool around the hairline (f) if the product is particularly runny.

13 If using heat, set for the correct time and check that the client is comfortable.

14 Set a timer for the processing time.

15 Rinse thoroughly when finished, avoiding roughing the hair too much. Note that treatments often take longer to rinse out than normal conditioners.

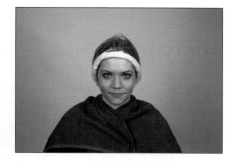

(f)

16 Put back any unused product in the original container. Only return product that has not been in contact with the hair.

17 Once finished, squeeze out the excess moisture before placing a towel around the front hairline. Wrap the hair in the towel before getting the client to sit up.

18 Check the towel and gown for wetness before taking the client over to the workstation.

19 Comb through with a wide-toothed comb.

20 Return to the shampoo area, clean up any mess, wash up your tools and ensure the basin is clean and ready for the next client.

Note: Always make sure all shampoo, conditioning and scalp treatment products are properly rinsed out of the hair. If any product is left in the hair, it can make the hair difficult to style and even cause a reaction when it dries.

Finishing

Once you have completed the shampoo and conditioning service, it's important to finish the process properly. On escorting a client to a cutting or technical station, ensure they are comfortable before checking that the shampoo area is clean, safe and ready for use.

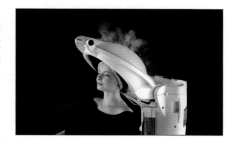

Micro Mist
Treatment processors often use moist heat to activate conditioning treatments as they won't cause further damage

After completing the shampoo and conditioning services, you may need to check:

> that the client's towel or gown is not wet or damp and needs to be changed

> that the client's hair is lightly towel-dried and combed through

> if the client would like a magazine or some refreshment, and ensure they are comfortable

> that the stylist or technician is aware that the client is ready for them

> the basin and shampoo chair to ensure that they are clean and dry

> that any tools you have used are clean and ready for the next use

> for and clean up any water or product spills in the shampoo area

> that the shampoo area is adequately stocked, and advise the relevant person if any stock needs to be ordered

> that your hands are clean and dried.

Aftercare advice

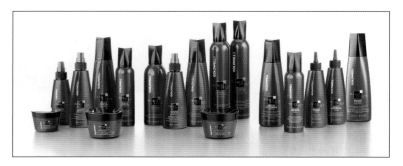

Always let clients know what shampoo and conditioning products you have used and why.

You should also advise them on:

> the availability of the shampoo and conditioner to purchase and use at home in order to maintain the condition of their hair

> how to use the products at home for the best results

> any effects of the long-term use of these or other shampoo and conditioning products

> how to avoid damaging their hair with heated tools, styling products or chemical services

> what, if any, conditioning or scalp treatments they should consider in the future.

Records

Not all salons record details of the shampoo on record cards – unless it's in relation to other services such as colour or perming. If you do need to record the shampoo details, you will need to make a note of information such as:

> the type of shampoo that was used

> the type of conditioner, how it was applied and how long it was left on

> the type of hair or scalp treatment that was used, how it was applied, how it was processed and how long it was left on

> specific skin and hair conditions

> any chemical services and pre-treatment products

> any retail products suggested/purchased

> notes for next time.

Over the following pages, you'll learn how to prepare for colour services, how to colour and lighten hair using a range of techniques, provide valuable aftercare advice to clients and, importantly, create amazing colour results effectively and safely.

You will learn to:

> **understand the different colour products and how they work**

> **prepare for colouring services**

> **change hair colour using a variety of techniques**

> **provide aftercare advice.**

You will be assessed against your knowledge and ability to:

1 Understand your salon's processes and procedures with regard to colouring services.

2 Understand your legal and health and safety responsibilities when carrying out these services.

3 Understand your personal obligations to other team members and know when and from whom you should seek advice and assistance.

4 Maintain effective and safe methods of working and carry out colouring in commercially viable time.

5 Consult with clients and consider key factors when deciding on the colouring service to suit their individual needs.

6 Communicate effectively with clients, using positive listening skills, body language and verbal communication.

7 Understand products and tools required for colouring.

8 Test and assess the hair, and prepare the client and their hair for colouring services.

9 Carry out various colouring techniques, including processing and washing off.

10 Recognise adverse results and deal with them effectively.

11 Provide aftercare and product advice.

Introduction

What is hair colouring?

Colouring is a permanent or temporary change to all or some sections of hair.

Why is hair coloured?

Hair colouring is incredibly versatile and is used to enhance styles, add detail and cover grey. Hair colour can also be used to completely change a look, without cutting or perming.

What colouring techniques will I need to know?

In order to qualify, you will need to know the most commonly used hair colour application techniques for men and women, as covered in Units GH9 and GB2. You will also need to know all the associated skills, such as sensitivity testing, colour selection and colour mixing.

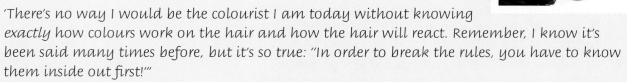

Case study
A colourful career

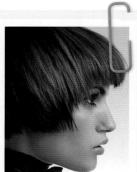

'Being a colourist can give you an amazing career, but to be a good colourist you need an eye for colour plus in-depth knowledge. No one can teach you to have a good eye for colour, but what you can learn is the technical aspects of colouring and the science behind it.'

'There's no way I would be the colourist I am today without knowing *exactly* how colours work on the hair and how the hair will react. Remember, I know it's been said many times before, but it's so true: "In order to break the rules, you have to know them inside out first!"'

'I know that the theory might be boring and difficult, with loads of chemical and technical information to learn – but believe me you will really need it in the future.'

Lisa Shepherd, Lisa Shepherd Salons, London, Sutton, Kidderminster and Birmingham

Three-times British Colourist of the Year

The amazing world of colour!

No other in-salon technical service has the same impact on the look and finish of a hairstyle as colouring. Whether you choose to specialise in colouring or not, understanding the range of technical possibilities that colour offers is a crucial skill for all hairdressers.

Modern hair colouring today is about more than covering grey hair with flat, bland colours; it's about creating natural tones or wild, striking colour statements. It's about adding subtle detail to enhance a hairstyle or adding a flash of vibrancy to create the look.

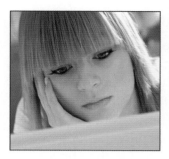 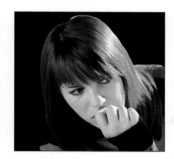 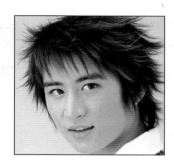

Hair colouring no longer means dry, brittle, lifeless hair. A vast range of high-quality hair colour products will enable you to create stunning looks, with shine, body and hair that's filled with life.

By learning the basic techniques for colouring hair, the limitless possibilities of hair colouring will be open to you, with a palette that's only limited by your imagination.

Colouring techniques

The main services offered by salons, and the ones you will need to learn to achieve Units GH9 and GB2, are as follows.

Full head

This is colouring of all the hair with a permanent colour. Full-head colouring can be used to lighten, darken, change the tone or cover grey.

Regrowth

This is colouring the new growth on clients who have previously had their hair coloured.

Highlights

Either by 'weaving' or by pulling hair through a highlighting cap, fine sections of hair are lightened with permanent colour or bleach, to create a softer, lightening effect.

Lowlights

Using the same techniques as highlighting, fine sections of hair are coloured darker or richer, with permanent colour. Lowlights are often used to add different tones to hair or to camouflage grey hair.

Semi-permanent

This is a non-damaging colour option that doesn't use strong chemicals or activators and slowly washes out of the hair. It cannot make hair lighter; it can only change the tone or darken hair.

Men's hair colouring

This involves carrying out male-specific hair colouring techniques.

Frosting/shoeshine

Sometimes called 'spot colour' or 'flashing', bleach or permanent colour is added to the hair tips, edges or other specific places on a hairstyle. These techniques are usually done freehand, using tin foil, a tint brush or a comb.

Colour science in a nutshell!

The colour of an object is defined by the light it absorbs and the light it reflects. White light is made up of different wavelengths of light, which each produce a colour. These colours make up the colour spectrum (colours of the rainbow) red, orange, yellow, green, blue, indigo and violet. The colour you see is the result of which colour is being reflected back to you. If a colour is green, then green light is being reflected. If a colour is a greeny-blue, then those light colours are reflected while all the others are absorbed.

White objects reflect nearly all the colours and black objects absorb them. The more white light that is reflected, the lighter and paler the colour. The more light that's absorbed, the darker the colour will become.

The principle behind hair colour is the same. The pigment in your hair absorbs and reflects light in the same manner, and it's the result of this reflection and absorption that dictates the colour of your hair.

Making colour

Pigments are what give objects their colour and all colour pigments are made up of the three primary colours: red, blue and yellow. By combining two of the primary colours, you get the three secondary colours: red and blue = violet; yellow and blue = green; yellow and red = orange.

Every painted or printed colour you see is a mixture of the three primary colours, with black or white used to increase or decrease the lightness or darkness of the shade.

What gives hair its colour?

The pigment in hair is called melanin. It is divided into two main types:

› eumelanin, which is the pigment that creates brown and black hair

› pheomelanin, which is the pigment that creates blonde and red hair.

The combination and density of these two main pigments results in the colour of your hair.

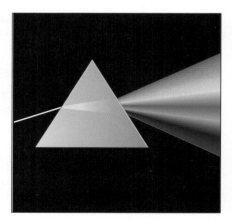

Activity Start to look at people and try to work out what colour service they have had. Next time you are out in public, look at the people around you and try to identify the type of colour service they have had. Look carefully at the shade range, placement of colour and any root regrowth to help you.

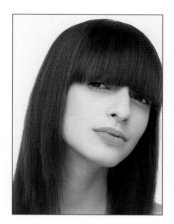

Dark hair

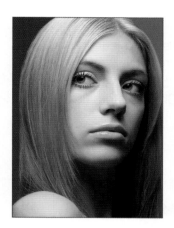

Blonde hair

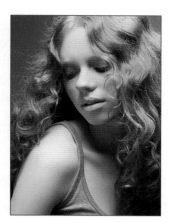

Auburn hair

Dark, oriental hair will have a high concentration of eumelanin, while light-blonde hair will have only a little pheomelanin. Warm-brown hair will have a combination of the two.

As well as the two more common pigments, bright auburn and vibrant red hair also contain an additional iron-rich pigment called trichosiderin; the higher the concentration of trichosiderin, the richer and more vibrant the colour. Trichosiderin is a strong pigment that can make it difficult to colour and lighten.

Hair that is white (often referred to as 'grey') is hair that has no pigment at all.

The two factors of hair colour

There are two elements to everyone's hair colour:

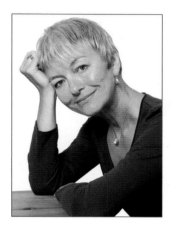

Grey hair

> depth – how light or dark the colour is
> tone – the hair's colour properties.

Depth

> Depth is how dark or light the hair is.
> Depth is measured from black to very light blonde.
> The more white/grey there is, the lighter the hair colour will appear.
> When colouring, it's important to work out the actual depth of the original natural colour, as this will affect your choice of colour.

Tone

> Hair tone is a combination of colour properties.
> Tones are split into cool tones, such as ash, mauve and blue, and warm tones, like copper, gold and red.
> Each tone has an underlying colour base: ash = green, mauve = blue, gold = yellow, red = red.
> It's important to be able to recognise these tones because, as with mixing paint, different combinations will create different results.

Shade charts

Shade charts are an essential tool for a colourist, and learning how to use them properly is crucial for a successful result.

While charts differ depending on the product or the manufacturer, they all tend to follow the International Colour Chart system (ICC).

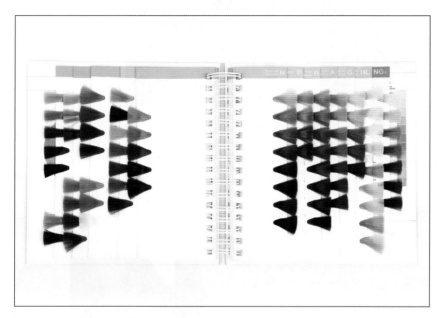

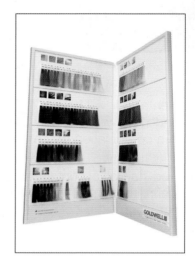

International Colour Chart system

Depth

Depth is listed vertically, usually in numbers from 1 to 10, with 1 being the darkest shade in the range (often black) and 10 being the lightest (very light blonde). With each increase in number, the colour is lighter. For example, 1 = black, 2 = very dark brown, 3 = dark brown, 4 = brown, 5 = light brown, 6 = dark blonde, and so on.

Tone

Tone is listed horizontally, usually in numbers from 1 to 8, although the tone options available in colour ranges vary. Each number denotes a base tone; the first numbers are usually ash colours, progressing through to the warmer tones that have a higher number. For example, 1 = ash, 2 = mauve, 3 = gold, 4 = copper, 5 = red, 6 = mahogany, and so on.

Each colour on a shade chart will have at least two numbers, separated by a dot or a forward slash; the first number is the depth and the second number is the tone. For example, 3.4 will be dark copper brown (3 = dark brown, 4 = copper). In some ranges, the colour will have two tones: a primary tone, which is the colour's main tone, and a secondary tone or 'flavour'. In these cases, there will be two second numbers. For example, 6.45 dark copper red blonde (6 = dark blonde, 4 = copper, 5 = red).

Activity Practise using a shade chart to work out hair colour. First find the depth, then work across to find the tone. Then try to work it out by sight first, and check your answers against the shade chart to see how well you did.

Types of hair colouring products

There are many different brands on the market and most salons will usually work with one colour 'house', such as L'Oréal, Wella, Goldwell, Schwarzkopf or one of the other brands available in the UK. This allows the salon team to learn the capabilities and individual characteristics of the products they are using. While each product line will have subtle differences and features, hair colour products fall into the following categories.

Permanent

Often referred to as 'tints', these products contain para-dyes that chemically alter the pigment (colour) of the hair. Permanent colour contains ammonia and this swells the hair, forcing open the cuticle and enabling the product to get to the melanin at the hair's cortex. It's this opening of the cuticle that can cause hair damage. When mixed with hydrogen peroxide, permanent colours create an oxidising process called polymerisation – it's this chemical reaction that fuses the para-dye pigments to those in the hair; if the hair has no pigment (white hair), the para-dye molecules combine together to become the hair's pigment. It is very important that a sensitivity test is carried out when using products with para-dyes as they contain the known skin irritant PPD (para-phenylenediamine). Permanent colours can be used to lighten, darken, change the hair's tone and cover grey.

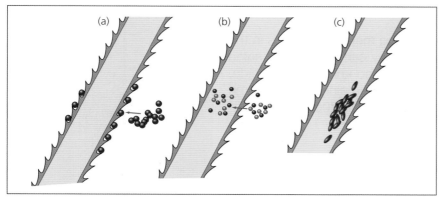

How hair colour works. (a) Large colour granules adhere to the cuticle layer; (b) Tiny colour granules are mixed with hydrogen peroxide – they pass through the cuticle layer into the cortex; (c) The granules join together, becoming permanently trapped when the cuticle closes.

Bleach

Bleach gradually removes the pigment of the hair until it is completely white. Bleach also swells the hair to open the cuticle and reach the cortex, so it will also damage the condition of hair. Also mixed with hydrogen peroxide, the strength of the bleach will depend on the percentage strength of the peroxide you use. Unlike permanent colours that stop when the chosen colour is achieved, bleach will continue removing pigment until it is washed off and can cause extreme hair damage.

Semi-permanent

As they don't contain a developer, these products 'stain' rather than chemically alter the hair. Semi-permanent colours fade over time. The durability of the shade will depend on the condition of the hair and how often it's shampooed. They have a limited ability to cover grey, but as no strong chemicals are used to alter the colour of the hair, a semi-permanent won't damage the condition. Also, as they fade out, they generally don't leave a regrowth line.

Quasi-permanent

These are essentially a semi-permanent colour with a small amount of hydrogen peroxide (or other oxidising agent), which enables some penetration into the hair.

Toners

Toners are used to blend coloured hair to create a uniform colour. Usually toners are permanent colours containing para-dyes and a weak peroxide solution. Toners are most often used after highlights or to 'tone down' a colour that's too light or bright.

Vegetable

Vegetable colours such as henna are natural pigments that have been used for hundreds of years to colour hair.

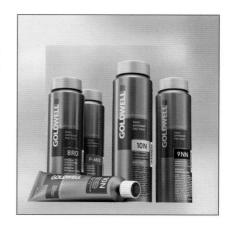

Non-permanent hair colour

Metallic

While you are unlikely to use surface-coating metallic hair dyes in the salon, you need to be aware of them as they can affect other salon technical services, like perms and colours. Also known as sulphide, reduction or progressive, metallic hair dyes are mainly used in home use products used to cover grey, such as Grecian 2000.

What colour service?

There is a lot to think about when deciding on the best method of colouring hair. Consider:

> **Result** – what result do you want to achieve?
> **Hairstyle** – what hairstyle does the client have and how could colour be used to enhance it?
> **Condition** – what is the condition of the client's hair?
> **Cost** – what is the service that best suits the client's budget and the commitment that they can make to maintaining their new hair colour?

By carefully considering these four factors, you will be able to choose a product and service perfect for each client. For example:

> **Result** – to cover a small amount of grey, even out the overall colour and add warmth and shine
> **Hairstyle** – the client has a layered haircut, worn smooth and brushed back with a slight fringe

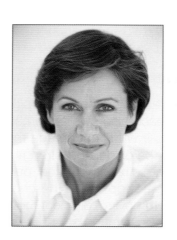

> **Condition** – the hair is dry and has been damaged by the sun and previous chemical treatments

> **Cost** – the client has a limited budget and doesn't want to spend too much.

Decision: semi-permanent.

Activity Use this method to practise selecting colour services for friends and family.

Preparation is the key to successful colouring

To get the right result, you've got to get your preparations spot on. Get it wrong and you could end up with a poor result, an injured client or even a lawsuit.

To ensure you do get it right, always follow these three simple rules:

1 **Test** – test the client's skin for sensitivity and test the hair for compatibility and condition.
2 **Select** – choose a product and colour that suits the client's hair and skin type, as well as their hairstyle and skin tone.
3 **Protect** – ensure the skin and clothes of both you and your client are protected.

Test

There are a number of tests that need to be carried out to ensure that colouring is suitable for the client and their hair.

First, however, you need to enquire into the client's history to find out if they have previously had hair colour and if they've ever had a reaction to it. You should also ask if they have any product or other allergies, skin disorders or if they have any medical conditions that could interfere with or be affected by the colouring process. Don't just think about how the colour may affect the skin or the scalp. If the client has a bad back, for example, they may not be able to sit for the length of time it takes to highlight or colour the hair.

Note: If you fail to carry out the appropriate test or those stipulated by the manufacturer, both you and your salon will be guilty of negligence if the client is injured or their hair is damaged. If your salon owner then shows that you have been trained and instructed to carry out these tests and you failed to do so, you could be guilty of gross negligence, which is a criminal offence. This could not only end your career, but you could end up with a criminal record.

Sensitivity testing

What is it?

Sensitivity tests (sometimes referred to as patch, skin or hypersensitivity tests) are used to check if a client will have an allergic reaction to a hair colour product.

How is it done?

Generally, a small amount of the product to be used is mixed and applied to a clean patch of skin behind the ear.

How long does it take?

The test takes moments, but it can take up to 48 hours for a reaction, after which time, if there's no reaction, the client can receive their colour treatment.

What reactions can occur?

Redness, itching, inflammation or general local soreness and discomfort. If the client experiences any of these reactions, the product should not be used.

Do I have to carry out a sensitivity test for all colour services?

No, only those that come in direct contact with the skin, but it's worth checking the instructions for all products to see if testing is recommended.

Do I have to carry out a sensitivity test each time the client has colour?

No, providing you are using the same product as previously used and there has been no change to the product or the client's health, you don't have to carry out the test again. Clients can, develop allergic reactions, however, and some manufacturers recommend periodic testing. You should always carry out a sensitivity test if you are using a new product or if you have any doubts.

Note:

> Testing requirements may vary from product to product, so make sure you check the instructions.

> Never take a client's word that they have been tested; they might be lying.

> If in doubt, always seek advice from a more senior colleague or from the manufacturer.

Hair colour sensitivity testing step by step

1 Mix a small amount of the product to be used with the appropriate percentage of peroxide or activator.

2 Select a small area behind the ear and ensure it is free from grease, hair product or make-up.

3 Apply a small amount of the mixture, slightly smaller than the size of a five pence piece (a).

4 Cover with a plaster or dressing (b).

5 Arrange for your client to return to the salon after the period stated by the manufacturer (usually 24 hours).

6 Ask if they suffered any discomfort or irritation and check the tested area for any swelling, redness or other reaction.

7 If there is any reaction, *do not carry out the service*.

8 If the result is inconclusive or you are unsure, retest behind the other ear.

9 Record the date, details and result of the test on the client record card.

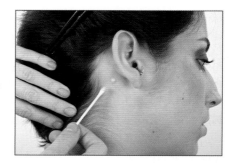

(a)

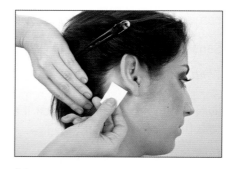

(b)

Incompatibility testing

What is it?

This tests how the actual hair will react to a particular product to make sure there will be no adverse reaction.

When should you carry out this test?

You only need carry out this test if you have been made aware or you suspect that the hair has been home-coloured using a product containing metallic salts (products such as Grecian 2000), or if you feel the hair may contain some product or coating that might react to hair colour.

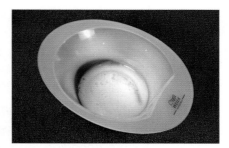
Incompatibility testing

How do you carry out the test?

Cut a small lock of hair and secure the strands using tape. Place the hair into a glass bowl containing a small amount of hydrogen peroxide and alkaline perm lotion.

How long will it take?

The hair should remain in the solution for approximately 30 minutes.

What will happen?

If the hair does not contain any metallic salts, nothing will happen. If however, the solution bubbles, fizzes, begins to give off heat or the hair changes colour or begins to dissolve, then perming lotions or hair colour products containing hydrogen peroxide should not be used on the hair.

Condition testing

Why do you need to test the condition?

The overall condition of the hair will affect how the pigment is absorbed. Porous, brittle and dry hair will be damaged further and may break, and can cause patchy or poor colour results.

What do you test?

You need to test the porosity and the elasticity to make sure that hair is in adequate condition to withstand the proposed chemical process.

When should you carry out the test?

You must assess the condition of every client's hair prior to any chemical process; this can be done during your consultation.

How is the test carried out?

Testing the condition is generally done visually and by touch.

> If the hair is overly porous, it will feel rough and coarse when you rub strands of it with the ends of your fingers. Also, it will remain heavy and saturated even after towel-drying.

> If the elasticity is poor, a hair held near the root and near the tip will be easily overstretched, have little or no tension and won't return to its original length. This will also determine if the hair is

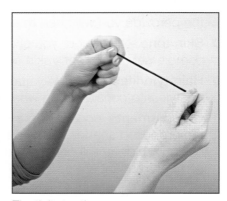
Elasticity testing

brittle. If it snaps too easily, it could be a sign of damage to the hair's inner cortex.

Any of these results are strong indicators of damaged hair. The condition can also be gauged by its general texture, sheen and tendency to tangle, which is a sign of damaged cuticle.

How do I decide if the hair is too damaged to proceed with the service?

Consider the additional damage that is likely to be caused by the service before proceeding and always take the most cautious approach.

What should I do if the hair is too damaged to proceed?

Recommend that your client book a professional in-salon conditioning treatment and advise on intensive home hair care to rehabilitate the condition.

Colour selection and mixing

The next step will be to select the colour. There are some very important factors you need to consider when selecting the shade, tone and strength of colour.

> **Hair type** – thick, coarse hair often requires stronger products and longer processing times than finer hair.

> **Hair length** – long hair may require three applications to cover and blend the roots, mid-lengths and ends. It will also require more products to be mixed.

> **Prior chemical processes** – virgin hair (hair that has not been chemically treated) can react differently to hair that has undergone a chemical process. Any colour from a previous application, whether it's permanent or otherwise, may also affect the result.

> **Grey hair** – base shades need to be considered when covering white (grey) hair.

> **Condition** – porous, brittle or dry hair will absorb the colour faster than virgin hair.

> **Tone** (ash, gold, red, etc.) – the colour you use will combine with that already in the hair to produce the new colour. It's important to know how different tones combine and what colours will result.

> **Shade** – the lighter the colour you want to achieve, the stronger the peroxide you will need to use.

> **Skin tone** – the colour you choose should match and complement the client's skin colour.

> **Hairstyle/lifestyle** – always take the client's overall look and lifestyle into consideration when choosing hair colour.

> **Commitment** – consider your client's willingness to commit to the proposed shades. The time and money needed to commit to platinum blonde will be far greater than that required to keep a semi-permanent shade looking good.

When selecting a colour, first use the shade chart to establish the client's exact hair shade and tone. Then, with the client, use the chart to select a new colour. (For more on consultations, see Unit G7.) By following the product instructions and taking into account the colour selection guidelines, you will be able to create a formula that will achieve the desired results.

Hydrogen peroxide H_2O_2

This colourless, odourless liquid is the principal oxidising agent used in hairdressing. Today, the strength of peroxide is predominantly measured as a percentage that relates to the total percentage of the solution that is pure H_2O_2. Peroxide can also be measured in volume (vol), although this is an older system and percentages are more widely used today. Hydrogen peroxide solution is water-based, although some solutions also contain conditioning agents.

Peroxide will remove colour from fabric and cause a burning irritation when in contact with the skin, so it should be used with care. If it does come into contact with skin or clothing, rinse immediately with cold water.

Peroxide strengths and uses

> **3% (10vol)** – a weak oxidant used to give the minimum amount of product activation. It is used for:
> > toners for highlights and full-head bleaches
> > colour washes to add depth to faded colours
> > when toning or colouring, to bring slight changes to damaged hair.

> **6% (20vol)** – a light oxidant, generally used for same-depth or darker colouring. It is used for:
> > covering white/grey hair
> > adding depth and deeper tones
> > lightening base colours by a shade (up to two shades on very fine hair)
> > on-scalp bleaching.

> **9% (30vol)** – a medium oxidant used when lightening hair by up to three shades. It is used for:
> > lightening dark hair by up to two shades
> > lightening mid-shade hair by up to three shades
> > bleach highlighting.

> **12% (40vol)** – the strongest peroxide on sale in the UK, 12% is a strong oxidant used for high-lift colouring. It is used:
> > with high-lift colours
> > to lighten hair by up to four or five shades
> > to bleach highlighting on strong, dark hair.

Being water-based, it is possible to dilute hydrogen peroxide to get the correct strength you need.

> 3 x part 12% (40vol) + 1 x part water = 9% (30vol)
> 1 x part 12% (40vol) + 1 x part water = 6% (20vol)

Activity Magazines and style books are a great help, as they show a full-head colour rather than a small swatch. Simply match the shade chart to the hair colour in the picture to find your target result.

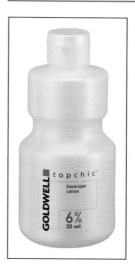

> 1 x part 12% (40vol) + 3 x part water = 3% (10vol)
> 2 x part 9% (30vol) + 1 x part water = 6% (20vol)
> 1 x part 9% (30vol) + 1 x part water = 3% (10vol)

Lightening hair colour

Lightening hair is achieved by dissolving the pigments within the hair by using bleaches or high-lift colours that contain alkaline chemicals. As with permanent colours, these products work by mixing them with hydrogen peroxide.

Hair lightening happens in stages, with the small molecules of pigment removed first, with reds and golds being the largest and therefore the last to be removed.

Here is an example of the colour-lifting sequence:

Dark brown – mid warm brown – light red brown – red blonde – copper blonde – golden blonde – light pale blonde – white.

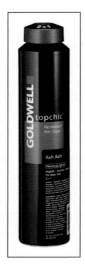

High-lift colours

High-lift colours combine the colour removal process with a tone by containing light-shade para-dyes. This means that once the hair has been lifted to a certain level, the para-dye pigment ensures the colour is even and stops it getting any lighter. In addition, the tone of a high-lift colour can be used to counteract a strong tone in the hair. Ash- and cool-toned high-lift colours are often used to counteract gold/yellow, as it's the hardest tone to remove when lifting.

High-lift colours are generally mixed with either 9% or 12% peroxide, dependent on the product or the amount of lift required.

The major benefits of high-lift colours over bleaches is that the results are much easier to predict. As they use a lower-strength peroxide and contain conditioning agents, they are far easier on the hair and cause less damage.

Bleach

Bleach gradually removes the pigment of the hair until it is completely white. As hair is a mixture of tones and shades, it lifts at different levels. This means that when using bleach it can be difficult to achieve an even result. For this reason, a toner is often used after bleaching to even out the colour and counteract any prominent tone. Care has to be taken when using bleach, as it will continue processing until it is washed off. Rinsing off bleach is carried out differently to other hair colour processes, and it's also recommended that anti-oxidising conditioners are used after the bleaching processes.

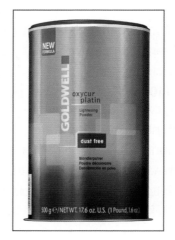

There are two different bleach types:

> Powder bleach – mixed with hydrogen peroxide up to a strength of 12% (40vol), powder bleach is used predominantly for highlighting, as it is generally not recommended for use on the scalp. While manufacturers will have mixing guidelines, it's often better to mix powder bleach on the thick side, to avoid leakage or seepage. Once mixed, powder bleach will slowly 'dry out'; if

this happens and it becomes too thick, simply add a little more peroxide. It's worth also noting that bleach will dry out completely and stop processing, especially under heat, so you will often need to cover bleach with a cap or cellophane while it's processing. Care should be taken when mixing powder bleach and it should only be carried out in a well-ventilated area.

> Powder bleach can be a bit tricky to wash off, as it sticks to the hair quite firmly. First, make sure you wet the entire head well, as this will stop the processing. Then take your time to carefully ensure that all the bleach is removed before shampooing and conditioning. Do not emulsify or scrub the hair too vigorously.

> Emulsion bleach (gel or oil bleach) – also mixed with peroxide, but emulsion bleach is specially formulated to be used on the scalp for full-head applications. Usually only mixed with 6% (20vol), these products often have 'activators' that help the lightening process; many also contain properties that help to even out the lifting process and reduce yellowing.

> When washing off full-head emulsion bleach, do not emulsify as you would a normal full-head colour. The bleaching process may have left the client's scalp sensitive. Wet the entire head with slightly cooler water than normal to stop processing, then rinse off gently, shampoo and condition.

Note: Lightening products are some of the strongest used in hairdressing and should be used with caution, especially with previously processed or coloured hair. High-lift colours can damage the condition and bleaches can even cause hair breakage.

Counteracting

Counteracting is the use of one colour to cancel out or to subdue another; it is one of the most important aspects of hair colouring you need to know. Each tone has an opposite that can be used to reduce its strength or to eliminate it all together.

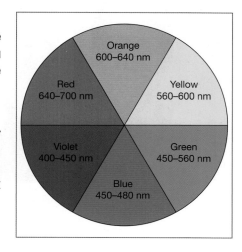

Colour wheel

The three primary colours – red, yellow and blue – are separated by the secondary colour that's created when the two colours are mixed, creating six shades – red, orange, yellow, green, blue and violet. Every colour on the wheel has an opposite, and that's the colour that will counter its tone.

> Red tones will reduce green tones; green tones will reduce red tones.

> Orange tones will reduce blue tones; blue tones will reduce orange tones.

> Yellow tones will reduce violet tones; violet tones will reduce yellow tones.

How does this work with hair colour?

By using a shade chart, you might find that your client's hair is mid ash blonde, with an ash tone and a green base. You client wants the same lightness but a warmer shade. You would choose a colour with a red tone base that's at the same depth, such as mid warm blonde.

The same measure can be used to counter warm colours. If you highlight a client's hair and the depth (lightness) is good, but the shade is a little too golden, select a violet tone of the same depth and use this as a toner. This will reduce the yellow.

Covering white (grey) hair

Covering grey is often where people encounter problems. The reason is that when colouring clients with grey, you are actually colouring two types of hair: hair that has pigment (natural colour) and hair that has no pigment (white hair). The pigmented hair will combine with the pigment in the hair colour to produce a particular result. As white (grey) hair has no pigment to react with, any colour you apply will produce that actual colour.

The result is that the tone of the colour will be far stronger and more prominent on white hair than on hair with pigment.

For this reason, when covering grey, you must always mix a base shade together with the tone shade you are using.

The amount of base shade you should use will depend on the amount (percentage) of white hair the client has – the more white, the more base you need.

As a rule of thumb, the percentage and amount of base you should use follows a simple pattern:

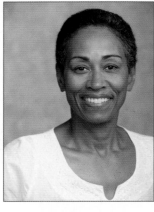
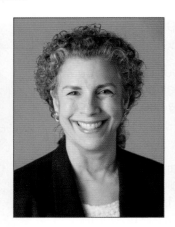
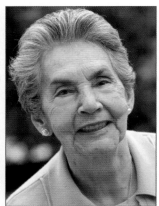

About 25% grey   About 50% grey   About 75% grey

> If 25% of the client's hair is grey – 25% – a quarter of your colour mix should be base shade.

> If 50% of the client's hair is grey – 50% – half of your mix should be base shade.

> If 75% of the client's hair is grey –75% – three-quarters of your mix should be base shade.

For example:

Target shade = light red brown 5.6 (depth 5, tone 6 – red)

> Client with 25% grey hair = ¼ base shade 5.0 + ¾ tone shade 5.6
> Client with 75% grey hair = ¾ base shade 5.0 + ¼ tone shade 5.6.

Tools and equipment

Using the right tools in the right condition will help to ensure that you achieve the best results and avoid possible problems. Below are listed the main tools you will need when providing various colour services.

Note: Some manufacturers produce specific tools for mixing or application. You must always use the correct tools and follow the manufacturer's instructions.

Standard (cutting) comb

This is used to section hair and for a number of colour application techniques.

Large, wide-toothed comb

This is used to comb colour through to the ends.

Pin-tail comb

This thin, mental-ended comb is used for woven highlighting.

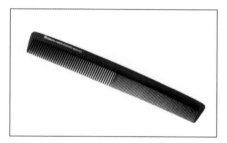

Standard cutting comb

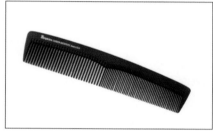

Large-toothed comb

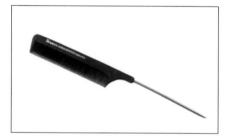

Pin-tail comb

Colouring tint brush

This is used for applying colour for a wide range of colour services.

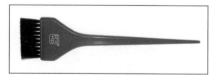

Colouring tint brush

Combination tint brush

This combined brush and comb can be used for a wide range of colour services.

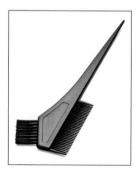

Combination tint brush

Tint bowl

This bowl is used to mix and hold colour for application. Good-quality tint bowls have measuring guides to help in mixing and a rubber base for stability.

Measuring jug

This is used to accurately measure peroxide and liquid colour products. Many manufacturers produce measuring tools designed to work specifically with their product.

Application bottle

Some products require application via a special bottle applicator.

Highlighting cap

A soft, rubber cap with fine holes that is placed over the client's head for highlighting services.

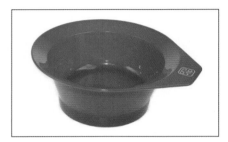

Tint bowl

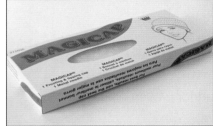

Highlighting cap

Crochet hooks

Metal or plastic hooks of various sizes that are used to pull hair through the highlighting cap.

Aluminium foil

This is used for woven highlights. Cut into strips and folded, foil is used to create an individual package of hair and hair colour. There are also custom products, such as Easi Meche™, that are used in a similar fashion.

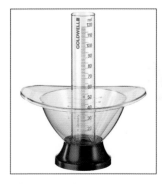

Measuring jug

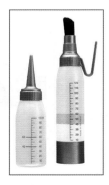

Application bottle

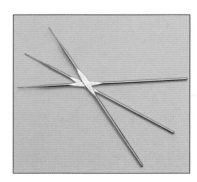

Crochet hooks

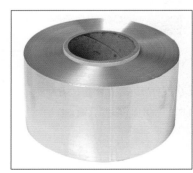

Aluminium foil

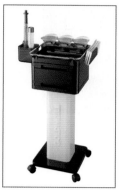

Trolley

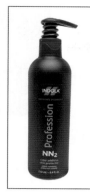

Barrier cream

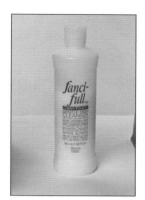

Stain remover

Trolley

A trolley is a mobile workstation. Tint bowls, products and other tools used during colouring work are placed on the trolley. Trolleys should be sturdy, with wheels (castors) free from hair.

Clips

Various different clips are used for colour services. Larger, 'grab' clips are used to keep large sections of hair out of the way, while smaller, 'pin-curl' clips can be used for finer sectioning.

Barrier cream

As its name implies, a barrier cream forms a barrier that stops the colour coming in contact with the skin and is used to protect skin around the hairline. Do not get barrier cream on the hair, as it will also stop the colour product penetrating the hair shaft.

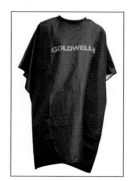

Clips

Stain remover

This is a specially formulated product, used to remove and reduce post-service skin discolouration and staining. (Careful application will help reduce the need for stain removers.)

Cotton wool

Cotton wool has many uses, including to protect clothes, remove access colour and stains, and check processing.

Gloves

Protective gloves for your hands should be used during all colour

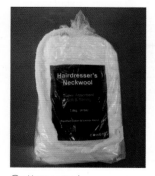

Cotton wool

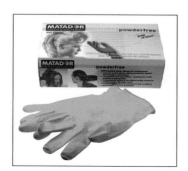

Gloves

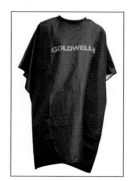

Gown

services. The current health and safety recommendation is for talc-free non-latex (nitrile) or vinyl gloves to be used for salon work.

Colour gowns

Dark-coloured gowns should be used to protect yours and the client's clothes.

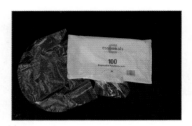

Plastic caps

Plastic caps/cling film

These are used to cover hair colour applications, to aid processing and to stop products drying out.

Timer

This is used to remind you when processing needs checking or is complete.

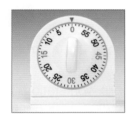

Timer

Client record card

This is used to record all technical services the client has and other relevant information.

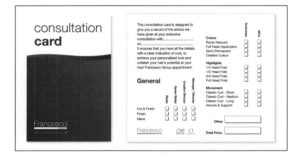

Accelerators

What are they?

Accelerators are used to speed up the processing time of a colour application.

How do they work?

As most hair colour products are processed by heat – the natural heat given off by the client's scalp – accelerators use heat to provide additional heat and therefore speed up the processing.

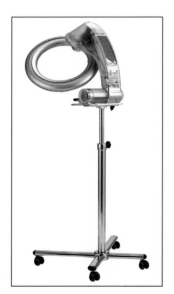

Accelerator

Are there different types?

Yes. Some use straightforward heat, others use infrared, while others also use a fan to produce 'hot air'. A hood dryer or a hairdryer can be used to accelerate processing times.

Are they easy to use?

Generally, yes, although as some require product and application information to be entered, it's important to be trained on how to use and position each machine individually.

Do I need to use an accelerator with all colour services?

No. They are useful for speeding up processing times or for targeting specific areas of the head in order to create an even result. Most products, however, will process perfectly well without them, and some products state that an accelerator should not be used, so always check the instructions.

Mixing

It's vitally important that you follow the manufacturer's instructions for each product you use, as they often differ. Mixing a product incorrectly may affect the result or could even cause hair damage or injury to the client.

Colour products are expensive, so take care to measure accurately and only the amount of product you need. Wasting product increases overheads and reduces a salon's profitability.

When mixing and preparing hair colours, you should always:

> ensure your hands and clothes are covered and protected

> make sure you have enough room to work on an even surface, and that the area is clean and clutter-free to avoid spillages or colour contamination

> the area where you mix colour should be well ventilated, especially if you are mixing bleaches and lighteners

> take care to select the correct products and check that they are not spoiled, out of date or contaminated

> only use professional tint bowls and brushes that are clean and in good order (if the product has its own special bowl or applicator, this should be used)

> take care to accurately measure out the correct amount of each colour to be used; failure to do so will affect the result

> use a clearly marked measuring jug to measure the correct amount of product and/or hydrogen peroxide; failure to do so will affect the result

> squeeze tubes from the bottom end and use opened products first; make sure that lids are replaced tightly on colour products and peroxides, as they will go off

> take time when mixing products together to avoid spilling and to ensure they are properly mixed

> replace all lids and caps straightaway and return products to the correct place.

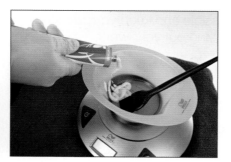

Activity When you see an accelerator being used, ask why it's being used and by how much it will speed up the processing. Also learn how to position it properly and how it should be stored when not in use.

Top Tip

When measuring colour products and peroxide, place measuring jugs and bowls on a flat surface rather than holding them up. Pour products in slowly and allow them to settle before adding more. This will help you to get an accurate measurement.

Note:

> You should never prepare hair colours or clean hair colour bowls and brushes in areas where food or beverages are stored, prepared or consumed.

> Take care not to inhale colour products like powder bleach. This can act as an irritant and cause breathing difficulties. It can also act as a trigger for allergies and chest complaints.

Protect

Hair colour products will stain skin and damage fabrics and furnishings, so ensure that you, your client and nearby surfaces are properly protected.

Whenever you carry out hair colour services, it's important to follow these steps relating to you, your client and your working area.

You

You should:

> wear gloves

> wear a tinting apron or gown

> ensure that your sleeves, hair and jewellery are out of the way and won't interfere with your work.

Your client

Your client should:

> wear a gown that covers their clothes

> remove any collars or high-necked clothing, or ensure these are turned down and adequately covered

> have barrier cream applied to the skin around the hairline (avoiding the hair) and on the ears

> be seated comfortably so that you are able to carry out the service.

Your working area

> The gown should cover the chair (if possible) or the chair should have a protective back cover.

> You should use a mobile trolley to keep the colour close to where you are working.

> Wipe up any spills as soon as possible and keep your working area as tidy as possible while carrying out your work.

Full-head colouring

What is it?

Full-head colouring is the process of changing the colour of all of the hair.

Top Tip

For clients with a low hairline at the nape, use cling film or a plastic cape tucked into the collar as additional protection.

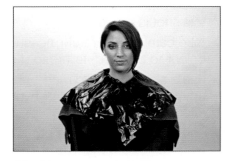

Client in gown and plastic cape

When is it used?

Full-head colouring is used to cover grey hair, to change the overall colour to suit a new hairstyle, or to create a new look on an existing haircut.

Why is it applied differently to regrowth colouring?

Due to the heat, the hair at the scalp will process quicker than that on the mid-lengths and ends. This means that full-head colours are applied in two or even three stages, in order for the colour to be even.

Preparation

The client

> All clients having full-head colouring must have had a sensitivity test. It is not necessary to carry out a sensitivity test each time the client has colour, providing you are using the same product as previously used. (See page 121.)
> Protect the client's clothes with a gown or cape and towels.
> Ensure that any earrings are removed and other jewellery is safely out of the way.
> Ensure that the client is seated comfortably and that you are able to carry out the service.
> Brush through the hair and check for broken or damaged skin.
> Hair that is excessively greasy or has styling product build-up should be shampooed before the colour application. A chelating shampoo is recommended, as it cleanses and rids the hair of residue and mineral deposits that may interfere with the absorption or colour coverage. Conditioners should not be used, as they will coat the hair and interfere with the colour process.

You

> Ensure that your hands are clean.
> Review the client record card and consult with the client, taking into account that the hairstyle may change after colouring. (For further details on consultation, see Unit G7.)
> Decide how you will apply the colour to the roots, mid-lengths and ends, taking into account that the roots and porous ends will take the colour quicker. Remember to take into account the time between the first-stage application and the second.
> Make sure none of your jewellery will get in the way while you are working.
> Protect your clothes with an apron and your hands with gloves.
> Make sure you have all the right tools and that they are clean and fit for purpose.
> Set out tools and a trolley.
> Mix and prepare the colour.
> Section the hair evenly, as this will help to create an even result.

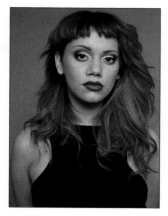

Full-head colouring

> Keep your working area as tidy as possible while carrying out your work.

> Make sure you know how to work safely, with the correct posture, and that you are wearing clothes and shoes that are suitable for the service you are carrying out.

Full-head colour step by step

Using permanent hair colour to change all the hair colour:

1 Ensure that all the proper preparations and tests have been carried out and that you and the client are protected.

2 Comb the hair through thoroughly.

3 Section the head into four quarter sections (a).

4 Starting at the crown, using the tail of your tint brush, take a horizontal section across the back left panel and apply colour to the mid-lengths and ends (b). If the hair is long, it may be easier to start at the bottom of the section.

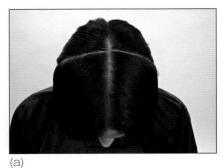
(a)

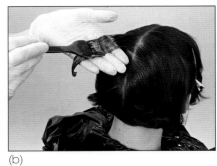
(b)

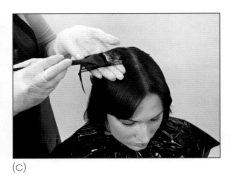
(c)

5 Continue working down the section and repeat on the right side before repeating the process on the front sections (c).

6 Once complete, allow the mid-lengths and ends to process for the estimated time. Use heat if needed and continually check progress (d).

7 When the colour has processed to the required level, again beginning at the back, lift the previously coloured sections and apply colour to the roots (e).

8 Continue this process in the same order as before.

9 When complete, check that all the hair is covered, especially at the hairline (f).

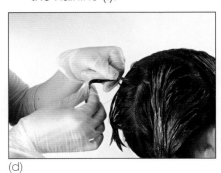
(d)

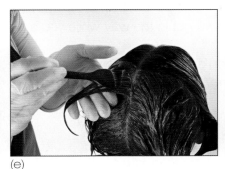
(e)

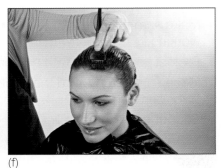
(f)

10 Remove any colour on the skin (g).

11 Place the client under an accelerator if required (h) and set a timer.

12 Check and wash off when ready (i).

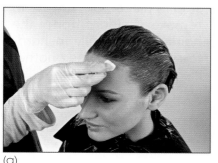
(g)

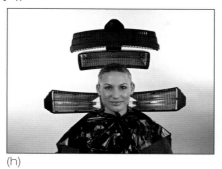
(h)

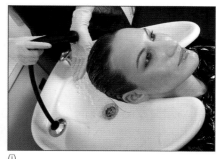
(i)

13 Discard any unused product and wash and clean tools.

Checking – strand test

The processing time will vary depending on the product and the result you are looking to achieve. Check the manufacturer's instructions for estimated processing times and set a timer for the earliest possible completion time.

Use the back of a comb or a piece of cotton wool to remove the colour product from a small section of the hair, to check if processing is complete. Check the progress of the colour separately at the roots, on the mid-lengths and on the ends.

Remember, the hair will be wet with product, so it may appear darker than it actually is.

If the colour is not yet ready, recover the checked hair with product and set the timer for a further five minutes. Continue to check until processing is complete.

Washing off

When washing off hair colour, it's important to ensure that all the colour is removed and to avoid splashing. Always check the manufacturer's instructions for rinsing and shampooing after a colour, as they may differ from product to product.

> Seat the client at the shampoo basin and make sure they are well covered.

> Lightly wet the hair with a small amount of warm water.

> Gently emulsify the hair colour by massaging the scalp. Pay particular attention to the colour around the hairline, as this process helps to remove the hair colour from the skin.

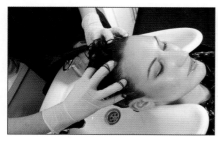

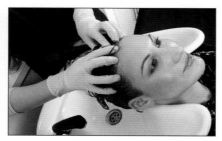

> Taking care not to splash, begin to rinse off the colour.
> Once the hair seems free from hair colour, shampoo and condition as normal or as directed in the instructions.
> Ensure that the client remains gowned and that you use dark-coloured towels, as the wet hair may still contain colour residue that can stain.

Regrowth colouring

What is it?

Regrowth colouring is applying permanent hair colour to new root growth to blend with previously coloured hair. Regrowth colouring or retouching colours in the new hair growth is carried out on clients with full-head colour.

When is it done?

Most clients will need their roots retouched every 4 to 6 weeks.

For most salons, regrowth colour accounts for the majority of hair colour services they provide. The need for regular retouching of colour is a regular source of salon income.

The goal of regrowth colouring is to create a seamless blend between the newly coloured and the previously coloured hair. It is also an opportunity to refresh the previously coloured hair that may have become dull or faded.

Preparation

The client

> All clients having regrowth colouring must have been sensitivity-tested. It is not necessary to carry out a sensitivity test each time the client has colour, providing you are using the same product as previously used. (See page 121.)
> Protect the client's clothes with a gown or cape and towels.
> Ensure that any earrings are removed and that other jewellery is safely out of the way.
> Ensure that the client is seated comfortably and that you are able to carry out the service.
> Brush through the hair and check for broken or damaged skin.
> Hair that is excessively greasy or has styling product build-up should be shampooed before the colour application. A chelating shampoo is recommended, as it cleanses and rids the hair of residue and mineral deposits that may interfere with the absorption or colour coverage. Conditioners should not be used, as they will coat the hair and interfere with the colour process.

You

> Ensure your hands are clean.

> Review the client record card and consult with the client, taking into account that the hairstyle may change after colouring. (For further details on consultation, see Unit G7.)

> Make sure that none of your jewellery will get in the way while you are working.

> Protect your clothes with an apron and your hands with gloves.

> Make sure you have all the right tools and that they are clean and fit for purpose.

> Set out your tools and a trolley.

> Mix and prepare the colour.

> Section the hair evenly, as this will help to create an even result.

> Keep your working area as tidy as possible while carrying out your work.

> Make sure you know how to work safely, with the correct posture, and that you are wearing clothes and shoes suitable for the service you are carrying out.

Regrowth colouring step by step

1 Ensure all the proper preparations and tests have been carried out and that you and the client are protected.

2 Comb the hair through thoroughly.

3 Section the top of the head from hairline to crown, down the back, and from the crown to just above each ear (a).

4 Apply colour, making sure you only cover the new growth (b). If the client has a definite parting, apply colour along the parting instead.

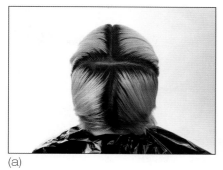
(a)

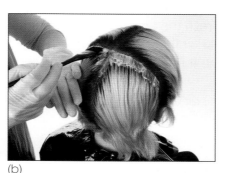
(b)

5 Starting with the top right panel, using the tail of your tint brush, take a section between the two coloured partings and apply colour to both sides. Take care to ensure that the section is not too big, so that no hair will be missed.

6 Continue working forwards to the hairline, then repeat on the left side (c).

7 Starting at the crown, follow the same method, working through the back panels.

8 Once the entire head is complete, check that all the hair is covered, especially the hairline.

9 Remove any colour on the skin (d).

10 Place the client under an accelerator if required (e) and set a timer. Remember, if the colour is to be refreshed (combed through), set the timer for when *this* should be done, rather than for the actual processing time.

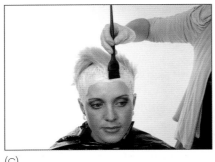
(c)

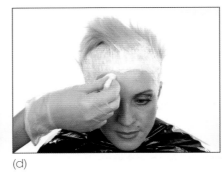
(d)

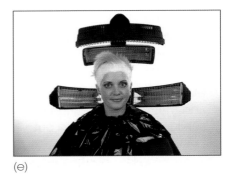
(e)

11 Comb through, if needed, and reset the timer for the remainder of the processing time.

12 Check and wash off when ready.

13 Discard any unused product and wash and clean tools.

Combing through

Combing through is where any remaining colour is applied to the mid-lengths of the hair (f), and then the colour is pulled through to the ends with a wide-toothed comb (g) and left, prior to the colour being washed off. This is done to refresh the previously coloured hair so that it is the same shade and tone as the roots.

> You need to decide if you will comb through colour before mixing, to ensure you will have enough.

> The more faded the lengths of the hair are, the longer the hair will need to be left combed through before rinsing.

> Take care not to comb colour off the root area if it is not fully processed.

> The hair will usually be drier nearer the ends and this will make it more porous, which means it will absorb the colour more quickly. Therefore, you may need to comb through the mid-lengths before it's combed through to the ends.

> If the hair colour only needs a slight amount of refreshing, you needn't comb through at all. Emulsify the colour with water at the basin and leave it for a few moments before rinsing off.

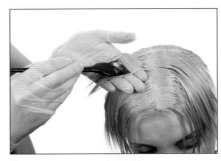
(f)

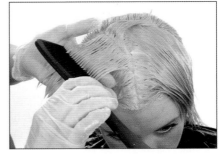
(g)

Checking – strand test

The processing time will vary depending on the product and the result you want to achieve. Check the manufacturer's instructions for estimated processing times and set a timer for the earliest possible completion time.

Use the back of a comb or a piece of cotton wool to remove the colour product from a small section of the hair to check if processing is complete. Check the progress of the colour separately at the roots, on the mid-lengths and on the ends.

Remember, the hair will be wet with product, so it may appear darker than it actually is.

If the colour is not yet ready, recover the checked hair with product and set the timer for a further five minutes. Continue to check until processing is complete.

Washing off

It's important when washing off hair colour to ensure that all the colour is removed and to avoid splashing. Always check the manufacturer's instructions for rinsing and shampooing after a colour, as they may differ from product to product.

> Seat the client at the shampoo basin and make sure they are well covered.

> Lightly wet the hair with a small amount of warm water.

> Gently emulsify the hair colour by massaging the scalp. This is a key part of the colour removal process. Pay particular attention to the colour around the hairline, as this process helps to remove the hair colour from the scalp and skin.

> Taking care not to splash, begin to rinse off the colour.

> Once the hair seems free from hair colour, shampoo and condition as normal or as directed in the instructions.

> Ensure that the client remains gowned and that you use dark-coloured towels, as the wet hair may still contain colour residue that can stain.

Cap highlights

What are highlights?

Highlights are small sections of hair that are lightened or coloured, to add a feature or to give the hair a lighter look.

What are cap highlights?

This is a method of highlighting where strands of hair are pulled through holes in a rubber or plastic cap.

Top Tip

Emulsifying the colour should enable you to remove it from around the hairline. However, if there is still some you've not managed to remove, add a small amount of shampoo to a flannel or small piece of towel to remove colour from the hairline, especially in hard-to-reach areas. Use another clean wet cloth to rinse.

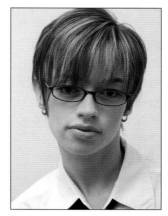

Highlights

When are they used?

Highlights are used to lighten or add light colour to the hair without having to colour the entire head. Cap highlights are generally used on shorter hair and when only one highlighting colour will be used.

When can't they be used?

You can't use the cap if you are using more than one colour. Also, if the hair is longer than the shoulders, or coarse and easily tangled, it can be hard to pull through and uncomfortable for the client.

Preparation

The client

> As the colour product should not come into contact with the skin, sensitivity testing is not required.
> Protect the client's clothes with a gown or cape and towels.
> Ensure that any earrings are removed and that other jewellery is safely out of the way.
> Ensure that the client is seated comfortably and that you are able to carry out the service.
> Brush through the hair and check for broken or damaged skin.
> Hair that is excessively greasy or has styling product build-up should be shampooed before the colour application. A chelating shampoo is recommended, as it cleanses and rids the hair of residue and mineral deposits that may interfere with the absorption or colour coverage. Conditioners should not be used, as they will coat the hair and interfere with the colour process.

You

> Ensure your hands are clean.
> Review the client record card and consult with the client, taking into account that the hairstyle may change after colouring. (For further details on consultation, see Unit G7.)
> Make sure that none of your jewellery will get in the way while you are working.
> Protect your clothes with an apron and your hands with gloves.
> Make sure you have all the right tools and that they are clean and fit for purpose. Check the cap for splits and tears, and select the correct size of crochet hook for the highlights you require.
> Set out tools and a trolley.
> Mix and prepare the colour.
> Keep your working area as tidy as possible while carrying out your work.
> Make sure you know how to work safely, with the correct posture, and that you are wearing clothes and shoes suitable for the service you are carrying out.

Putting on the cap

Using a good-quality highlighting cap and putting it on correctly is crucial to getting the best results.

1 Ensure all the proper preparations and tests have been carried out and that you and the client are protected. Ensure you have the right-sized cap and that it is in good condition.

2 Brush the hair through thoroughly. You may want to apply a small amount of talc to the hair to make it easier to pull through.

3 Ask the client to hold the front of the cap and pull it firmly over their head.

4 Pull the cap down at the sides and make sure that the ears are not folded over.

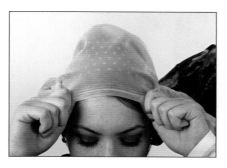 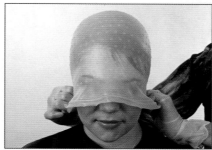

5 The cap should be as tight to the head as possible, with no bubbles or wrinkles.

Pulling through the highlights and applying the hair colour

The size of crochet hook you use will determine the thickness of the highlights, so for fine highlights use a finer hook. Remember, you can always pull more through, but you can't push hair back under the cap!

Cap highlights step by step

1 Start at the nape, gently pushing your crochet hook through the holes in the cap at an angle and pulling out sections of hair (a). Don't push the hook in straight and take care not to push it in too hard.

2 Work systematically up the head, working from left to right. Ensure that you are taking even amounts of hair that match the look you want to achieve (b).

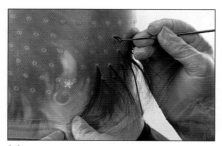 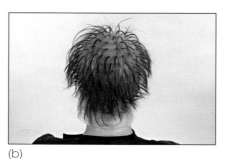

(a) (b)

Top Tips

The highlight cap will be easier to stretch over the head if it's warm. Use a hairdryer to warm up the cap slightly before putting it on the client, especially if it's cold.

Think about the shape and look of the finished hairstyle and use this to decide on areas of the head that may need a few more or a few less highlights.

Top Tip

Make sure the product mixture is not too runny – especially with bleach. If it's too liquid, it could cause seepage.

3 Continue up and across the head, taking particular care around the ears and the hairline.

4 Once complete, check for balance and even distribution and make sure all the pieces of hair are fully pulled through.

5 Apply the product to the hair, making sure that every hair is covered (c). The product should not be too runny, as it may leak through the cap.

6 Place the client under an accelerator if required (d) and set a timer.

7 Check and wash off when ready (e).

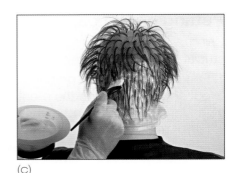

(c)

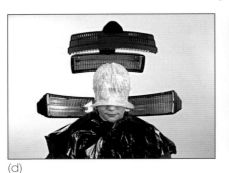

(d)

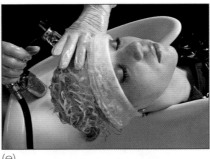

(e)

8 Discard any unused product and wash and clean your tools.

Removing the highlighting cap

> Seat the client at the shampoo basin and make sure they are well covered.

> Do not emulsify, but rinse off the colour product as quickly as possible, taking care not to splash the client. As a precaution, ask the client to close their eyes while you do this.

> Once all the colour product has been removed from the hair and the cap, lightly towel-dry. Apply a small amount of conditioner and, particularly for longer hair, gently comb through with a large-toothed comb if the hair is tangled.

> Starting at the front, gently ease the cap from the head. You may need to use your fingers to free the hair from the cap.

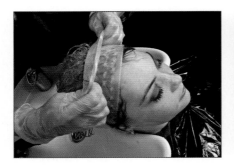

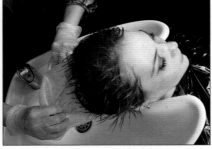

> Once the hair seems free from hair colour, shampoo and condition as normal or as directed in the instructions.

> Ensure that the client remains gowned and that you use dark-coloured towels, as the wet hair may still contain colour residue that can stain.

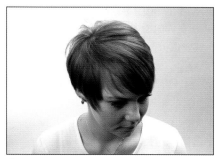

Cap highlights, completed

Woven highlights

What are highlights?

Highlights are small sections of hair that are lightened or coloured, to add a feature or to give the hair a lighter look.

What are woven highlights?

Often called foil highlights, this is a method of highlighting where strands of hair are woven from a main section and coloured by placing them in aluminium foil or purpose-made plastic pouches.

When are they used?

Woven highlights enable the use of more than one colour, and they enable the operator to place the highlight more accurately. They are also more comfortable for the client.

Do most salons offer both cap and woven highlight services?

No. While nearly all salons offer woven highlights, many salons, especially high-end salons, have stopped offering the cap method.

Preparation

The client

> As the colour product should not come into contact with the skin, sensitivity testing is not required.

> Protect the client's clothes with a gown or cape and towels.

> Ensure that any earrings are removed and that other jewellery is safely out of the way.

> Ensure that the client is seated comfortably and that you are able to carry out the service.

> Brush through the hair and check for broken or damaged skin.

> Hair that is excessively greasy or has styling product build-up should be shampooed before the colour application. A chelating shampoo is recommended, as it cleanses and rids the hair of residue and mineral deposits that may interfere with the absorption or colour coverage. Conditioners should not be used, as they will coat the hair and interfere with the colour process.

You

> Ensure that your hands are clean.

> Review the client record card and consult with the client, taking into account that the hairstyle may change after colouring. (For further details on consultation, see Unit G7.)

> Make sure that none of your jewellery will get in the way while you are working.

> Protect your clothes with an apron and your hands with gloves.

> Make sure that you have all the right tools and that they are clean and fit for purpose. Ensure you have adequate foils or plastic meshes for the entire process.

> Set out tools and a trolley.

> Mix and prepare the colour.

> Section the hair evenly, as this will help to create an even result.

> Keep your working area as tidy as possible while carrying out your work.

> Make sure you know how to work safely, with the correct posture, and that you are wearing clothes and shoes suitable for the service you are carrying out.

Deciding how much hair to weave

The thicker the pieces of hair you weave out of a section, the thicker the highlights will be. For natural-looking results, you should keep the weaves fine, approximately 1 mm or thinner. To create a stronger effect or 'streaks' of colour, take thicker pieces of hair of 2–3 mm.

The thickness of the hair should also be taken into account. The same thickness of weave will be strong and prominent on fine hair, and hardly noticeable on thick hair.

> **Activity** Watch other hairdressers when they highlight hair, taking note of the size and thickness of the weaves and the results they achieve.
>
> Practise weaving and putting in foils (without product) on a friend or on a block. Put in three rows of foils – one to achieve a natural result, one for a more prominent look and the last for streaks. Try to keep the weaves uniform in each section. Ask a senior technician to check and judge the result.

Making and folding foils

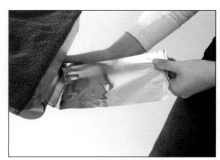

(a)

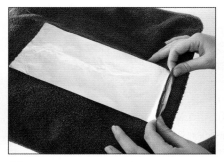

(b)

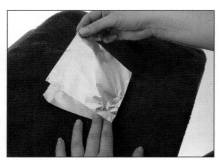

(c)

There are different ways of making and folding foils and each salon will have its preferred method. There are also machines on the market that cut and fold the foils for you.

Generally, they are made from rolls of foil found at the wholesalers, and are cut and folded using the following method.

> Cut the length of foil to roughly the length of the hair to be coloured (a).

> Fold the end of the foil over about 0.5 cm (b).

> Make sure that the line is straight and don't flatten the edge; keep a slight lip.

> Repeat on the opposite end.

> Fold the foil in half so that both ends meet (c).

> First close the foil, ensuring that all the hair and product is inside.

> Use the end of your tail comb to 'bend' the edge of the foil in about 1 cm on both sides.

> Again using your tail comb, bend the package in half and fold the bottom part upwards, taking care not to squeeze the package too much.

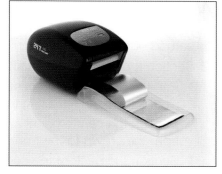

Automatic foil cutting and folding machines are able to make foils of varying lengths and types

Removing the foils

> Seat the client at the basin and ensure that they are well covered.

> With the client sitting upright, but leaning slightly back, begin at the nape. Gently unwrap and pull the foil from the hair, so you don't pull the client's hair.

> Continue up the head until you reach the crown.

> Now recline the client in the basin, ensuring that all the hair is inside.

> Continue removing the foils, working towards the front and making sure each section is falling backwards, away from the face.

> If you are unable to reach the front hairline from the back, go round to the front, but keep the hair in the basin.

> Once all the foils have been removed, clear them from the basin, check the temperature of the water and rinse the hair as soon as possible.

> Ensure that all the colour is properly rinsed from the hair before shampooing.

Note: In some cases, you may need to remove some sections of highlights while leaving others to process. If you need to do this, carefully remove the foils from the processed area and rinse carefully with water, taking great care not to disturb or wet the other foils. Water can dilute the product, and if you move them you can cause the product to leak. Don't shampoo at this stage; just make sure all the product has been removed. Gently towel-dry with an old towel and return the client to the accelerator if required, making sure the hair is not dripping.

Woven highlights step by step

1 Ensure that all the proper preparations and tests have been carried out and that you and the client are protected.

2 Section the hair into nine sections.

> Part the hair from the recession line (temple) to the nape on each side of the head, ensuring that each panel is the same width.

> Section the centre panel at the crown and secure the hair from the crown to the front in a clip.

> Section the back of the central panel in two, just above the occipital bone, and secure the two sections with clips.

> Divide the two side panels into three, following the guidelines of the central section, and secure with clips.

> Once completed, you should have nine sections; these should be wound in order, as they are numbered above (a).

3 Beginning at the nape, take a narrow section across the bottom of the first section and clip the rest of the hair out of the way.

4 Holding the section near the roots, use the end of your pin-tail comb to move up and down across the section, taking small sections of hair (b). Lift these pieces of hair off the tail comb and drop the remainder of the hair.

5 Lift the hair up and place a foil in at the roots (c). You may choose to place the pin of the tail comb in at the root, so that it forms a guide.

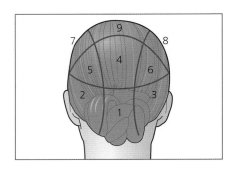

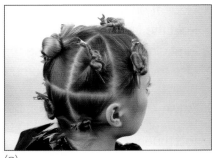

(a)

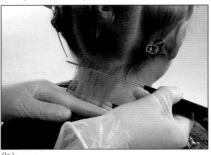

(b)

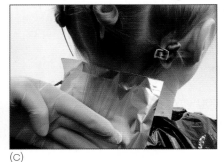

(c)

6 Pull the hair down so that it clamps the foil to the head and hold firmly.

7 Apply the colour, using it to 'stick' the hair to the foil (d). Taking care not to go over the edge of the foil, cover all the hair (e).
Note: As the colour processes, it will swell, so make sure you have not put the colour too close to the roots.

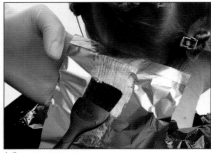

(d)

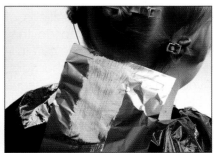

(e)

8 Close the package using your tail comb, taking care not to squeeze it too much (f).

9 Work through the nine sections to ensure that you keep the weaves even (g) (h) (i).

10 If during the process the colour thickens, add a little peroxide to refresh it.

11 Once the entire head is completed, place the client under an accelerator if required and set a timer. **Note**: you may only need to use heat on the last sections you have completed.

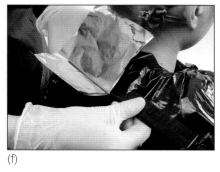
(f)

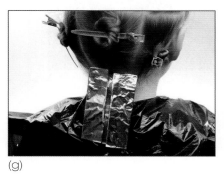
(g)

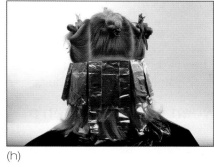
(h)

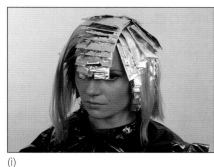
(i)

12 Check and wash off when ready (j).

13 Discard any unused product, wash and clean your tools and dispose of the used foils appropriately.

Activity Look at hair that has been highlighted and decide how it was done. Also look at hair that is one colour and think about how highlights could be used to soften or change the colour.

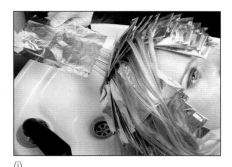
(j)

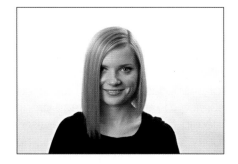

The objectives in changing men's hair colour are the same as noted at the beginning of this colour chapter. Earlier we covered the science, tools and general application methods; here we look at the additional and specific things you need to know for Unit GB2 and to successfully carry out men's colouring.

Introduction

What is it?

Changing men's hair colour covers the techniques and information relevant to the permanent or temporary colouring of men's hair.

What is the difference between colouring men's and women's hair?

There is very little difference. The science, products and preparations are all exactly the same, as are the application methods. There is a difference in the colours men have and the ways they are applied, to achieve results more in keeping with men's hairdressing.

For example, men's hair colouring tends to be less subtle, and colour application techniques generally focus on adding feature to a hairstyle. Also, while there are exceptions, men tend to use colour as a fashion statement rather than as a practical service to cover grey.

A growing service

Men's hair colouring is big business and is getting bigger all the time. Colour in men's hair was first seen on the punk rockers of the late 1970s, when it was a sign of rebellion and non-conformity. It remained the badge of the rebel or the eccentric for nearly 30 years, until fashion-conscious, so-called 'real men', like footballers, started adding colour to enhance their hairstyles. Since then, hair colouring for men has gained a social acceptance that has opened up the service to men from all age groups and walks of life. Dress codes for men in the workplace have also relaxed, further opening the opportunity for hair colour. All of this has led to a new and lucrative market for the hairdressing industry. To meet this demand, many salons have looked at male-specific hair colouring and initiated a dedicated service menu and price list.

But in order to reap the benefits of this growing market, you need to know how to meet its demands.

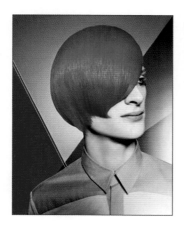
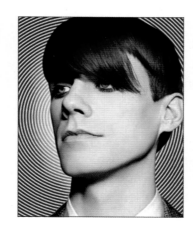
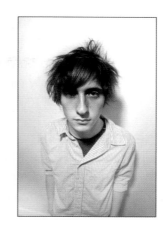

Spot the difference

It's important not to approach men's hair colouring with the idea that there are separate methods and techniques for men and women – there aren't. There's no reason why all the creative and exciting methods of colouring you'll learn can't be used on either men or women. Hair colouring is hair colouring: the science is the same; the need for testing, care and preparation is the same; the colour selection process and the way colour is applied are the same.

There are, though, general rules on colour selection and application that apply more commonly to men, and it's important to be able to identify these in order to meet the needs of your male clients.

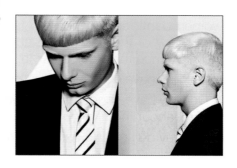

The general rules are:

> Men rarely have a single-shade all-over colour, preferring highlights or spot colour.

> Colour is added to make a feature of a particular hairstyle, whereas women will have their hair coloured as an ongoing service, regardless of their style.

> Men's hair colouring is usually prominent and obvious, rather than subtle and natural-looking.

> Lighter colours and bleaches are most often used to add highlights.

> Sheen, warmth and colour richness are generally not key targets of men's hair colouring.

> Men tend to have quicker colouring services, like frosting or spot highlights.

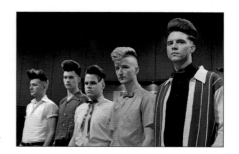

> Men tend to be more 'spur of the moment' and irregular with hair colouring.

> Generally, men are not be prepared to spend as much on hair colouring as women.

But remember, these are general rules, so don't use them to predetermine and restrict how you will provide colour services.

> Some men do have full-head colouring to cover grey.

> Some men do have full-head foil highlights.

> Some men do have rich plum and burgundy hair colours.

Fashions change, and what seems weird and unacceptable today could be the height of fashion in six months' time.

Matching men's colour

When deciding on the type of service and the colour to use on male clients, you need to take a number of factors into account:

> **Lifestyle** – how hair colour will combine with the client's work and social activities.

> **Hairstyle** – the cut, and how and where colour can be used to enhance or add feature to the style.

> **Budget** – what the cost of the service will be and if the client will be comfortable paying for it.

> **Time** – how long it will take and if the client is prepared to spend the time having it done.

> **Upkeep** – if the client will be prepared to commit to the upkeep of a colour or if they want something done as a one-off.

Lifestyle

As in all consultations, it's important to pay attention to your client's lifestyle. There are still dress code rules men have to follow that women don't, so you need to take into account the work they do. Plus many of the sports and activities more often enjoyed by men may influence their chosen style.

> Do they have a job with rules on hair colour?

> Do they have concerns about what their friends and peers will think about them colouring their hair?

> Do they do sports where coloured hair could be a problem, like swimming?

> Do they have a hobby or a pastime, like playing in a band, where they need their hairstyle to be versatile?

Peer pressure – reassuring your clients

Although more acceptable than ever, peer pressure can still be a major concern with men considering hair colouring for the first time. Many men worry that their friends will tease them for being 'girly' if they have hair coloured. There are some things you can do to put their mind at rest and to make sure they are comfortable with what you are going to do.

> Remind them of actors, sports stars and other well-known men who have hair colour, especially those who are seen as manly or tough.

> Let them know that, unlike those who may tease them, they are up to date and fashionable.

> Start small – suggest only adding a small amount of colour to the tips or the fringe, for example, that will soon grow out if they decide they don't feel comfortable with it.

> Reassure them that if they really don't like it, you can easily change it back.

Hairstyle

Look at the hairstyle and think about where colour will help to enhance the look.

> Will highlights help to emphasise the longer sections on the top or at the fringe?

> Will colour help to define or create definition between long and short areas?

> Will colour add feature and interest to a simple, basic haircut?

> Will colour help to add texture or movement?

Budget

As men's haircuts are still generally cheaper than women's, and hair colouring is still a relatively new service for men, the additional cost can be a shock and an obstacle. It's important to keep this in mind when suggesting colouring for men.

> For the first time, suggest a relatively inexpensive service, like spot colouring or frosting, that uses little product and doesn't take long. They can always have more done next time.

> Be clear about the cost so they know exactly what the price will be. If it's too expensive, suggest cheaper alternatives.

> Remind them that you have gift certificates (if your salon has them) and that a friend or family could pay for or towards the service as a present.

> Never pressure clients to have a service they can't really afford; this will make them regret it in the long term and they will begin to distrust your motives.

Time

As a rule, men don't like sitting around all day in hairdressing salons. Women find the experience relaxing, while most men find it an inconvenience that has to be endured to look good.

If you are suggesting colour to enhance a new haircut, find out how much time the client has, and if they haven't time for the full service, offer quicker alternatives, suggesting that they have the full service next time.

Note: Be honest and give realistic times for treatments. If the service takes longer than you said, it will not only inconvenience the client, but it will also make them question your judgement and reasons. If they suspect that you misled them in order to get them to spend more money, they are unlikely to come back.

Top Tip

Versatility – think of ways to make the hair colour versatile, so that it suits different aspects of your client's life. For example, if they work in an office but also play in a band, look at ways in which you could add colour that's not noticeable if they wear it one way, but becomes visible if they style their hair differently. Colouring the underside of the fringe is a good way of doing this. When flat, you can't see the colour, but if you spike the fringe section up, it becomes noticeable.

Activity

Look at your male friends and family and think about how colour could be used to enhance their existing haircut. If you can, write down your notes and consider them with a fellow student or work colleague. You could even ask a senior technician or manager to assess your ideas.

Upkeep

Not all men are as committed to looking after their hair as most women are, so it's important that you take into account the need and their desire to redo their hair colour periodically. Not all hair colour services require regular upkeep; some can simply be left to wash or grow out unnoticed. Make sure you find out how committed they are to keeping up the colour and suggest a look and a service that suits the individual.

Men's hair colour services

As has been clearly stated, there are no specific hair colours or colouring services for men; there are only those that are more commonly used on men.

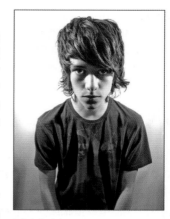
Highlights

Highlights

Highlighting is popular with men. It tends to be concentrated on the top of the head, although men with longer hair will have all-over highlights. Cap highlights are still popular with men; this is due to cap highlights being cheaper than woven (foil) highlights. It's also an easier technique, generally favoured by male-only barbering salons.

Frosting/shoeshine

This is a technique where bleach or permanent colour is added to the hair tips. This is usually done by applying colour to a strip of tinfoil and mimicking the motion used to shine shoes. Colour is gently rubbed on to the ends.

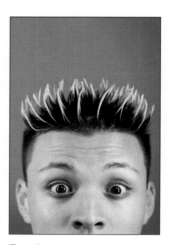
Frosting

Spot colouring

Also called flashing, hair colour is applied to the hair freehand, using a tint brush or the fingers. The hair is cut and styled, and then hair colour is added to key areas to add interest and feature. This is generally the easiest, quickest and cheapest method of colouring hair.

Section colouring

This technique is sometimes called spot colouring, because colour is applied to one spot. A section of hair – for example, the underside of a fringe or two panels down the sides of the head – is coloured. This technique is sometimes used to add detail to clipper patterns and designs.

Full head

While some men will have full-head colouring as a fashion statement, it's still not that popular a service for men. More men are however beginning to use this service to cover grey.

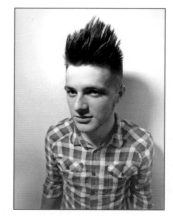
Spot colour

Lowlights

A few men are beginning to use lowlighting to add different tones or to camouflage grey hair.

Semi-permanent

This is not really a service previously associated with men's hairdressing, because semi-permanents tend to be all-over colours that add rich colours and shine. The advances and developments in semi-permanents mean that they are being used more often in men's hairdressing, especially some of the darker colours.

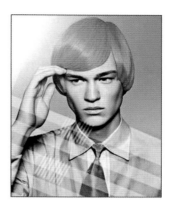

Full head colour

Preparation is the key to successful men's colouring

As with all services, preparation is the key to successful colouring, so it's important that you take the time to prepare properly.

Note: There may be a more casual approach to men's colouring in that men may make decisions about hair colour more on the spur of the moment, and may opt for the simpler and quicker colour services, but this doesn't mean you can take a more casual approach to your preparation.

You must follow the same rules and procedures that apply to all hair colouring, regardless of the type or cost of the service you are carrying out.

To ensure you get it right, always follow these three simple rules:

Test – test the client's skin for sensitivity and test the hair for compatibility and condition.

Select – choose a product and colour that suits the client's hair and skin type as well as their hairstyle and skin tone.

Protect – ensure that the skin and clothes of both you and your client are protected.

Testing

There are a number of tests that need to be carried out to ensure that colouring is suitable for the client and their hair.

First, you need to enquire into the client's history, to find out if they have previously had hair colour and if they've ever had a reaction to it. You should also ask if they have any product or other allergies, skin disorders or any medical conditions that could interfere with or be affected by the colouring process. Don't just think about how the colour may affect the skin or the scalp. If the client has a bad back, for example, they may not be able to sit for the length of time it takes to highlight or colour the hair. (For details on the colour testing procedures, see page 121.)

Note: While some services, such as shoeshining and spot colouring may not be intended to come into contact with the skin, as there is no physical barrier between the colour and the skin (as in cap highlights), you might find it advisable to carry out a sensitivity test just in case – especially if the hair is short or you are colouring long sections that could fall onto the skin.

Colour selection and mixing

As with colouring women's hair, there are some very important factors you need to consider, in addition to lifestyle, when selecting the shade, tone and strength of colour.

> **Hair type** – thick, coarse hair often requires stronger products and longer processing times than finer hair.

> **Hair length** – long hair may require three applications to cover and blend the roots, mid-lengths and ends. It will also require more products to be mixed.

> **Prior chemical processes** – virgin hair (hair that has not been chemically treated) can react differently to hair that has undergone a chemical process; any colour from a previous application, whether it's permanent or otherwise, may also affect the result.

> **Grey hair** – base shades need to be considered when covering grey (white) hair.

> **Condition** – porous, brittle, dry hair will absorb the colour faster than virgin hair.

> **Tone** (ash, gold, red, etc.) – the colour you use will combine with the colour already in the hair to produce the new colour. It's important to know how different tones combine and what colours will result.

> **Shade** – the lighter the colour you want to achieve, the stronger the peroxide you will need to use.

> **Skin tone** – the colour you choose should match and complement the client's skin colour.

When selecting a colour, first use the shade chart to establish the client's exact hair shade and tone. Then, with the client, use it to select a new colour. (For further details on consultations, see Unit G7.) By following the product instructions and taking into account the colour selection guidelines, you will be able to create a formula that will achieve the desired results. (For further details on colour and product selection, refer back to pages 124–8, where it is covered in more detail.)

Protecting

Hair colour products will stain skin and damage fabrics and furnishings, so even if you are only applying a small amount of colour to the fringe or top sections, ensure that you, your client and nearby surfaces are properly protected.

You

You should:

> wear gloves

> wear a tinting apron or gown

Activity Whenever you see an image in a magazine or newspaper of a man who has hair colour, see if you can figure out what colour and what colour service has been used. Always check your thoughts with a colour technician to see if you are right.

> ensure that your sleeves, hair and jewellery are out of the way and won't interfere with your work.

Your client

Your client should:

> wear a gown that covers their clothes
> remove any collars or high-necked clothing, or ensure they are turned down and adequately covered
> have barrier cream applied to the skin around the hairline (avoiding the hair) and on the ears
> be seated comfortably, so that you are able to carry out the service.

Your working area

> The gown should cover the chair (if possible) or the chair should have a protective back cover.
> You should use a mobile trolley to keep the colour close to where you are working.
> You should wipe up any spills as soon as possible, and keep your working area as tidy as possible while carrying out your work.

Partial colouring

What is it?

Partial colouring is adding colour to certain sections of the hair or certain parts of the head.

What types of partial colouring are there?

Shoeshining, frosting, spot colour and flashing are the terms normally used. All of these are methods to completely colour or highlight certain sections or just add colour to the ends of the hair.

How is it done?

There are a number of ways. You can use a tint brush or a piece of tin foil. You can also use a highlighting cap to pull through a few highlights or add some foil weaves.

When is it done?

Usually this type of colouring work is carried out after the style has been created, so it's easier to see where the colour should go.

Preparation

The client

> All clients having colour that will or may come into contact with the skin must have been sensitivity-tested. It is not necessary to carry out a sensitivity test each time the client has colour, providing you are using the same product as previously. (See page 121.)

Top Tip

For clients with a low hairline at the nape, use cling film or a plastic cape tucked into the collar as additional protection.

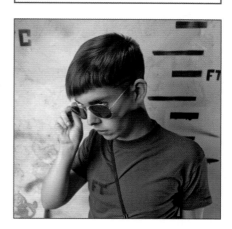

> Protect the client's clothes with a gown or cape and towels.

> Ensure that any earrings are removed and that other jewellery is safely out of the way.

> Ensure that the client is seated comfortably and that you are able to carry out the service.

> Brush through the hair and check for broken or damaged skin.

> Hair that is excessively greasy or has styling product build-up should be shampooed before the colour application. A chelating shampoo is recommended, as it cleanses and rids the hair of residue and mineral deposits that may interfere with the absorption or colour coverage. Conditioners should not be used, as they will coat the hair and interfere with the colour process.

You

> Ensure that your hands are clean.

> Review the client record card and consult with the client, taking into account that the hairstyle may change after colouring. (For further details on consultation, see Unit G7.)

> Decide how and where you will apply the colour, taking into account that the roots and porous ends will take the colour quicker.

> Make sure that none of your jewellery will get in the way while you are working.

> Protect your clothes with an apron and your hands with gloves.

> Make sure you have all the right tools and that they are clean and fit for purpose.

> Set out tools and a trolley.

> Mix and prepare the colour.

> Section the hair evenly if needed, as this will help to create an even result.

> Keep your working area as tidy as possible while carrying out your work.

> Make sure you know how to work safely, with the correct posture, and that are wearing clothes and shoes suitable for the service you are carrying out.

Shoeshine/frosting step by step

This is a technique to add colour or highlight the ends of the hair on a spiky hairstyle.

1 Dry the hair into its finished style, so that it is sticking up as it will do normally (a) (b). *Do not use styling products, as they may interfere with the colour products.* (If you do need to use styling products to get the hair to stand up, only applying them to the roots and avoid the ends.)

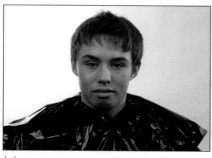
(a)

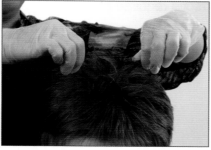
(b)

2 Tear off a strip of tin foil approximately 30 cm long and fold over both ends about 1 cm or so from the edges.

3 Use a tint brush to apply the colour product to the centre of the tinfoil.

4 Starting at the crown and holding the edges of the foil, gently move the foil left and right, rubbing the colour onto the tips of the hair (c) (d).

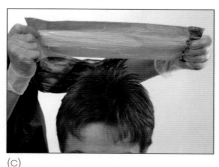
(c)

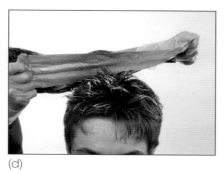
(d)

5 Take care not to press too hard, and avoid overloading the hair with colour.

6 Add more colour to the foil as needed and continue moving along the top of the head towards the front.

7 When you reach the front section, ask the client to lean their head slightly backwards, so that if any product is splashed it won't fall on their face.

8 Use the mirror to continually check for balance and that the application is even (e).

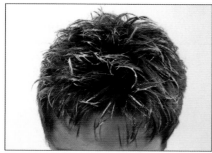
(e)

9 If you need to, use the tint brush to gently add colour to any small sections that were missed.

Top Tip

When shoeshining, mix the bleach or colour a little bit thicker than you would normally, so that it doesn't run.

10 Place the client under an accelerator if required and set a timer.

11 Check and wash off when ready.

12 Discard any unused product and wash and clean your tools.

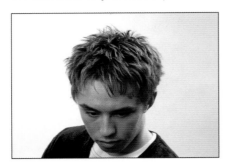

Checking – strand test

The processing time will vary depending on the product and the result you are looking to achieve. Check the manufacturer's instructions for estimated processing times and set a timer for the earliest possible completion time.

Use gloved fingers or a piece of cotton wool to remove the colour product from a small section of the hair to check if processing is complete.

Remember, the hair will be wet with product, so it may appear darker than it actually is.

If the colour is not yet ready, recover the checked hair with product and set the timer for a further five minutes. Continue to check until processing is complete.

Washing off

It's important when washing off hair colour to ensure that all the colour is removed and to avoid splashing. Always check the manufacturer's instructions for rinsing and shampooing after a colour, as they may differ from product to product.

> Seat the client at the shampoo basin and make sure they are well covered.

> Do not emulsify, but rinse off the colour product as quickly as possible, taking care not to splash the client. As a precaution, ask the client to close their eyes while you do this.

> Once the hair seems free from hair colour, shampoo and condition as normal or as directed in the instructions.

> Ensure that the client remains gowned and that you use dark-coloured towels, as the wet hair may still contain colour residue that can stain.

Other colour services for men

As part of unit GB2, you also need to know how to carry out a full-head application on virgin hair and a regrowth application. For

> **Activity** Practise shoeshine and freehand colouring methods by using conditioning treatments. Pour a small amount of a conditioning treatment into a bowl (choose a treatment that is fairly thick and has the consistency of hair colour) and apply it to friends and colleagues, as you would colour. Practise using tinfoil to shoeshine and a tint brush to apply spot colour. Ask a senior technician to review what you have done. By using this method, you can practise various different ways of applying colour. Remember that treatment products are expensive, so only use a small amount.

information on how to carry out these techniques, follow the step by step processes for colouring women's hair (see pages 134–9). The processes are the same; just remember to take into account male lifestyle factors and characteristics when selecting the colours you'll use.

Post-colouring problems and how to deal with them

By careful preparation and concentration, you should avoid unsatisfactory results. Sometimes things may not go the way you planned, so it's important to quickly identify the source of the problem so that it can be corrected or addressed next time.

In all cases of poor results, seek the advice of a senior member of the salon or the manager.

Problem	Possible cause	How to deal with it
Poor, weak coverage	• Not enough product used • Peroxide or product gone off • Poor application – not all hairs covered • Under-processed (washed off before ready) • Product or chemical barrier on the hair.	• If particularly bad, reapply when condition permits • Spot-apply to missed areas • Use a toner to even out the result.
Colour too bright	• Wrong shade selection • Peroxide too strong • Not enough base shade • Over-processed (colour left on too long) • Under-processed (washed off before ready).	• Use a toner to tone down the shade • If particularly bad, reapply when condition permits.
Colour too dark	• Wrong shade selection • Over-processed (colour left on too long) • Under-processed (washed off before ready) • Too much base shade • Bad porosity.	• Use colour removers if condition permits.
Colour too red or gold	• Wrong shade selection • Peroxide too strong – too much lift • Not enough base shade • Over-processed (colour left on too long) • Under-processed (washed off before ready).	• Use a toner to counteract and tone down the shade. • If particularly bad, reapply when condition permits.
Colour fades quickly	• Hair in poor condition • Client overstyling the hair at home • Swimming or effects of the sun.	• Apply toner to reinvigorate the colour • Condition and treat the hair.
Highlight cap has leaked, leaving spots or stripes at the roots	• Highlight cap is too old • Crochet hook too large • Highlight cap is split.	• Use spot colour to correct • Discard highlighting cap.
Woven highlights have leaked, leaving spots or stripes at the roots	• Foils not fastened properly • Too much product used • Foils squeezed or pressed to the head.	• Use spot colour to correct.

Problem	Possible cause	How to deal with it
Too much root between scalp and highlights	• Highlight cap not fitted correctly • Foils not put in close enough • Product not put close enough to the lip of the foil.	• Use spot colour to correct • Redo highlights, only colouring unprocessed hair • Offer a reduction in cost and redo the highlights sooner than usual.
Skin or scalp irritation	• Peroxide too strong • Accelerator/dryer too hot • Over-processed (colour left on too long) • Product not washed off well • Client allergic to chemicals.	• If residue product found, rewash hair • Seek advice from manager • Advise client to seek medical advice.
Hair breakage	• Over-processed (colour left on too long) • Peroxide too strong • Accelerator/dryer too hot • Hair in poor condition • Too many chemical treatments.	• Use reconstructing treatment • Seek advice from manager • Advise client to seek medical advice.
Skin or scalp staining	• Colour applied too far over the hairline • Inadequate application of barrier cream • Colour ran due to too much being applied • The cap or foils leaked.	• Use a skin stain remover with cotton wool and gently rub clean.

Problems, causes and actions

Finishing up

As well as being unsightly, dirty tint bowls and colouring tools left lying around can damage clothes and surfaces, and even cause injury if they come in contact with skin or are ingested. They can also contaminate other products or mixed colours, so it's important to dispose of unused colour product and clean tools as soon as possible after use.

Note: If, because you are busy, you are not able to deal with dirty tint bowls and tools straightaway, make sure that all used colour tools are put safely out of the way until you have a chance to deal with them. Never leave them lying around on a counter or in the shampoo basin. As well as being unsightly, they can contaminate other products or stain clothes and skin.

> Wash away any unused colour in a shampoo basin or dispensary sink – never in a sink used for the washing of cups or in an area where food or drinks are prepared.

> Carefully and thoroughly wash bowls, tint brushes, combs, clips and anything else that may have come into contact with the colour. Take particular care with dark-coloured tint brushes and bowls.

> Sterilise any tools that require it.

> Make sure that no colour product is left in the sink.

> Dry bowls, brushes and other tools and put them away.

> If you have used plastic caps, cotton wool or aluminium foil, dispose of these correctly, noting that some may be recyclable or reusable.

> Put dirty towels and gowns in the appropriate bins.

> Wipe trolley tops and counters and check the floor for spillages.

> Check and wipe your apron or gown.

> Wash gloved hands (if reusable gloves) and dry properly before removing. Make sure that your hands are clean and dry.

> Advise the relevant person of low stock or items that need to be ordered.

Aftercare

Always advise your client on how best to maintain their hairstyle and how to achieve the same look at home. It's worth noting that most men's product ranges don't have colour-protecting shampoos or conditioners. So if you've carried out men's colour services, you may need to suggest a product from another range that will help to maintain the colour and condition.

> Give advice on shampoos and conditioners that will help keep the hair looking good.

> Give advice on and show the client how to use styling products and tools to get the best results.

> Inform clients how best to protect their hair from damage by heated stylers or other electrical tools, to maintain condition and keep their colour looking good.

> Also let them know how sunlight, swimming and other lifestyle activities can affect or change the colour and how the hair could be protected.

> Advise the client on when they should or could have the colour done again or retouched.

> Suggest additional services, such as treatments that will improve the look or ability to maintain the style.

Finally, before the client leaves, let them know that if they have any problems with the colour, they can always come back to have it adjusted. Clients are often embarrassed about coming back if there is something that they are not altogether happy with, and sometimes they will even go elsewhere. So always make sure they know that it's part of the service and included in the price!

For the record...

It's important that you maintain accurate and up-to-date client records. It ensures that you can repeat the same colour if the client wishes, and provides a valuable record of the processes and chemical treatments the client has had, which is all important information that should be considered when deciding future technical services or treatments.

It's also important to record the details of the service just in case there are any future problems that may lead to legal action. If your client has an adverse reaction to the colour and decides to sue your salon, you need to be able to prove that you carried out all the

> **Top Tip**
>
> To make reordering easier, keep the packaging of any product you use up and give it to the person who orders the stock. This will enable them to order the correct item.

required tests, asked the appropriate questions and did everything possible to avoid a reaction. Even if the client has not told the truth or did not give you the correct information at the time, if you fail to make proper records, you will not be able to prove that you weren't at fault.

Always record:

> the results of sensitivity or other tests
> any relevant information learned during the consultation (it may be significant for a future service)
> the date of the service
> the service details – foil highlights, regrowth, etc.
> the products used; be sure to note carefully the product codes, amounts and strength of the peroxide
> how the product was applied (e.g. roots first, then mid-lengths and finally ends)
> processing – time and method
> shampoo, conditioning and treatment products used, how they were applied and any processing information
> the result – the colour, the coverage and if you achieve the desired result (was the client happy?)
> notes on the hairstyle
> retail products purchased
> any information that would be of use for next time.

Top Tip

Be honest when writing client records. If you thought the colour could have been better, say so and why. This will help you to improve the result next time.

Case study

Hair colouring is crucial to a modern salon

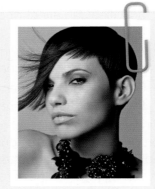

'Almost every single client in our salon has colour; it is a huge part of the business. It is my passion and I have passed this passion onto my team. It is the finishing touch, the chance for you to add your own creative signature to a look and create a focal point within every haircut. Every single one of my clients has colour, so I know that they will look great from every angle, 24:7.'

'Blonde clients know what shade they want and are always seeking the perfect tone and finish so getting it right is crucial. If you can get this right every time then they will return – get your blonde services right and watch your profits grow. Blonde is now 60 per cent of my salon business!'

'Colour can act as an advertisement for your salon. When they meet their friends after you've done their hair, you want their friends to say "Wow! Who did your hair? It's fantastic!"'

'And one really important piece of advice – don't just use your eyes, use your ears and listen closely to what the client wants. It takes a great listener to make a great colourist.'

Mark Leeson, Mark Leeson Hair, Body & Mind, Mansfield

Styling hair is a combination of interchangeable skills that allow you to change looks, control hair and create hairstyles. Here you'll learn those skills and how to use them to suit your client's individuality and ever-changing needs. So whether it's for a wedding, a night out or just a day at the office, the skills and techniques in this chapter will enable you to show your expertise and meet and exceed the needs of a demanding clientele.

You will learn:

> **prepare for a wide range of styling services**
> **blow-dry and style hair, using your hands, brushes and electrical tools**
> **set, dress and finish hair**
> **French twist and plait hair in a variety of ways**
> **attach permanent and temporary hairpieces**
> **understand and use styling tools and products**
> **provide quality aftercare.**

You will be assessed against your knowledge and ability to:

1 Understand your salon's processes and procedures with regard to promoting styling products and services.

2 Understand your legal and health and safety responsibilities when carrying out all styling services.

3 Understand your personal obligations to other team members and know when and from whom you should seek advice and assistance.

4 Maintain effective and safe methods of working and carry out all styling services in a commercially viable timeframe.

5 Consult with clients, consider key factors and choose looks and styles that suit their individual needs.

6 Communicate effectively with clients, using positive listening skills, body language and verbal communication.

7 Blow-dry, set, plait and put hair up, using a variety of basic styling techniques.

8 Attach and remove permanent and temporary hairpieces.

9 Use and understand a broad range of styling tools, styling products and accessories used in styling services.

10 Recognise adverse results and deal with them effectively.

11 Provide aftercare and product advice.

Introduction

What is it?

Hair styling and finishing is the art of drying, shaping and completing your client's hairstyle, and using your talents to create exciting looks that clients could never achieve at home.

What does it include?

It includes the skills of blow-drying, finger-drying, setting and dressing. It also covers the use of styling products and tools.

Why are all the styling and finishing units put together in one chapter?

In hairdressing, especially in styling, it's about using your talents and imagination to combine skills and techniques to meet the needs of your clients. While the specific elements relating to each unit are separate, by learning styling and finishing as one, you'll have a better grasp of where and how the techniques can be used for best results.

What does this chapter cover?

This chapter covers all the styling and dressing skills that you need to know for NVQ Level 2, including:

> GH10: Style and finish hair
> GH11: Set and dress hair
> GH13: Plait and twist hair
> GH15: Attach hair to enhance style.

The value of your skills

Finishing your style is where you highlight all your talents as a hairdresser. Well-finished hair will show your skills as a colourist, your technical expertise in hair cutting and your creative vision. This is also where you show the value of your craft, by creating a look that's crisper, sleeker or smarter than the client can ever achieve at home. Well-styled and finished hair completes a client's visit and encourages them to come back regularly, not just for a haircut, but also for special occasions.

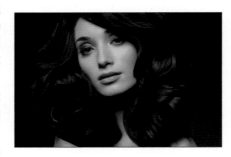

A walking advertisement for your work, a well-finished haircut or a stunningly dressed look will get noticed and will bring recommendations!

There are many valuable skills and techniques that can be utilised to finish and style hair. All great hairdressers can finish hair, and many award-winning and iconic looks have been created using traditional core styling techniques.

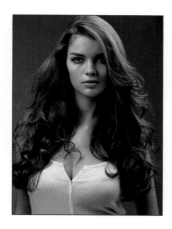
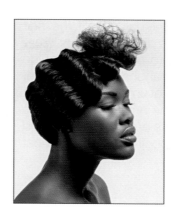
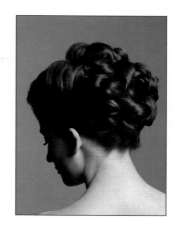

Most innovations in hairdressing are simply new explorations of old looks and techniques and many young hairdressers mistakenly think that certain styling and dressing skills are unimportant as they are old-fashioned and not used in today's modern salon. Fashions constantly change and return and what's not popular today may be in Vogue *magazine tomorrow. And also if you want to work on photo shoots or fashion shows, you must be able to create a wide range of finished looks.*

(Mark Woolley, Electric Hairdressing)

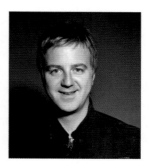

How styling hair works

Left to dry naturally, the haircut, texture and growth patterns will dictate how the hair will fall. This shape and direction can only be changed in three ways:

1 By placing or holding wet hair into a shape and drying it.
2 By using products to coat the hair and hold it into a shape.
3 By physically fastening hair into a shape with elastics, clips and pins.

All styled hair has been manipulated in one or more of these ways.

Drying

One of the chemical bonds that give hair its strength and shape is the hydrogen bond. There are more hydrogen bonds in the hair than the stronger disulphide bonds. The hydrogen bonds account for approximately a third of the hair's strength, but they are weak and easily broken by water. Hair's ability to absorb water, its *hydroscopic porosity*, means that these bonds are easily broken. When hair dries, the hydrogen bonds re-form, and if the hair is set in a new position when this happens, it will hold this shape until the hydrogen bonds are again broken by moisture. Alpha keratin is the term used for when hair is in its natural state. Once forced into a different shape – blow-dried straight or curled by setting – it becomes known as beta keratin.

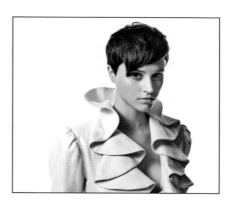

Mark Woolley for the Five Point Alliance

While this breaking and re-forming of the hydrogen bonds enables us to transform and shape hair, the result only lasts until the hair gets wet. Although fewer in number, the hair's disulphide bonds are far stronger and, unless chemicals are used to alter the disulphide bonds, the hair will always return to its natural shape and texture. Whether it's caused by shampooing, rain or even humidity or mist in the air, hair will always absorb moisture. The amount of moisture will determine how quickly the hair returns to its natural state. Humid air will have a gradual effect, while shampooing will be almost instantaneous.

Products

Styling products work in two ways:

> They coat the hair in a substance that hardens when dry.
> They stick hair strands together and use weight to hold and control the hair's direction.

Most products use one or a combination of these two ways to help create and maintain a style. There has been an increase in styling products that are also designed to protect the hair from heat and the damaging effect of styling. Some products will have an additional function of giving the hair a moisture-resistant coating that helps to protect the finished look. Apart from waxes, all styling products are generally water-soluble, however, and will lose their functionality when wet; all can be removed by shampooing.

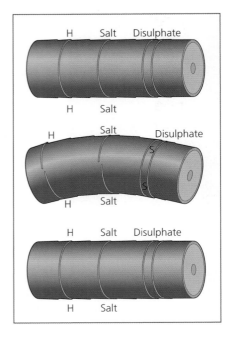

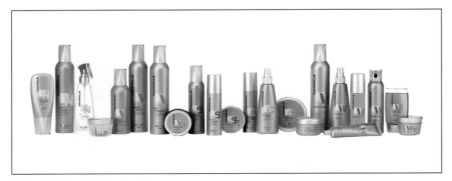

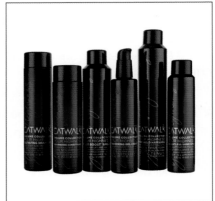

Grips, elastics, clips and pins

Unlike drying or using products to style hair, moisture will not affect a look created using clips, elastics, grips or pins. A well-secured, finished look will remain in place until they are removed. Pins, elastics, clips and grips can be used invisibly to create a style, or used as accessories to enhance a finished look. The world of photographic and session styling largely relies on the use of these tools to create some of the amazing looks we see on catwalks and in fashion pages.

Preparation

During the consultation process, you will already have decided on the final finished look; now you need to prepare the client and gather the correct tools and products to create the look.

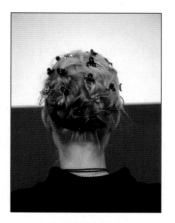

The client

> Ensure the client is gowned to protect their clothes and that there is a towel around their shoulders to absorb any dripping water.

> Make sure the client is positioned correctly and comfortably, and that they are relaxed.

> The client's hair should be shampooed to remove any grease, dirt or product build-up and should have been conditioned if needed.

> Blot, squeeze and gently towel-dry the hair well to remove excess water. Try not to rub the hair too much, as this will roughen the cuticle and make the hair more difficult to manage.

> The hair should be combed through and tangle-free. (You may need to gently blot the ends again after combing through.)

> Make sure the client is sitting upright and is comfortable.

> Ensure that any earrings are removed and that other jewellery is safely out of the way.

> Always ask if the client has any allergies to certain products and check the scalp for abrasions or sores.

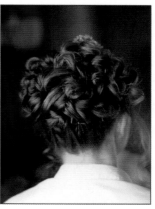

You

> Ensure your hands are clean.

> You may need to wear an apron or protective gown if the hair has recently been coloured.

> Make sure your jewellery will not get in the way while you are working.

> Make sure you have all the right tools and that they are clean and fit for purpose.

> Make sure you have selected the correct styling products for the client's hair type and desired result.

> Keep your working area as tidy as possible while carrying out your work.

> Make sure you know how to work safely, with the correct posture, and that you are wearing clothes and shoes suitable for the service you are carrying out.

Styling products

There are thousands of professional styling products on the market. It's always important that you know how each of the products in your salon should be used and the results they each produce. While generally using the wrong product or the wrong amount will not result in injury to the client or damage to the hair, it will affect the finished result. Using too much of a product or using the wrong product may mean that you will need to re-shampoo the hair and start again, which may be embarrassing for you and inconvenient for the client.

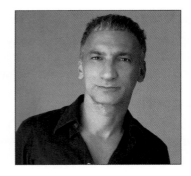

When it comes to styling products I always start small and build the product into the hair. It allows you to 'read' the results you are getting without overburdening the hair and ruining the look you want to achieve.

(Akin Konizi, British Hairdresser of the Year, International Creative Director, HOB Salons)

The styling products you use will depend on the client's hair and the result you are trying to achieve. Four simple factors should help you to decide on the best products for your chosen style:

> condition
> volume
> hold
> texture.

Condition

Consider the condition of the client's hair and how it will be affected by the styling methods you are planning to use.

> Will a leave-in conditioner make styling easier?
> Are you planning to use hot curling irons, straighteners or stylers? And if so, should you use a heat protector?
> Will a serum or smoothing cream help to smooth and protect the cuticle?

Volume

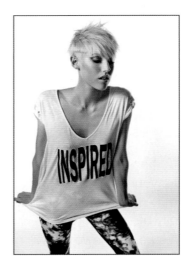

Consider the type of hair, the thickness and the amount of volume the style should have.

> Does the style require any root lift? If so, how much, and would a mousse or spray gel be best?
> If you want to keep the hair flat and smooth, will you need a frizz or volume reducer?

Akin Konizi for the Five Point Alliance

Hold

Think about the hair type, length and condition and how it will hold the style. Also consider how much movement the style should have and how long the client needs the style to last.

> Is the hair soft or fine, and will it need a blow-dry spray, mousse, gel or setting lotion to hold the style?
> Are you dramatically changing the direction or texture of the hair and, if so, do you need a gel or moulding paste to keep it in place?
> Is the hair heavy and do you need to use a mousse or styling lotion to stop the weight pulling out the style?

> Will you need a hairspray to hold the finished look and help to protect against moisture?

Texture

Finally, consider the texture of the hair and finished style. Think about whether you need to change the texture of the hair and what texture you want the complete look to have.

> Do you need to control frizz, curl or flyaway hair?

> Will a mousse or spray gel help to generate curl?

> Will a serum or smoothing cream help to create a smooth, sleek finish?

> Will a shine spray be needed to enhance the gloss finish?

> Will you need to create or accentuate detail using gel, moulding paste or styling spray?

> Will you need a wax or pomade to 'break up' and add texture to the ends?

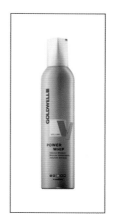

You should also bear in mind how you plan to style the hair – finger-drying, blow-drying straight, curling, setting, and so on – as some products work better with certain styling methods.

Types of styling products

Gel, setting lotions and mousses

> Applied to the hair before the styling service to give hold and support.

> Vary in strength, from very firm gels that can be 'sticky' and hard to work with, to light mousses.

> The results vary, from firm styles that don't move, to hair with movement and light control.

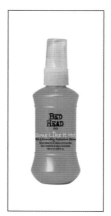

Serums, styling sprays, heat protectors and leave-in conditioners

> Applied at the beginning of the styling service or as the style is taking shape, to make the hair easier to manage or to protect it while styling.

> Vary in strength and texture, from thick and oily, to light and hardly noticeable.

> The results vary from sleek, glossy finishes to free-flowing movement.

Waxes, moulding pastes and finishing creams

> Applied towards or at the end of a service, to add sheen, texture and definition to the style.

> Vary in thickness and consistency, from hard, solid wax, to light creams.

> The results vary from hard spikes and defined ends, to the slight break-up of flat shapes.

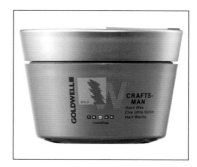

Hairspray and fixing products

> Applied when the look is completed to hold the look in place.

> Vary in strength and consistency, from firm-hold aerosol or liquid pump sprays, to lighter, misting products.

> The results vary, from fixing the hair into a solid, immoveable shape, to light hold that still allows movement.

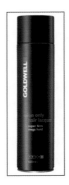

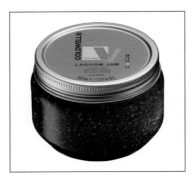

Styling gel

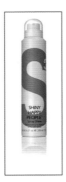

Shine spray

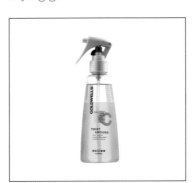

Curl-enhancing lotion

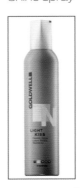

Lite hold styling spray

Top Tip

When applying styling and finishing products, apply small amounts at a time and see how they affect the hair. It's easy to add a little more as you need it. If you apply too much, it's not only a waste of expensive product, it can also make the hair hard to style or even mean you have to re-shampoo it and start again.

Tools

Blow-drying and styling tools account for the vast majority of tools in a hairdresser's tool kit. Next to your scissors, they can be the most costly to buy, so you want to make sure you buy the right tools. You also want to make sure you buy good-quality tools that will last and that you take good care of them.

Styling tools fall into three categories:

> brushes and combs
> electrical tools
> pins and accessories.

Brushes and combs

New brushes and combs are continually launched to help create certain textures and finishes more quickly and easily. When starting in hairdressing, it makes financial and practical sense to concentrate on putting together a kit of a few key tools and learning how to use them to create different results.

Below are listed the main tools you will require for hair styling and dressing, their primary uses and also alternative tools that could be used to get the same or a similar result.

Brushes

Vent brush

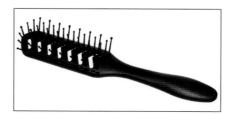

> Description: A lightweight brush with broad-spaced teeth, often with a semi-open back to allow increased airflow.
> Usage: To move hair around the head while drying, to remove moisture and to blow-dry with little tension, to create light, free-moving styles.
> Options and alternatives:
>   > tunnel vent brush for more airflow
>   > Denman free-flow
>   > paddle brush.

Denman classic D3

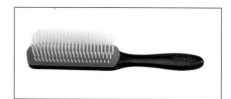

> Description: A versatile, seven-row, toothed, cushion, nylon brush that can be used in a wide range of blow-drying and dressing techniques.
> Usage: Good for brushing out, generating tension, creating root lift, bend and smoothness.
> Options and alternatives:
>   > larger, nine-row version for thicker, longer hair
>   > smaller, five-row version for shorter, tight areas
>   > Denman free-flow.

Large bristle brush

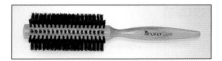

› Description: Large, often wooden-handled, radial brush, with natural or synthetic bristles.

› Usage: The tight bristles grip the hair firmly, so it is used primarily to straighten and smooth hair, especially coarse, wiry hair. It can also be used to create volume and curl. Radial brushes with pointed handles make it easier to take sections. Thermo-ceramic, heat-retaining brushes help to set the hair, creating stronger curl.

› Options and alternatives:
  › nine-row Denman classic
  › large, thermo-ceramic, heat-retaining brush.

Small round brush

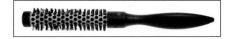

› Description: Narrow-barrelled radial brush, with natural, nylon or plastic bristles.

› Usage: To create tight bend and curl. The size of the barrel will determine the size and tightness of the curl, so it's worth having two or three of different sizes.

› Options and alternatives:
  › thermo-ceramic, heat-retaining brushes will help generate a stronger set
  › well-spaced, nylon-bristled versions will help avoid tangling
  › natural bristle versions will give more tension and a smoother result.

Paddle brush

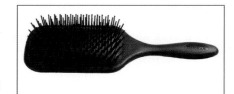

› Description: Large, flat, square-cushioned brush, with short or medium-length, fine, flexible bristles.

› Usage: To brush out hair prior to shampooing, and to brush through after setting, using hot rollers or curling irons, or to loosen finished styles. Also used when dressing formal hair, to smooth and finish. Can also be used when blow-drying, to move the hair around the head, to reduce moisture and smooth.

› Options and alternatives:
  › cushioned 'grooming' brush
  › Denman classic D3
  › flat bristle brush.

Combs

There are a number of combs that will help you to create various styled and finished looks. While some are interchangeable, others are designed for a specific purpose and will make certain tasks easier.

Large-toothed comb

Description: A heavy-duty comb, with large, widely spaced teeth, used primarily to comb through hair after shampooing, for sectioning and for combing through styling products to ensure that they are evenly distributed.

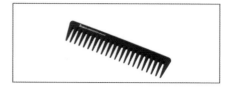

Standard comb

Description: Standard cutting comb, with wide and narrow teeth, used for more detailed sectioning, when using straighteners, curling irons or other electrical styling aids, and for general finishing.

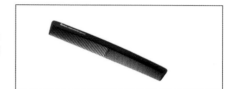

Tail comb

Description: Narrow-toothed comb, with a long, tapering, pointed tail that is used in setting and dressing hair.

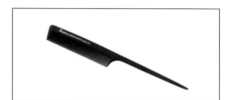

Backcomb

Description: The teeth on the backcombing comb are usually alternate long and half-length. Often the shorter teeth are also barbed. One end of the comb is split into four thin spikes. The shorter teeth and barbs make it easier for the hair to be backcombed, while the spikes can be used to 'pick' and dress the hair.

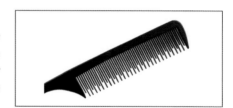

Pick comb (afro comb)

Description: Comprising of about six long, widely spaced teeth, the pick or afro comb is use to tease out and add volume to curls.

Note: Make sure you clean, disinfect or sterilise your tools between clients, and as and when they need it. This will help to keep them in good working order and prevent cross-infection.

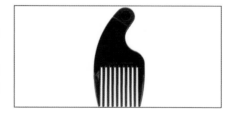

Electrical tools

The improvement in quality and the reduction in cost has meant that there are a large number of specialist electrical tools available to today's hairdresser. It's worth investing in and learning to use one or two key items, and adding to these as and when you can.

Dryer (hairdryer)

> Description: Hand-held hairdryer, used primarily in blow-drying, but can be used to speed up processing colours.

> Important features: A dryer should have varying speed and heat settings; it should also have a removable nozzle and an easily cleanable filter.

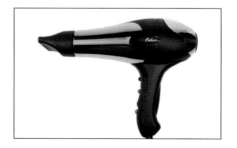

> Additional features: A 'cool shot' button can be useful to instantly cool and set sections while blow-drying. Long-nosed dryers can be used to support sections while blow-drying. There are also ionic dryers that add negative ions when drying.

> Nozzles: Most professional dryers come with a detachable nozzle that concentrates the airflow into a narrow and more controllable jet. As this concentrates the airflow, it's far easier to scald the scalp than when you are not using one. Some hairdressers always use them, while others never do. Although a few salons may have a strict policy on nozzle use, the choice is usually up to you. Best practice is to use the dryer both with and without, so you can learn when best to use a nozzle and when not to.

> Diffusers: A diffuser is an attachment (usually cup-shaped) that fits onto the end of a hairdryer and diffuses the airflow, so drying the hair without blowing it around. With the dryer on a slow setting, diffusers are used to dry hair naturally, especially to enhance natural curl.

Straightening (styling) irons

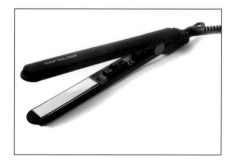

> Description: Flat, heated plates that sandwich hair and are slowly pulled along the lengths of the hair. Used mainly to smooth and straighten hair, they can also be used to create bend, although as the exterior of the straightener is cooler, they are not efficient at creating even curls.

> Important features: Safety cut-offs, ceramic and tourmaline plates for even temperatures, smooth surfaces to prevent cuticle snagging, changeable crimping plates.

> Additional features: Curved edges will help create bend.

Curling irons (curling tongs)

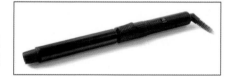

Description: Heated metal cylinder with a fitted metal clamp to hold the hair in place. Used to create strong bend, long even curls and root lift.

Important features: Curling irons should have a free rotating electrical cord and a built-in stand to stop them from rolling and to keep the heated barrel off counters, and so on.

Additional features: Some models have a spring-loaded clamp that makes it easier to secure the hair, while others have an unheated tip that allows both hands to be used.

Crimping irons

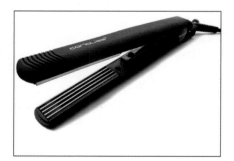

Description: Similar to straightening irons, except that heated surface is corrugated, which creates a ridge-wave effect. Available in different sizes to allow fine crimps and larger crimps.

Heated rollers

Description: Rollers that are heated and used on dry hair to add curl and volume. Hot rollers should be various sizes and should have a temperature indicator on each roller.

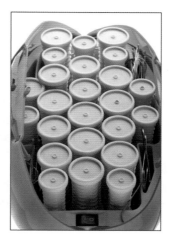

Waving (finger-waving) irons

Description: A cross between a crimping and a curling iron, where the hair is clamped between two undulating, heated metal plates to create a soft wave.

Note: When using heated electrical tools, it is important to keep the following points in mind.

> Ensure that they are kept away from the scalp.

> Make sure that you use them carefully, to avoid the heated parts coming into contact with your client's skin or you. Take care around the hairline and ears.

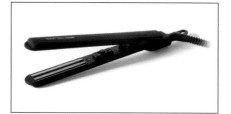

> Make sure the hair is in good enough condition and avoid damage through lengthy contact.

> Always take the right amount of hair for each section to be styled: too much and it won't deliver the result; too little and the hair could be damaged.

> Ensure that all electrical tools are CE marked and have been PAT tested (Portable Appliance Testing) where necessary.

> Never use any electrical tool that's faulty, has loose wires or is damaged.

> If the styling tool you are using does not have a 'ready for use' indicator light, do not test on your skin to see if it's hot enough. Try it on a section of hair and assess the result. (Most heated styling products will have one maximum operational temperature, and the instruction manual will tell you how long it will take to reach it and be ready for use.)

> Blocked filters, hair and product build-up will affect the performance and safety of electrical tools, so keep your electrical tools clean and free from product build-up. Always follow the manufacturer's recommendations for cleaning and maintenance.

> Hot styling tools can damage counters and upholstery. Never put hot tools down on chairs, fabrics or plastic counters. Always use a heat-protective mat or stand.

Pins and accessories

As you become more experienced, you will collect lots of accessories to add to your tool kit to help with styling, dressing and finishing work. A few key items are described below that you will find in most hairdressers' tool kits and session bags, forming the foundation of a practical and versatile accessories kit.

Top Tip

Keep your pins, clips and accessories together in a separate case in your tool kit bag. This will make it easier and quicker to find what you want.

Large 'grab' clips

Description: Spring-loaded, toothed clip for general sectioning.

Kirby grips

Description: Sprung metal grips, with one straight and one corrugated side. Kirby grips should have sealed ends, slightly forked open, and are a great styling aid, used when dressing hair to secure it firmly in place. They are available for blonde and brunette hair.

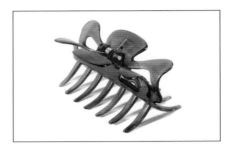

Grab clip

Straight pins

Description: Sturdy, oval, open, straight metal pins that have a variety of uses, including to secure rollers when setting, putting hair up in twists and chignons, and securing curls for sectioning.

Fine pins

Description: Small, thin, corrugated metal pins, used to tidy and secure small amounts of hair.

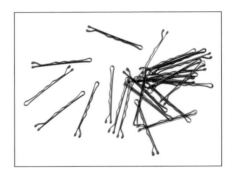

Kirby grips

Pin-curl clips

Description: Flat, usually aluminium, sprung, two-pronged clip, generally used as a working tool to secure curls and detail while drying or before finishing. Also used for fine and detailed sectioning.

Elastic ties

Description: Fabric-covered elastic ties for tying back hair and making ponytails. Available in transparent rolls or as individual bands. Always use professional standard bands and ties, as they are stronger and won't damage the hair.

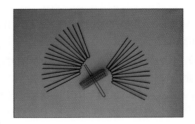

Straight pins

Barrettes, clips and decorative combs and accessories

Description: Various ornate clips and accessories that can be used both to create and to enhance a look. You needn't buy lots of these in one go; simply pick them up when you see them.

Items such as setting rollers, wefts, doughnuts and hairpieces are also styling tools, but generally the salon would supply them. If, however, you move into freelance hairdressing or you start to do session work, you will need to incorporate these and other tools into your tool kit.

Hair types

The type of hair you are working on will affect your choice of service, tools and products. You need to take into account the hair type as well as the desired finished look.

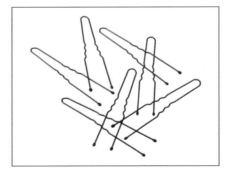

Fine pins

Curly hair

> To straighten, blow-dry or set on large rollers.
> May need to be blow-dried straight for plaiting or French twists.
> A diffuser or finger-drying will keep the natural curl.

Straight hair

> Blow-dry to add sheen or soft movement.
> Set for stronger curl.
> Finish with hot stylers to straighten or add bend.

Short hair – above the shoulders

> Finger-dry for soft and natural looks.
> Blow-dry with round brushes for curl.
> Use cornrows to plait the hair.

Long hair – below the shoulders

> Set on rollers for strong curl.
> Blow-dry with large, round, bristle brush to smooth.
> French or fishtail plait or French twist.

One length

> For shoulder-length bobs, use a Denman for a classic bob shape.
> For curl, set using larger rollers on top and smaller at the nape.
> Use stylers or tongs to add bend to the ends.

Layered hair

> Finger-dry to create texture.
> Use small, round brushes for bend and volume.
> Set using universally sized rollers for even result.

Key factors to consider when deciding how to style and finish a look

When deciding on which styling technique to use and what result you want to achieve, you need to consider certain key factors.

> **Purpose** – Where is the client going and why are they getting their hair done?
> **Duration** – How long does the look need to last?
> **Haircut** – How is the hair cut and what are the options and limitations?
> **Look and lifestyle** – What style will match the client's image and suit their head and face shape?
> **Growth patterns** – Are there strong growth patterns that need to be counteracted or taken into account?
> **Condition** – How will the condition and elasticity affect the way you style the hair, and the tools and products you use?
> **Texture** – What techniques and products will you need to work with the texture of the hair?
> **Hair length and thickness** – What styling methods and products will work best with the length and thickness of the hair?

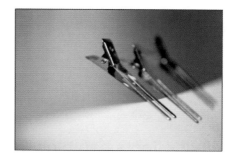

Pin-curl clips

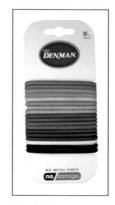

Elastic ties

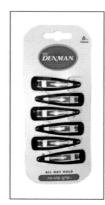
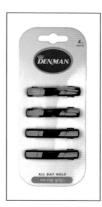

Decorative clips and barrettes

GH10: Blow-drying – style and finish hair

Introduction

What is it?

Blow-drying is the skill of using a hand-held dryer to dry, shape and finish a hairstyle.

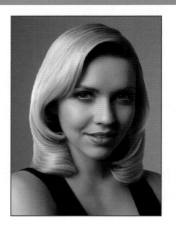

What effects can blow-drying create?

It's your most versatile tool, so practise and experiment! The blow-dryer can create hair that's straight and smooth, waved and curled, full and spiky, as well as every possible combination of these effects.

How does it differ from setting?

With blow-drying, you build the finished look by drying and styling sections one after another. With setting, you place wet hair in the shape and direction you want, and dry it in one go, finishing it by brushing and combing it into place.

What are the advantages over setting?

Blow-drying tends to create a softer, looser result that suits contemporary haircuts. Blow-drying is a very versatile and portable skill, and it's also a more personal process than setting, as you work one-on-one with the client to create the look.

Preparation

During the consultation process, you will already have decided on the final finished look. Now you need to prepare the client and gather the correct tools and products to create the look.

The client

> Ensure the client is gowned to protect their clothes and that there is a towel round their shoulders to absorb any dripping water.
> Make sure the client is positioned correctly and comfortably and that they are relaxed.
> The client's hair should be shampooed to remove any grease, dirt or product build-up, and should have been conditioned if needed.
> Blot, squeeze and gently towel-dry the hair well, to remove excess water. Try not to rub the hair too much, as this will roughen the cuticle and make the hair harder to manage.
> The hair should be combed through and tangle-free. (You may need to gently blot the ends again after combing through.)
> Make sure the client is sitting upright and is comfortable.
> Ensure that any earrings are removed and that other jewellery is safely out of the way.
> Always ask if the client has any allergies to certain products and check the scalp for abrasions or sores.

You

> Ensure your hands are clean.

> You may need to wear an apron or protective gown if the hair has recently been coloured.

> Make sure your jewellery will not get in the way while you are working.

> Make sure you have all the right tools and that they are clean and fit for purpose.

> Make sure you have selected the correct styling products for the client's hair type and desired result.

> Keep your working area as tidy as possible while carrying out your work.

> Make sure you know how to work safely, with the correct posture, and that you are wearing clothes and shoes suitable for the service you are carrying out.

What you will need

> Gowns and towels

> A multi-speed hairdryer with nozzle

> A selection of brushes

> A standard (cutting) or backcombing comb

> Styling and finishing products

> A water spray.

Using a blow-dryer

Core blow-drying skills

> Placing moussed hair in a diffuser and drying it on a slow setting will create soft, natural curl.

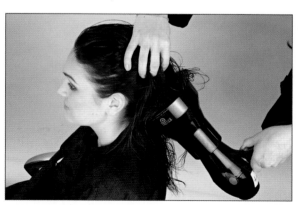

> Pulling hair tight through a bristle or large-barrelled brush while drying will straighten and smooth the hair.

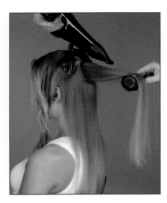

> Elevating the hair while drying will generate volume.
> Rolling a Denman classic or round brush on the ends of the hair will create bend.

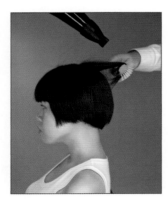

> Tightly rolling a heat-retaining or round brush into the hair and leaving to cool will create curl.

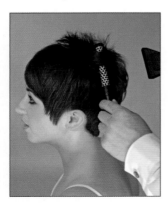

> Using a larger round brush in the same fashion will create soft movement (see next photo).

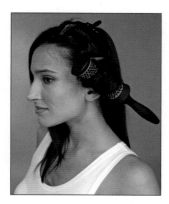

> Push-drying the hair into place with the fingers will create a soft, natural, unfinished result.

Key points to remember when blow-drying

> Always make sure the hair is clean. Greasy or dirty hair will be hard to style and the look won't last.

> Hair only takes shape when it goes from damp to dry, so remove excess moisture by rough-drying before styling.

> The direction in which you dry the roots will dictate the direction of the hair.

> Only use workable sections that fit on or around the brush.

> Always section off the hair, so that you can dry key areas properly, especially at the nape.

> Damp hair will not hold its shape! You must dry it completely and thoroughly.

> Dry the roots as well as the mid-lengths and ends. Damp roots will make the hairstyle fall very quickly.

> Generally, try to keep the airflow from the dryer directed down the hair from above, for better control and finish.

> Keep the dryer moving to avoid scorching the hair or the scalp.

> Use the right tool for the right job to get the best results.

> Keep the hair moist with a water spray if needed.

> Once dried, you can't change hair. If you keep on blow-drying, it will become static, frizzy and over-dried. To change the result, you need to wet the hair, so mist with a water spray and start again.

> Take your time! Think about the tools and products you'll need and how best to build and create your look.

> Finally, keep your tools clean and well maintained.

The modern crop blow-dry step by step

This modern take on the crop shows textured style with plenty of volume.

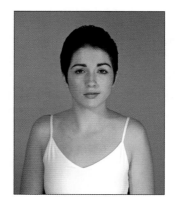

1 Ensure the client is gowned, with a towel round their shoulders, and that the hair is cleansed and conditioned. Towel-dry the hair to remove excess water and add styling products.

2 Work without tension by following a paddle brush with the dryer (a). This brush eliminates static and allows the hair to fall naturally. Begin moving the top sections, blow-drying from side to side, without tension.

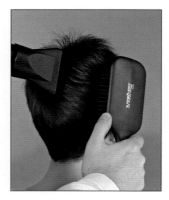

(a)

3 Switch to a Denman classic for more control and polish. Work from the centre nape towards the front hairline. Blow-dry each section forward and follow the brush carefully with the nozzle of the dryer (b).

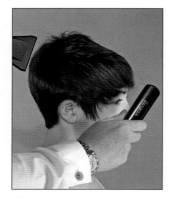

(b)

4 As you progress, move the hair in alternating directions, wrapping the sections around the head and working with the natural growth patterns. Repeat this technique for the opposite side.

5 Concentrate on the crown and nape, following each section with the flow of the dryer and alternating in a forward and back motion (c) (d). Swap hands with your tools to achieve balance.

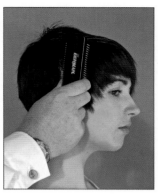

(c)

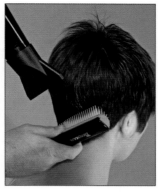

(d)

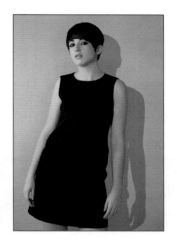

6   Now use a vent brush to create texture and direction. Begin working on the fringe, taking one section at a time. Place the brush in at the root, pull backwards and lift. Using the brush, push the hair back towards the dryer by about 1 cm, then pull the hair forward. Follow the top sections in this manner towards the front hairline.

7   Change to a small, heat-retaining brush at the crown. Take brush-sized sections, using the dryer to heat the barrel to create additional lift and curl. Vary the direction of your sections for height and movement. Repeat for the opposite side. Accentuate the texture with your fingers.

Long, one-length blow-dry step by step

Long hair can be so expressive, giving the wearer the opportunity to express both their mood and the occasion. This one-length look has slight soft graduation through the sides, and is styled straight to frame the face or in soft sensuous waves.

1   Ensure the client is gowned, with a towel round their shoulders, and that the hair is cleansed and conditioned. Towel-dry the hair to remove excess water and add styling products.

2   Begin by moving the hair around with a free-flow or vent brush, allowing the air to flow over the sections. Follow each section down with the nozzle of the dryer, from root to tip. Brush the hair alternately forward, then back (a).

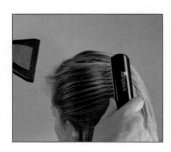

(a)

> **Activity** When you are free or watching, practise rolling a brush (a Denman classic) until you can do it smoothly and it doesn't make your hand ache.

3 Section the hair along a centre parting and from the crown to the back of the ear (b).

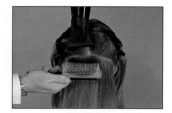

(b)

4 Begin working with a seven-row or nine-row Denman classic brush, rolling the brush in at the root to pick up the hair (c). With firm tension, lift and pull the brush through the section, keeping the airflow aimed down the hair shaft (d). Draw the brush down through the lengths to the tips. Continue working in this manner, keeping the tension even and drying from root to tip.

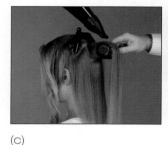 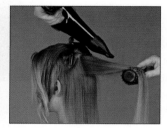

(c)   (d)

5 When the section is almost dry, take a radial heat-retaining or bristle brush and rework the section. Using the barrel of the dryer to hold the section, place the brush in at the root. Draw the brush down the lengths to create a smooth, polished finish (e). Continue taking horizontal sections in this manner and work up towards the crown. Work in horizontal sections up through the sides towards the centre parting.

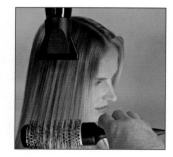

(e)

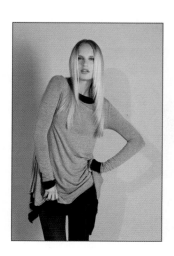

6 At the front hairline, roll the brush into the root and pull the section forward. Heat the barrel of the brush with the dryer and pull through the lengths. Hold the heat on the ends to set a bend into the hair. Lastly, working without heat, push the hair into place using a paddle brush, keeping the hair flat and sleek.

Using ceramic stylers or curling irons

What are they?

These are heated electrical tools used after blow-drying to enhance or finish a style.

How do they work?

Heat is used to 'dry out' any remaining moisture in the hair and set it in a particular way.

What can they do?

Stylers or straightening irons have flat ceramic plates that smooth the hair and flatten it. They can also be used to give the hair a loose curl. Curling irons, or curling tongs, are cylindrical and the hair is wrapped round to create a tighter curl.

Are there different types?

Loads! As well as different manufactured versions with various features, they come in different sizes and allow you to create a wide variety of finishes.

Stylers, curling irons and other electrical tools are very hot and need to be handled with great care, as they can burn you or your client, and melt fabrics and counters. Also, they can cause electric shock, so they should be continually checked to make sure they are in good working order. Never use electrical tools if they are damaged or not in good working order.

Using straighteners, stylers or curling irons step by step

1 Prepare by turning on the appliance so that it will be ready for use. Make sure it's safe and can't cause injury or damage.
Note: Do not leave electrical tools on indefinitely when not in use. This wastes energy and can lead to injury or damage.

2 Ensure the hair is dry and tangle-free and apply heat-protecting products if required.

3 Section the hair to be worked on into manageable sections (a).

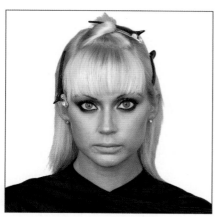

(a)

4 Beginning at the back of the head and at the bottom of the section, take a section of hair approximately 1 cm thick and no wider than the appliance you are using.

5 Place the styler or iron close to the roots, placing your comb under the appliance to protect the scalp (as shown in (c)).

6 For straightening, slowly pull the iron down along the hair, keeping the tension consistent and taking care not to stop in one place, as this can damage the hair (b) (c).

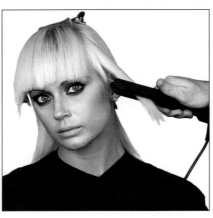

(b)

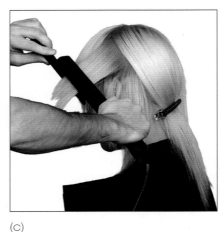

(c)

7 Once you reach the ends, lay them flat, ensuring the hair does not touch the skin, and allow it to cool. Repeat the process if needed, taking care not to overheat and damage the hair.

8 For curl, slowly pull the styler or iron down the length of the hair until the ends. Keeping the appliance closed on the ends of the hair, roll up the length of the hair until it is close to the roots. Again, place the comb between the appliance and the scalp.

9 Hold for a few seconds and then slowly unwind and leave the hair to cool.

10 Continue working in this method throughout the head, reviewing the look and the style as you go.

Activity Practise using your stylers on yourself, your colleagues or even a block. See how many different shapes and textures you can create – straight, slight bend at the ends, wavy roots, tight and loose curls. See if you can create ten different styles!

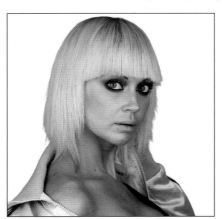

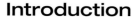

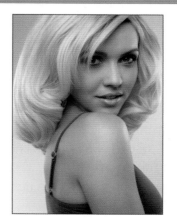

Introduction

What is it?

Setting is the technique of using rollers, pins and clips to dry hair in a particular style or shape.

How does the result differ from blow-drying?

While it's possible to get the same effect with both techniques, setting generally creates a stronger, firmer, more durable result.

What are the advantages over blow-drying?

It can be easier to create volume and a strong result with setting, and it is a good foundation for hair-up and bridal styles. Setting can also increase the number of clients a hairdresser can accommodate, and some clients enjoy relaxing under the dryer.

Many young hairdressers mistakenly believe that setting is an old-fashioned technique that has no place in modern hairdressing. Wrong! Even if your salon only ever does blow-drying, setting hair is a crucial skill for any session or catwalk hairdresser. Plus, setting hair, in many cases, is still the best way to prepare hair for up-styles and dressing.

Setting hair is still carried out as a regular service in many UK salons and also remains popular in many salons around the world. It is a valuable and important skill for any hairdresser to learn. And remember, fashions change…

Preparation

During the consultation process, you will already have decided on the final finished look. Now you need to prepare the client and gather the correct tools and products to create the look.

The client

> Make sure that the client is gowned, to protect their clothes, and that there is a towel round their shoulders to absorb any dripping water.

> Ensure that the client is positioned correctly and comfortably, and that they are relaxed.

> The client's hair should be shampooed to remove any grease, dirt or product build-up, and should have been conditioned if needed.

> Blot, squeeze and gently towel-dry the hair well, to remove excess water. Try not to rub the hair too much, as this will roughen the cuticle and make the hair more difficult to manage.

> The hair should be combed through and tangle-free. (You may need to gently blot the ends again after combing through.)

> Make sure the client is sitting upright and is comfortable.

> Ensure that any earrings are removed and that other jewellery is safely out of the way.
> Always ask if the client has any allergies to certain products, and check the scalp for abrasions or sores.

You

> Ensure your hands are clean.
> You may need to wear an apron or protective gown if the hair has recently been coloured.
> Make sure your jewellery will not get in the way while you are working.
> Make sure you have all the right tools and that they are clean and fit for purpose.
> Make sure you have selected the correct styling products for the client's hair type and desired result.
> Keep your working area as tidy as possible while carrying out your work.
> Make sure you know how to work safely, with the correct posture, and that you are wearing clothes and shoes suitable for the service you are carrying out.

What you will need

> Gowns and towels
> Tail comb
> Brushing out or grooming hairbrush
> Backcombing comb
> Rollers (and straight pins)
> Pin-curl clips
> A hairnet
> A hood dryer
> Styling and finishing products
> A water spray.

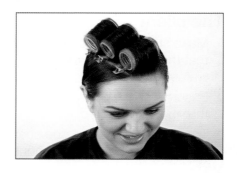

Setting hair

Core setting skills

> Directional winding dictates the way the hair will go when dry and can be used to change or compensate for natural growth patterns.

❯ Winding the roller so that it sits on top of the section base will maximise lift and volume.

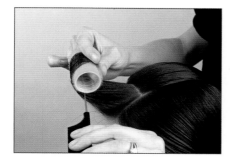

❯ Brick winding helps to eliminate channels and breaks in the hairstyle.

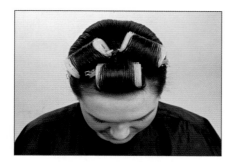

❯ Dragging the roots so that the roller sits behind the section 'off base' will create a flatter look.

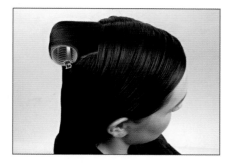

❯ Barrel and clock-spring pin curls are used to set small areas or add detail.

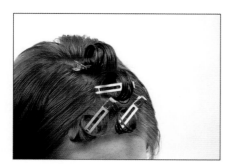

> Stand-up pin curls add volume, while flat pin curls give movement.

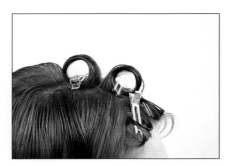

> Finger-waving creates undulating waves that are flatter to the head.

> Spiral winding, starting at the root and winding the hair as a strand along the length of the roller, creates corkscrew curls.

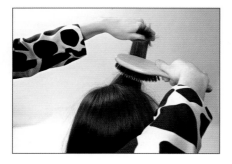

> Back-brushing gives the hair volume and more hold, enabling you to create shapes.

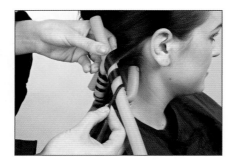

> Backcombing forms tighter, stronger support at the roots, for stronger results and bigger shapes.

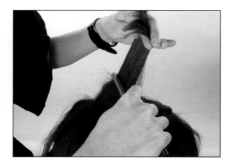

> Carefully brushing the outside, visible layer of the hair smooths and tailors the hairstyle, without disturbing the internal backcombing or back-brushing.

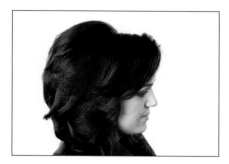

Key points to remember when setting hair

> Always make sure the hair is clean. Greasy or dirty hair will affect the look and how long it will last.

> Take care not to injure the client when using pins and clips.

> Don't put rollers and clips in too tightly, as this will become uncomfortable for the client while they are drying.

> Take sections appropriate to the size of the roller.

> Ensure sections are uniform and neat, and that you use even tension throughout.

> The bigger the roller you use, the more volume and open curl you will create.

> The smaller the roller you use, the tighter the curl and the more 'rolled' effect you will create.

> Rollers sitting on top of the roots (base) will create vertical lift. Dragging or over-directing roots will influence the direction of the hair.

> Ensure the hair is kept damp during winding.

> Make sure the client is seated correctly and comfortably under the dryer, so that all the rollers will be dried evenly.

> Check and set the temperature that's comfortable for the client and hand them the controller if there is one.

> Drying takes around 25 minutes – less for fine hair and more for thick hair.

> Check on your client while they are under the dryer to make sure they are comfortable and that the style is progressing as planned.

> Check various rollers for dryness – front, crown, side and nape. All the hair must be completely dry before you remove the rollers and pins. Hair that's even the slightest bit damp will lose its shape and style very quickly.

> Once dry, allow to cool before removing the rollers and pins carefully.

> Finally, ensure rollers, pins and clips are kept clean and tidy, and that combs and brushes are clean and well maintained. Product build-up will affect future results and contaminate clean hair.

Brushing out

Once your set is dry and you've taken out the rollers, it's easy to think that the hard work is over. It's not. Brushing out is not as easy as it seems, and many hairdressers waste all the effort put into winding and drying the hair by not brushing out properly.

The worry is often that if you brush the hair too hard, you will brush out the set – you won't. If the hair is dry and has been set well, only wetting it down will destroy it. If you don't brush it out properly, the hair will re-form into the roller sections' 'set marks' and look bitty and separated.

> Using a paddle or a grooming brush, brush the hair hard and well. Do this for a good minute or so, brushing the hair with and against the direction of the set.

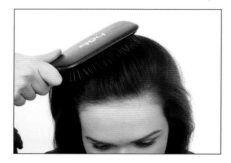 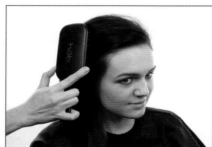

> Starting at the nape, ensure all the roller sections are blended.

> Begin to brush the hair into place. Once in place, leave it and move up the head to the next section.

> Once you have completed the entire head, use a standard comb or a dressing/backcombing comb to tease and finish the hair.

> To create more volume, backcomb or back-brush the hair by holding a section of hair near the tip and pushing the comb or brush down the length towards the root. The more you do this, the more the hair will 'tangle' and form a matted lump at the roots.

> Disguise any backcombing or back-brushing by gently combing or brushing smooth the outside of backcombed sections. (Take care not to comb out what you put in!)

> Take care not to 'over-dress' the hair. Once it is in place, leave it. If you continue to brush, comb and fiddle with the hair, it will begin to lose its curl and become fluffy or frizzy.

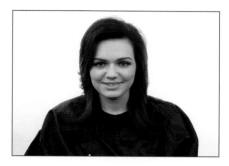

Setting step by step

Creating a styled look using setting rollers and pin curls.

1 Ensure that the client is gowned, with a towel round their shoulders, and that the hair is cleansed and conditioned. Towel-dry the hair to remove excess water and add styling products (a).

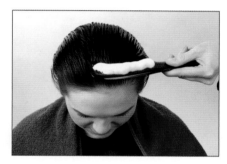

(a)

2 Decide the size and direction of the rollers. Comb the hair into the direction it is to be set. Starting at the centre front hairline, take a section of hair, approximately the same size but slightly narrower than the roller.

3 Comb the hair straight up and slightly forward so that it's smooth. Hold the tips of the hair between your thumb and forefinger and place the roller in front of the tips.

4 Place the tips of the section in the centre of the roller and, while holding in firmly against the roller, roll into the hair evenly, making sure that short or wispy hairs are included. Roll down so that it sits in the required position (b). Use a pin through the roller to hold it in place.

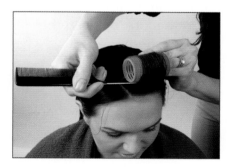

(b)

5 Take a follow-on section, continuing the same line, and roll as before. Use a pin to secure the roller to the first. (Remove the pin in the first roller if it is against the skin or scalp.) Continue working backwards, following the direction of the style.

6 At the sides of the hair, use pin curls to set shorter hair or to set the hair flat (c).

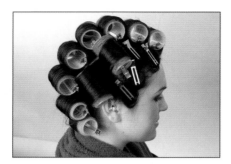

(c)

7 Continue through to the nape, where you may need to use smaller rollers for a tighter curl.

8 Once complete, cover with a net if needed (d), before drying (e).

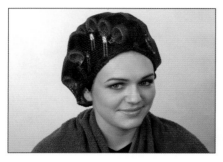

(d)

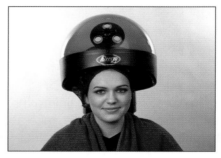

(e)

9 Once dry, remove the rollers and brush and comb into shape.

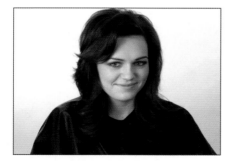

Activity Try achieving the same result by setting a blow-dry style. Think about how you blow-dry the hair and where you create volume or bend, and use rollers to achieve the same result. Once finished, look at how the two finished looks differ. Also, compare how the look holds in the two finished looks.

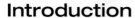

Introduction

What is it?

Hair dressing is the techniques used to create looks and styles by weaving the hair together (plaits) or twisting and pinning it into place (twists).

When are these techniques used?

In the salon, most often to create looks for special occasions or to transform hair quickly into a new look. They are also key techniques for session styling, catwalk and film work.

Are these techniques difficult?

While more elaborate looks may require a high level of technical skill, basic plaits and twists are very easy and, with practice, you can master them quite quickly.

Case study

Dressing hair: a timeless skill

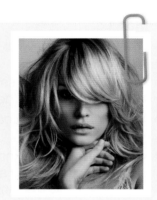

'Dressing hair is an essential part of every hairdresser's job – it's the essence of what we do. I always emphasise how important a good grounding in classic techniques is and this includes dressing, perming and setting hair. Education in these and other classic techniques builds the foundation of a hairdresser's skill and can be built on and used in conjunction with more contemporary techniques.'

'It's important to have fun with hair and experiment with textures. Keep the passion and motivation in your team alive with weekly training nights – challenge them to interpret a look from magazines or the catwalk. Total image is vital for editorial work – you need to have the final goal in mind and remember your target audience. Make sure make-up, styling and photography work seamlessly to produce your final look.'

'On my "The Business of Blondes" tour with Goldwell, using setting and dressing techniques, I created a vanilla-blonde Louis Vuitton-inspired "poodle-pony" editorial look, which was both eccentric and beautiful.'

Mark Leeson, Mark Leeson Hair, Body & Mind, Mansfield

Preparation

During the consultation process, you will already have decided on the final finished look. Now you need to prepare the client and gather the correct tools and products to create the look.

The client

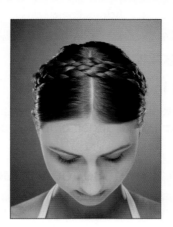

> Ensure that the client is gowned to protect their clothes, and that there is a towel round their shoulders.

> Make sure the client is positioned correctly and comfortably, and that they are relaxed.

> The client's hair should not be overly greasy, dirty or have product build-up.

> The hair should be brushed through and tangle-free.

> Make sure the client is sitting upright and is comfortable.

> Ensure that any earrings are removed and that other jewellery is safely out of the way.

> Always ask if the client has any allergies to certain products, and check the scalp for abrasions or sores.

You

> Ensure your hands are clean.

> Make sure your jewellery will not get in the way while you are working.

> Make sure you have all the right tools and that they are clean and fit for purpose.

> Make sure you have selected the correct styling products for the client's hair type and desired result.

> Keep your working area as tidy as possible while carrying out your work.

> Make sure that you know how to work safely, with the correct posture, and that you are wearing clothes and shoes suitable for the service you are carrying out.

What you will need

> Gowns and towels

> Brushing or grooming hairbrush

> Tail comb

> Backcombing comb

> Assorted pins, grips and clips

> Covered ties and/or barrettes

> Styling and finishing products

> A trolley.

Using hair dressing

Core plaiting and French twisting skills

> A French twist can be created without using a row of grips. The hairstyle is secured using long, straight pins.

> When plaiting, keeping the sections uniform in size and using smaller sections will make the plait appear more intricate.

> Reversing the plaiting process – crossing the sections under rather than over each other – will create an external plait that sits on top of the hair.

> Starting the plait at the nape, with the head upside down, can be used when putting hair up, especially if the hair is short.

Key points to remember when plaiting or twisting hair

> Ensure the client understands the length of time the service will take and the cost.

> Ensure the client understands how the finished style will look and that they are happy for you to continue.

> Hair needn't be clean for either method of styling, but overly greasy or dirty hair will be hard to secure when twisting.

> Make sure your hands are clean and your fingernails are smooth, and that you're not wearing any jewellery that will catch the hair.

> Always make sure the hair is well brushed through.

> Use strong hands and don't be afraid to hold the hair firmly.

> The closer to the head you keep your hands when plaiting hair, the tighter the finished result.

> When plaiting, keep your sections even.

> Take care when using pins that they don't scratch or stab the skin or scalp.

> A few well-placed, well-secured pins will hold a twist – adding more pins won't necessarily make it stronger.

> Pins are used to hold and secure hair in place; hairspray should only be used to finish.

> Always section off and clip away hair not being worked on.

> Make sure everything is to hand before you start and that you have someone to hand things to you if needed.

> Always check to make sure that the look is secure by getting the client to move and shake their head. If it is not, secure it or start again – it's better that it falls out in the salon than on the way to a party!

> Finally, make sure all your tools and accessories are clean and tidy.

French pleat step by step

Creating the classic up-style.

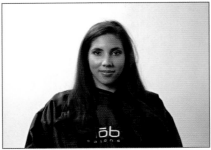

(a)

1 The hair should be dry and well brushed through (a). If the hair is too clean or flyaway, spray with hairspray.

2 Starting at the front hairline, take sections of hair and lightly back-brush the lower and root sections (b). For finer hair, you may need to add more back-brushing or backcombing. Work through to the back until you have covered the entire head.

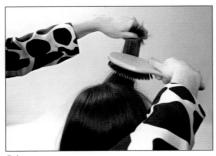

(b)

3 Place the parting and begin to brush the hair to the back, brushing out excess back-brushing and smoothing the sides and front as you go.

4 Brush the hair at the back of the head over to one side and place a row of grips slightly to one side, up from the nape to just below the crown (c). Ensure the grips are tight into the hair and interlocked in a criss-cross fashion.

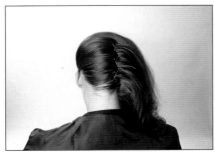

(c)

5 Check that the client is comfortable.

6 Brush the hair smooth, avoiding disturbing the grips. Holding the hair in your hand, bend the hair in on itself over the line of grips (d).

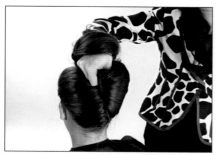

(d)

7 Use straight and fine pins to secure the pleat. Place the pins on the inside edge of the pleat so that they won't be seen (e).

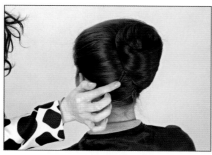

(e)

8 Tuck the remaining hair inside the pleat and secure, or leave out of the top and curl or style to add detail.

9 Use a tail comb to smooth and refine the look before adding styling and finishing products.

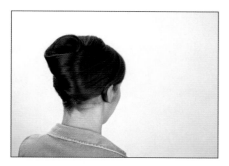

Fishtail plait step by step

Plaiting the hair using two pieces – a simple skill that can be used in many ways to create or add feature to either a daywear or a special-occasion look.

1 The hair should be clean, dry and well brushed through.

2 Take a section of hair at the centre of the front hairline, approximately 4 cm wide and 3 cm deep. Comb through and, while holding it in one hand, push the index finger of your other hand up through the section to create two even pieces (a).

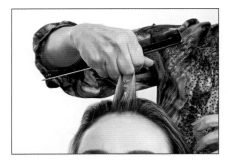

(a)

3 Cross the right piece over the left (b).

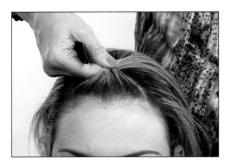

(b)

4 Holding the centre of the plait firm with your right hand, use the little finger on your left hand to scoop a small section of hair from the hairline to the centre. Cross this section over and combine it with the right piece.

5 Holding the centre of the plait firm with your left hand, use the little finger on your right hand to scoop a small section of hair from the hairline to the centre (c). Cross this over and combine it with the section on the left side.

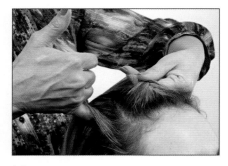

(c)

6 Continue working back along the head in this fashion, taking even sections and making sure you keep your knuckles close to the scalp and a firm grip in the centre of the plait (d).

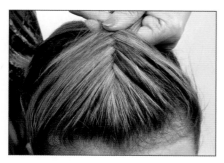

(d)

7 Check that the client is comfortable.

8 Once you have reached the nape hairline and there is no more hair to be brought into the plait, take a similar-sized section of hair from the outside of each section and continue to plait as before. When you reach the end, secure with a covered elastic.

9 You may leave the hair down or tuck the end of the plait up inside the hair and secure with grips or pins.

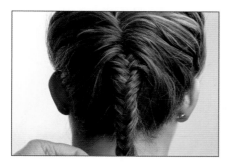
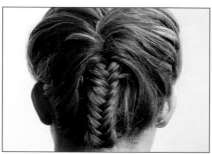

French plait step by step

Plaiting the hair using three pieces that can be used in many ways to create or add feature to either a daywear or a special-occasion look.

1 The hair should be clean, dry and well brushed through.

2 Take a section of hair at the centre of the front hairline, approximately 5 cm wide and 3 cm deep. Comb through and, while holding it in one hand, push the index and forefinger of your other hand up through the section to create three even pieces (a).

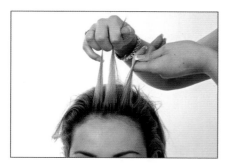

(a)

3 Cross the left piece over to between the centre and the right – you now have two pieces on the right. Then cross the right piece over to between the centre and left – you now have two pieces on the left (b).

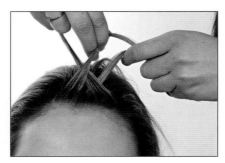

(b)

4 Holding the centre of the plait firm with your right hand, use the little finger on your left hand to scoop a section of hair from the hairline to the centre (c). Combine this new section with the section on the left and cross over to between the centre and right pieces.

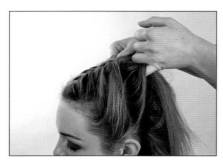

(c)

5 Holding the centre of the plait firm with your left hand, use the little finger on your right hand to scoop a section of hair from the hairline to the centre. Combine this new section with the section on the right and cross over to between the centre and left pieces.

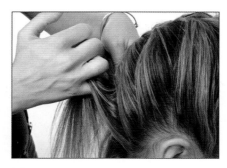

(d)

6 Continue working back along the head in this fashion (d), taking even sections and making sure you keep your knuckles close to the scalp and a firm grip in the centre of the plait.

7 Check that the client is comfortable.

8 Once you have reached the nape hairline, continue to plait the three pieces until you reach the end of the hair and secure with a covered elastic.

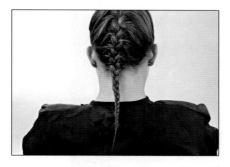

9 You may leave the hair down or tuck the end of the plait up inside the hair and secure with grips or pins.

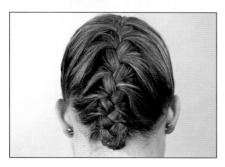

To create a plaited strand or section such as a ponytail, simply divide the section into three pieces and cross as before, but don't take any new hair from the scalp.

> **Activity** Practice, practice, practice! The key to successful plaiting and pleating is practice.
>
> For one week, before you leave work, leave college or go out for the evening, practise doing a fishtail plait. Don't leave until you've done it! By the end of the week, if you can do it, well done. If not, start again the following week.
>
> Once you have mastered the fishtail plait, the others will be fairly easy to learn.

Scalp plaits – cornrows

What are they?

Scalp plaits, cornrows or cane rows are narrow rows of French plaits that are used to create designs and patterns on the head. Twists are similar, but rather than plaiting the hair, it is twisted onto the scalp.

Can they be left in the hair?

Yes. The hair can be shampooed with the cornrows in and they are often left in for many weeks.

How long can they be left in the hair?

After about six weeks the hair will have grown and they will have become loose. They shouldn't be left much longer than this and should be removed.

How often can they be done?

As often as the hair or the scalp can remain undamaged, but it's best to give the hair a rest between times.

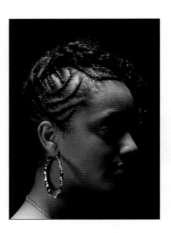

What you will need

> Gowns and towels
> Brushing or grooming hairbrush
> Tail comb
> Covered ties and/or barrettes
> Styling products
> A trolley.

Core cornrow and scalp-plaiting skills

> Creating a design that has balance and looks attractive.
> Ensuring each row is uniform in size and width.
> Ensuring the tension remains constant.
> Being able to work with short, often coarse hair.
> Concentrating and working for long periods of time.

Key points to remember when creating cornrows or scalp-plaiting hair

> Ensure that the client understands the length of time the service will take and the cost.
> Always plan and prepare your design before you start, and ensure that the client is happy with the way it will look.
> The hair must be properly conditioned and prepared in order to carry out the service.
> Some styling products will make the hair more manageable, but others may make it greasy or slippery, so choose products carefully.
> Traction alopecia can be caused by cornrows or twists that are too tight.
> If there are signs of hair breakage or traction alopecia, the service should not be carried out until the hair has recovered.
> If the plaits are too tight, they can also cause scalp soreness and headaches.
> Section the hair carefully, ensuring balance and evenness.
> If you or the client becomes uncomfortable or stiff at any time during the service, stop and take a break.

> Advise the client that they should return to the salon if there is any hair loss, breakage or discomfort.

Note: Traction alopecia is bald patches and broken hair, caused by the hair being wound or plaited too tightly. It's most commonly seen on the hairline and can give the appearance of a receding hairline. It's fairly easy to spot, as the affected area won't be completely bald; it will be a mixture of bald skin and broken hair. If you see signs of traction alopecia, you should not carry out a plaiting service; you should release any plaits or cornrows that are in the hair and seek advice from a senior colleague.

Traction alopecia

Creating cornrows step by step

French plaiting the hair in rows to create intricate designs and styles that can be left in the hair.

1 Make sure that the hair is clean and conditioned and that the appropriate styling products are applied.

2 Starting at the front, make a clean, even section on the scalp that follows the pattern you want to create.

3 Clip away all the other hair so that you have a clear working area (a).

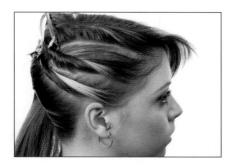

(a)

4 At the front of the section, take a small square of hair and divide it into three even pieces (b).

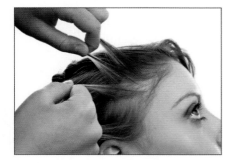

(b)

5 Cross the left piece over to between the centre and the right – you now have two pieces on the right. Then cross the right piece over to between the centre and left – you now have two pieces on the left.

6 Holding the centre of the plait firmly with your right hand, take a small piece of hair from the left side of the section and combine

it with the piece on the left, and cross over to between the centre and right pieces.

7 Holding the centre of the plait firmly with your left hand, do the same on the right side, crossing it over to between the centre and the left pieces (c).

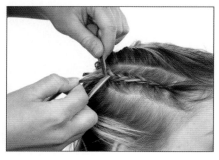

(c)

8 Continue working back along the section in this fashion, taking even sections and making sure you keep your knuckles close to the scalp and a firm grip in the centre of the plait (d).

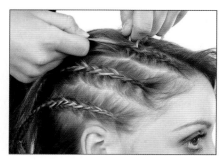

(d)

9 Once you have reached the end of the section, continue to plait the three pieces until you reach the end of the hair and secure with a covered elastic (e).

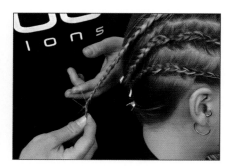

(e)

10 Take further sections, following the pattern, ensuring that they remain even in size and thickness, until the style is completed.

11 If short ends pop out from the plaits, use the end of a tail comb to gently poke them back inside.

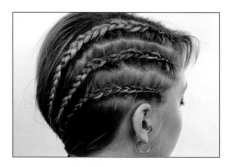

Twists

What are they?
Twists are sections of hair that are twisted rather than plaited to create styles.

Can they be left in the hair?
For a short time, yes, but they are not as secure as plaits and cornrows, so they will likely fall out with wear.

What types are there?
There are a number, but the two main ones you need to cover for NVQ Level 2 are flat twists and two-strand twists.

How often can they be done?
Twists can be done as often as you like. You just need to make sure that the hair is clean and that there is no sign of hair breakage or traction alopecia.

What you will need
> Gowns and towels
> Brushing or grooming hairbrush
> Tail comb
> Covered ties and/or barrettes
> Styling products
> A trolley.

Core twisting skills
> Creating a design that has balance and looks attractive.
> Ensuring that each twist is uniform in size and width.
> Ensuring that the tension remains constant.
> Concentrating and working for long periods of time.

Key points to remember when scalp-twisting hair
> Ensure the client understands the length of time the service will take and the cost.
> Always plan and prepare your design before you start, and ensure that the client is happy with the way it will look.

> The hair must be properly conditioned and prepared in order to carry out the service.

> Some styling products will make the hair more manageable, but others may make it greasy or slippery, so choose products carefully.

> Traction alopecia can be caused if twists are too tight.

> If there are signs of hair breakage or traction alopecia, the service should not be carried out until the hair has recovered.

> If the twists are too tight, they can also cause scalp soreness and headaches.

> The narrower the sections, the slimmer the twists and the more you'll have to put in.

> Section the hair carefully, ensuring balance and evenness.

> If you or the client becomes uncomfortable or stiff at any time during the service, stop and take a break.

> Advise the client that they should return to the salon if there is any hair loss, breakage or discomfort.

Flat twist step by step

Flat-twisting the hair in rows to create intricate designs and styles that look very similar to cornrows.

1 Make sure that the hair is clean and conditioned, and that the appropriate styling products are applied.

2 Make sure you have decided on the look and how you will place the twists in the hair for the desired effect.

3 Brush the hair through so that it's tangle-free and smooth.

4 Starting at the front, take a clean, even section, approximately 1 cm wide, from the hairline to the crown, along the scalp, that follows the pattern you want to create.

5 Clip away all the other hair so that you have a clear working area.

6 Comb through so that it is smooth.

7 Starting near the head, twist the hair in one direction so that it follows the line of the section and is tight to the scalp (a). Take care not to make the twist too tight and check that the client is comfortable.

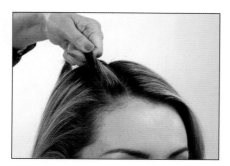

(a)

8 Twist the hair until the root section forms a single row (b) and secure where the twist ends with grips.

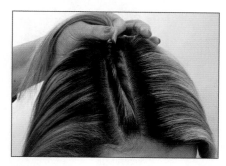

(b)

9 Continue in this method around the head (c), always twisting away from the hairline towards the crown, until all the sections of your design are complete.

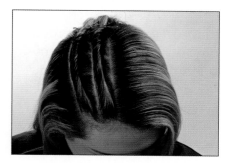

(c)

10 Once all the twists rows are complete, curl or style the ends of the hair, taking care not to dislodge the grips holding the twists in place.

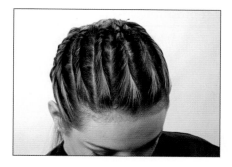
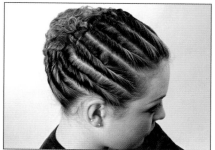

Two-strand twist step by step

Two-strand twisting is carried out in much the same way as flat twisting. The difference is that each section to be twisted is divided into two and the hair is twisted up to the ends. The effect looks quite similar to a plait.

1 Make sure that the hair is clean and conditioned, and that the appropriate styling products are applied.

2 Make sure you have decided on the look and how you will place the twists in the hair for the desired effect.

3 Brush the hair through so that it's tangle-free and smooth.

4 Starting at the front, take a clean, even section, approximately 1 cm wide, from the hairline to the crown, along the scalp, that follows the pattern you are wanting to create.

5 Clip away all the other hair so that you have a clear working area.

6 Comb through so that it is smooth.

7 Divide the section in two so you have two equal pieces of hair. Cross the two pieces over each other and continue criss-crossing until you reach the ends. Take care not to make the twist too tight and check that the client is comfortable.

8 Continue in this method around the head, always making sure that all the sections are the same size and twisting each section in the same fashion.

9 Once all the twists are complete, pin or clip the ends together to finish the style.

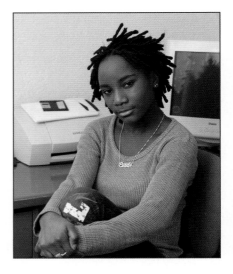

Activity Take a close look at the fashion spreads in your favourite magazine and think carefully about what techniques and tools might have been used to create the styles you see. Check out the catwalk images from the season's key London Fashion Week shows on www.vogue.com and imagine how you would recreate those looks.

Introduction

What are they?

This is the technique of adding real or synthetic hair to increase length or to add volume, colour or texture.

Today, enhancements generally refer to extensions, but can also mean wigs or hairpieces, traditionally called postiche.

How is it done?

Hairpieces and wigs are usually clipped or pinned in. There are many different extension systems, from simple clip-in or stick-in enhancers, to methods where they are woven in and secured using heat, rings or special glues.

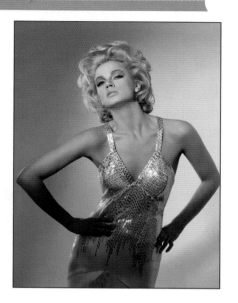

How long do they last?

Pieces that are clipped or pinned in tend to be used for a day, while extensions that use heat and glues can last up to four months.

When are they used?

Until recently, this type of work was used primarily for bridal and evening styles, catwalk, session and film work. Today, it is more widely used to add length and to accessorise and enhance hairstyles.

Adding hair and hairpieces is a great skill in your repertoire. It enables you to transform hair in so many ways that clients can't achieve at home. You can create beautiful bridal and evening looks, or add length and colour without the need to wait or damage the hair. Today, extensions are an important income-generating service for salons, and most salons will offer extensions. There are many different extension systems on the market and technology in constantly changing and improving, allowing you to create ever more amazing hairstyles.

But this chapter is not just about extensions. While they may be the most common hair enhancement process that salons use, they are not the only one. Whether it's for salon work or for sessions and catwalk shops, being able to attach hairpieces is a valuable and key hairdressing skill that enables you to take your creativity to a whole new level.

Extensions – permanent enhancements

What are they?

These are pieces of hair that are weaved or bonded into the hair and remain in the hair.

How long do they last?

Different systems recommend different lengths of time before they should be removed; some say four weeks, but others can be left in much longer. Leaving them longer than recommended could cause damage to the hair or scalp.

What are they made of?

Some are natural, 'real' hair, while others are synthetic.

Where does the real hair come from?

Real hair is sourced from different places, often from developing countries. Most companies have ethical and Fairtrade standards in place for sourcing their hair, but you should always check if you have any concerns.

How are they fixed to the hair?

There are many different systems. Some use weaving, while others use glues or other bonding methods.

Are they safe?

There is no reason why they shouldn't be safe. As long as it's a reputable extension brand and the process is carried out by a trained hairdresser, who has been properly instructed by the manufacturer, there shouldn't be any problems.

Note: There have been a number of high-profile cases where a client or their hair has been damaged by extensions. These have been due to poor-quality extension systems or lack of proper training for the hairdresser. Only ever use a reputable extension brand and never carry out extensions unless you have been properly trained to do so.

Types of enhancement extension systems

Thermal heat bonding

Also referred to as keratin bonding or micro bonding, extensions are secured to the hair with resin that is applied with a glue gun or heat clamp. Thermal bonding can last on average four months or longer and needs to be removed by the salon. It's great for adding length, volume and highlights, and the bonds are so tiny they are very hard to detect.

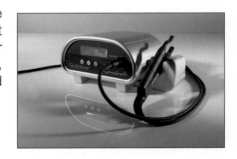

Cold bonding

There are two types of cold bonding:

> One uses ultrasound to activate the glue in a system similar to thermal bonding. These can last on average four months or longer and need to be removed by the salon. These extensions are also hard to detect and, as cold bonding doesn't use heat, it is kinder to the hair.

> The second method uses a cold adhesive to attach the extension to the client's hair. These extensions don't last as long – a maximum of a week, depending on how often the hair is washed

– and also need to be removed by the salon. This is great for adding temporary volume, length or colour.

Ring bonding

This is a glue-free bonding method that uses tiny rings to encircle the natural hair and the extension to fasten them together. Ring-bonded extensions also last up to four months and must be removed professionally.

Weave bonding

Extensions are woven or plaited into the natural hair so there is no need to use glue or a ring to secure them. There are a number of different systems or methods of weave bonding, which can be used to add length, colour and volume. This method often requires two operators, but the client can usually remove these extensions themselves or have them taken out in the salon.

Clip-in bonds

This is a temporary extension method where extensions are simply clipped in to change or enhance a hairstyle. They can be cut to blend with any style and are available in many colours. As the clips can be safely removed at home, the extensions can be reused. There are also similar systems that use strips of adhesive tape to secure the extension. Clip-in or adhesive-tape extensions are only designed for temporary 'day' use.

Note: For NVQ Level 2, you will only be assessed on extensions that are non-permanent (only last 24 hours) or those that last up to four weeks. Longer-lasting extensions are covered in Level 3.

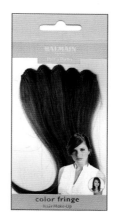

Clip-in extension

Preparation

During the consultation process, you will already have decided on the final finished look. Now you need to prepare the client and gather the correct tools and products to create the look.

Before adding extensions, the hair should be cut into the style that the extensions will enhance.

The client

> The client's hair must be long enough to attach extensions safely.

> Make sure you have carried out all pre-testing and questioning in accordance with the manufacturer's instructions.

> The client should be made aware of their personal care obligations for having extensions, and how their lifestyle can affect the condition and longevity of the extensions.

> Ensure that the client is gowned to protect their clothes and that there is a towel round their shoulders.

> Make sure that the client is positioned correctly and comfortably, and that they are relaxed.

> The client's hair should shampooed to ensure that it is not greasy, dirty or has product build-up. Some systems have their own pre-extension shampoos.
> Conditioners may interfere with the bonding process of some systems, so check rules on usage.
> Make sure you apply any protective or pre-extension products as set out in the manufacturer's guidelines.
> Pre-cut the client's hair to help with blending and to achieve the best results.
> The hair should be completely dry, brushed through and tangle-free.
> Make sure that the client is sitting upright and is comfortable.
> Ensure that any earrings are removed and that other jewellery is safely out of the way.
> Always ask if the client has any allergies to certain products, and check the scalp for abrasions or sores.

Note: Some systems recommend that the hair is left for around 20 minutes after it has been dried, to allow the cuticle to settle before the extensions are added.

You

> Ensure that your hands are clean.
> Make sure that your jewellery will not get in the way while you are working.
> Make sure that you have all the right tools and that they are clean and fit for purpose.
> Take into account the hairstyle, growth patterns, hair density and other factors when deciding on how to apply the extensions.
> Make sure you have enough extensions, or wefts, and that they are of the right colour, prepared and set out, ready to use.
> Keep your working area as tidy as possible while carrying out your work.
> Make sure that you know how to work safely, with the correct posture, and that you are wearing clothes and shoes suitable for the service you are carrying out.

What you will need

> Gowns and towels
> A brushing-out or grooming brush
> Attachment system tools (heat gun, rings, protective shield, etc.)
> A tail comb
> Enhancers or hair attachments
> A trolley
> Assistant (if needed).

Working with extensions

Key points to remember when extending or adding hair

> Many different systems are used to add hair, so make sure you've been properly trained in the one you are using.

> Always follow the manufacturer's instructions, both in preparing the hair and in the application.

> If hair or skin testing is required, make sure that it is carried out according to the manufacturer's instructions, and record the details on the client record card.

> Check if the client has any history of allergic reactions, scalp or hair disorders, or is currently taking medical advice that should be considered.

> The condition and elasticity of the hair must be properly assessed to check that it is suitable for extensions.

> Make sure the client knows how long the enhancers will last in the hair and how they should be removed.

> Follow the instructions on the width/size of extensions and the width/size of the natural hair that they will be attached to.

> Some extensions have special aftercare stipulations and products, so make sure you know what they are.

> Always ensure that you have enough hair to complete the look before you begin.

> Make sure that you work with clean, appropriately sized and even sections, to allow you to see where you are working.

> Know the salon pricing structure for enhancers so that you can easily advise on the cost of enhancing a style.

> Adding hair often requires two people, so make sure you have help if you need it.

> Take care to avoid injuring the client or damaging their clothes when using heated systems or systems that use glues.

> New versions and systems are being launched all the time, so try to keep up with current product developments.

> Ensure that you record the details of the service on the client record card, noting the system used and the type and amount of extensions used.

> Finally, make sure that you keep all extension equipment and hair additions clean, tidy and easy to use.

Note: Poorly applied or 'heavy' extensions can cause scalp soreness, headaches and even traction alopecia. Also, if the hair is in bad condition, they can cause breakage. If you are unsure about the suitability of the hair or the client for permanent extensions or the amount to use, always seek the advice of a senior technician or manager. If there is any doubt, always call the manufacturer for support. (For more details on how to spot traction alopecia, see page 206.)

Testing

Most extension services require some level of testing, so make sure that you carry out the required tests and record the results.

Pull test

Use this to test if the hair would be pulled out by the weight of the extensions.

Take a small clump of hair just above the root, approximately 20 strands or 0.5 mm wide, and gently but firmly pull your fingers through to the ends. If more than one or two strands come out, you should seek the advice of a superior.

Elasticity test

This tests how stretchy the hair is. If elasticity is poor, the extensions may cause breakage.

If the elasticity is poor, a hair held near the root and near the tip will be easily overstretched, have little or no tension and won't return to its original length. This will also determine if the hair is brittle. If it snaps too easily, it could be a sign of damage to the hair's inner cortex.

Skin test

Some extensions require a skin test to check for allergic reactions or skin/scalp sensitivity. These tests should be carried out according to the manufacturer's instructions.

Selecting the enhancement extension hair

During the consultation process, you will have agreed and decided on the style and look the client wants. Use this information, together with other key factors, to decide on the amount, position and direction of the extensions you will use to blend with the client's natural hair.

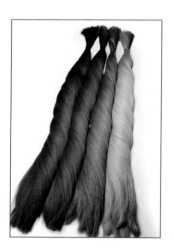

> Colour – Are the wefts to match the natural hair colour or are you using them to enhance or create a colour feature?
> Texture – Will the wefts match the client's hair texture or will you need to cut or style it?
> Length – Are the wefts to add length, and, if so, how much?
> Width – How think or thin is the client's natural hair and what thickness and density of wefts do you need to use?
> Curl – Does the client want the extensions to have waves or curls?
> Head shape – How will the look suit the client's head and face shape?

Note: While it is possible to perm some extensions, you must check with the manufacturer's instructions before doing so. Also, if perming can be done, it should be carried out before the extensions are added, unless otherwise stated by the manufacturer.

Where to attach enhancement extensions

The versatility of extensions means that they can be attached almost anywhere to change or enhance a hairstyle. They can be added to give length to a particular area of the head, like the back or the top, or they can be added to increase overall volume. For this reason, there is no set way to apply extensions. Each system will have its own recommendations, on how to section the hair and where to start, that best suit their individual product. It is important that you know and follow these recommendations.

Permanent enhancement step by step

The following step by step uses the Great Lengths classic extension system, as it is a good example of a thermal heat-bonding system.

1 Turn on the activator machine, allowing enough time for it to warm up before starting.

2 Section off the area where you are going to attach the extension and clip the rest of the hair out of the way.

3 Take a small rectangular section of hair – slightly less than the thickness of the extension you want to apply – and place it inside the protective shield. Clip the protective shield securely to the head, ensuring that it is straight and in the correct position (a).

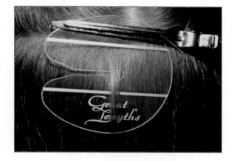

(a)

4 Place the extension underneath the natural hair so that the bond is no less than 2 cm from the scalp. Hold it in place between your finger and thumb (b), making sure that you maintain even tension, as this will keep the extensions uniform.

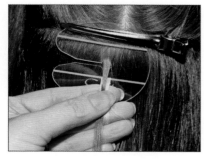

(b)

5 Ensure that the section of the client's hair is held downwards as it falls naturally and check that the extension is in line with the hair.

6 Hold the arm of the activator at a 90° angle to the bond and hair join, with the bulbous part underneath.

7 Close the arm around the bond (c) and wait until it becomes soft.

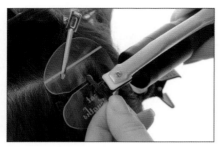

(c)

8 Allow a few seconds for the bond to begin to cool, but before it sets, use your fingers to spread the bond along and around the join (d), to create a 'flat' bond.

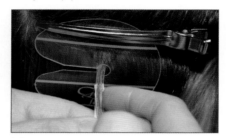

(d)

9 Apply the arm again and repeat the process at least twice, to make sure the bond is smooth and without bumps.

10 Once the bond is cool and set, check with the client that it's comfortable before moving on to the next section.

11 Repeat the process throughout the head until complete, checking periodically that the client is happy with how things are going.

12 Once finished, check that all the extensions are comfortable.

13 Put away unused extensions, turn off the machine, clean the machine as recommended, and clean and sterilise tools as required.

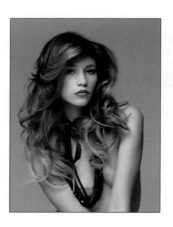

Note: The bond can also be cylindrical, so that it doesn't lie flat to the head. This method is used to create additional volume.

Finishing the hairstyle

You will often need to blend and tailor the extensions after you have finished attaching them. This is done by trimming hair that is too long and using pointing to texturise and soften any hard lines.

Allow the hair to rest for 5 to 10 minutes after you have finished adding the extensions, to give the bond time to really set. Use this time to review the look and discuss with the client the result so far and any areas they think need attention.

Brush the hair through carefully, using a bristle brush to remove any loose hair and tangles. Take care not to catch the bonds or pull too hard.

Cut the hair dry and, using your scissors and comb, slowly finish the hairstyle.

Note: Avoid blunt, club-cutting, as you may create lines in the hair. Instead, use pointing for a softer blend. If you need to blow-dry the hairstyle, lightly dampen the hair from the mid-lengths to the ends. Section off the hair and use a bristle or paddle brush to style the hair. Take care not to brush or comb the bonds.

Check the manufacturer's instructions for rules and recommendations on using heated stylers, hot rollers or curling irons.

Note: The glue bonds on the extensions are at their weakest and most vulnerable when they are wet, so avoid overly wetting or pulling the hair when blow-drying.

Removing extensions

When your client has decided or you have advised them that the extensions should be removed, arrange for them to come into the salon for a removal consultation. This will enable you to take a look at the extensions and discuss how the client would like their hair once the extensions have been taken out. It will also enable you to estimate how long it will take to remove the extensions and book an appointment for the appropriate time. The time needed will depend on the number of extensions in the hair and how well they have been maintained. If the hair is tangled, it will take longer to remove them.

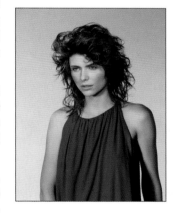

You client may wish to have a new set of extensions put in, so you will need to carefully assess the condition of the hair and scalp to see if this will be okay. You may also want to check the manufacturer's instructions, as they may recommend that the hair is left for a period of time to recover between extension services.

Each permanent extension system will have its own removal method, often using specialist tools and products. You must only use the removal tools and products for the system used to put in the extensions, as mixing products could cause hair damage or injury.

Most extension removal is carried out using a liquid or gel that is applied to the bond to break it down. There may also be a heated or electrical tool that is applied to the bond to aid the process.

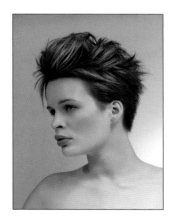

When removing extensions you should ensure that they are removed properly, without damaging the hair or leaving any residue.

Many extension systems also have specially formulated cleansing and conditioning products, designed to be used with extensions, and these should be used, as they will help to ensure the best results. Also, make sure that you advise your client on any specific products that they should use.

Once removed, the extensions should be discarded appropriately. Extensions should never be reused.

Non-permanent enhancements

What are they?

These are clip-in extensions, ponytails or false hairpieces that are pinned into the hair.

When are they used?

They are used to add a temporary feature to the hair or to create a particular look for a special occasion, for session work or for fashion and catwalk shows.

What shapes and styles do they come in?

There are many shapes and styles, from simple, thin, clip-in extensions, to long pieces with full-bodied curls. Some come pre-shaped and styled, while others can be tailored to suit the style of the client.

How are they used?

Some are simply attached to add length or movement for a particular look, while others are worked into the hairstyle to give body and shape.

The use of temporary enhancements and hairpieces differs from permanent extension work in that you are only using the hairpieces to create a one-off look. They give you fantastic creative versatility and enable you to create looks on clients, and for show and photographic work, that would be impossible with the natural hair alone.

All great hairdressers understand the potential of using hairpieces and you would be amazed at how often they are used, especially in session and photographic work.

There is no right or wrong way to use temporary hairpieces, so you are limited only by your own imagination...

> **Activity** Find a hairpiece (either buy one or use one from your salon or from one of your colleagues) and use it to create three different looks on a block or on a friend or colleague. Use the piece to change the length, the volume and/or to add a feature to a French twist or up-style. Ask a senior member of the team or your manager to review your work. Time yourself to see how long it takes you to create each look. Finally, get your model to shake their head, or shake the block hard, and see how well the hairpiece stays attached and the style remains intact.

Note: Working with wigs and hairpieces is an area of hairdressing called postiche. Wigs are still worn by men and women, especially by people who are undergoing medical treatments such as chemotherapy that cause the hair to fall out. It's important that over your career you learn how to work with wigs and hairpieces, and also how to treat the clients who wear them with tact and understanding.

Key points to remember when extending or adding hair

> Always follow the manufacturer's instructions for preparing the hairpiece.

> All hairpieces should be clean, well maintained and fit for purpose.

> Make sure that the client knows how long the style will last in their hair and how any hairpieces should be removed.

> Before you begin, always make sure that you have enough hair or the right-sized piece to complete the look.

> Make sure that you have all the pins, grips, and so on that you may need.

> Make sure that you work with clean, appropriately sized and even sections, to allow you to see where you are working.

> Know the salon pricing structure for enhancers so you can easily advise on the cost of enhancing a style.

> Adding hair often requires two people, so make sure you have help if you need it.

> Make sure that any pieces you add are secure and won't fall out easily.

> Always take care when adding hairpieces that you don't injure the client with clips or pins.

> Make sure that you record the details of the service on the client record card.

> Keep tools and hair-dressing trays clean and ready for future use.

Note: Many hairpieces are reusable, and salons will charge the client for the hairpiece so that they can keep it afterwards and reuse it themselves. At other times, the client may not need to use the hairpiece again or the salon may want it back. Make sure you know your salon's policy on hairpieces and that the client is also made aware of either the additional cost of keeping the hairpiece or their obligation to return it.

Non-permanent hair enhancement step-by-step

This sequence shows how to use clip-in hairpieces to add temporary length to a hairstyle.

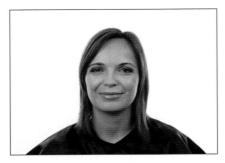

(a)

1   Select the correct number and colour of hairpieces that you will need and place them on a trolley.

2   Ensure the client's hair is clean and dry (a).

3   Smooth the hair using straightening irons if needed. Straightening the hair will make it easier to attach the hairpieces and help them 'blend in' with the natural hair.

4   Start at the back and section the head in half; take a horizontal section at the occipital bone (b). (You generally don't need to add any extensions from the nape to the occipital bone, as they won't be seen.)

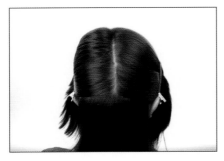

(b)

5   Take a section of hair in the centre of the head, roughly the same size as the extension, and backcomb the root area (c).

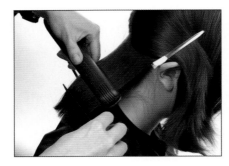

(c)

6   Either clip in the extension at the root (d), or attach it 2 to 3 cm away from the scalp, if it is secured by an adjustable tie.

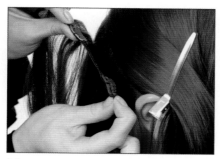

(d)

7   Test that the hairpiece is secure and is not uncomfortable before moving onto the next section.

8   Working towards the outside hairline, continue to add extensions along the section. Keep the hairpieces close together, as spaces will result in gaps in the finished look.

9   Once the section is complete, review for balance.

10   Move up the back, taking a further section across the head approximately 2 to 3 cm above the previous one and repeat. For thicker results, reduce the thickness of the sections so you'll add more.

11   Continue up the head as far as required, making sure you leave enough natural hair on the top of the head to comb down and hide the hairpiece attachments.

12   Follow the same process on the sides of the head if required, ensuring that both sides are evenly balanced.

13   Once complete, gently brush the hair into place, being careful not to pull too hard and to avoid catching the clip or tie.

14   With the hair in place, trim and tidy the ends of the hair.

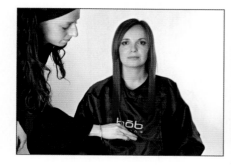
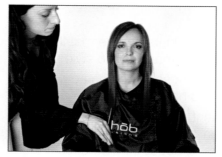

15   Check that the client is happy with the look and that none of the hairpieces are uncomfortable.

16   Finally, advise the client how and when the pieces should be removed and whether they are to be returned to the salon.

Note: Always check returned pieces for damage or infestations.

Care of hairpieces

With care, many hairpieces can be used over and over again, to create lots of different looks. Therefore, it's important that they are looked after and stored properly.

225

> Check the hairpiece for damage, pins, clips or infestations.

> Read the manufacturer's care instructions.

> Brush the piece through thoroughly before washing.

> Most real hairpieces can be shampooed and conditioned as normal hair.

> Pat the hairpiece dry between towels to remove the excess water.

> Comb into shape and allow to dry naturally, or set on rollers as required.

> Store hairpieces by hanging up if possible. If this is not possible, store flat, ensuring that they don't become crushed or tangled.

Aftercare

Always advise your client on how best to maintain their hairstyle and how to achieve the same look at home.

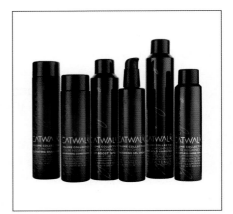

> Offer advice on shampoos and conditioners that will help to keep the hair looking good.

> Tell the client how to re-create the look at home, with tips on what tools, brushes and products to use.

> Advise and show the client how styling products should be used for best results and to avoid wastage. Also, tell the client what products should be avoided as they won't work with the style.

> Give advice on and show the client how to use styling products and tools to get the best results at home, and how to avoid hair damage or personal injury.

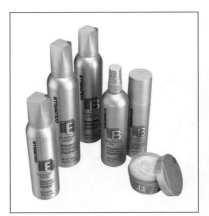

> Inform your client how to take down or undo any up-styles and plaits.

> Let your client know how extensions should be cared for and when they should be removed.

> Suggest additional services, such as colours and perms, that will improve the look or the client's ability to maintain the style.

> Advise on how the client's lifestyle, work and sporting activities can influence and affect their hair and hairstyle.

Finally, before they leave, let the client know that if they have any problems with the hairstyle, they can always come back to have it adjusted. Clients are often embarrassed about coming back if there is something that they are not altogether happy with, and sometimes they will even go elsewhere. So always make sure they know that it's part of the service and included in the price!

For the record...

It's important that you maintain accurate and up-to-date client records. It provides a valuable record of services and treatments the client has had, which is all important information that should be considered when deciding future technical services or treatments.

Case study

Dressing up!

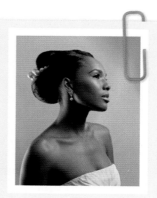

'I'm always surprised that some salons don't promote or publicise their hair "dressing" skills and services. They think it has a negative impression on their business, which is crazy. A good salon has a real balance of services that can meet the many and various needs of their clients, and dressing hair is an important service to offer. And as a good hairdresser, dressing hair should be part of your repertoire.'

'Clients may not need their hair dressed in a stunning evening style all the time, but when they do, you need to be ready. Around 18 per cent of the work in our salon is dressing hair and our work has become a draw for clients whose own salons either don't do or don't promote this service. This is great for us, as once they've visited the salon, they become regular clients for their cut and colour work.'

'Dressing hair is also the main skill you need for sessions and catwalk shows. In fact, 90 per cent of the session work we do involves dressing or putting hair up. But to do good up-styles and dress hair well, you must learn the basics: how to plait, how to backcomb, how to pin hair up and how to set. For example, we never use traditional setting in the salon, but we are always using rollers on shoots and for shows, and the basic principle is exactly the same.'

'Unlike other skills, dressing hair is unique. If you can do it well, you will be in demand in the salon, for weddings and even for shows and photo-shoots. Plus it's a service that you can charge extra for and can be a great way to increase your earnings.'

Errol Douglas MBE, Errol Douglas Salon Knightsbridge, London

Over the following pages we will explain the details of basic cutting, and show you the skills and knowledge you'll need to complete Unit GH12 and to learn the techniques you'll need to progress in your hairdressing career.

You will learn to:

> **understand the basic techniques, tools and terms used in cutting hair**
> **cut hair to achieve a variety of looks**
> **provide aftercare and advice.**

You will be assessed against your knowledge and ability to:

1 Understand your salon's processes and procedures with regard to promoting products and services.

2 Understand your legal and health and safety responsibilities when carrying out these services.

3 Understand your personal obligations to other team members and know when and from whom you should seek advice and assistance.

4 Maintain effective and safe methods of working and cut hair in a commercially viable timeframe.

5 Communicate effectively with clients, using positive listening skills, body language and verbal communication.

6 Consult with clients, consider key factors and choose looks and styles that suit their individual needs.

7 Cut hair using a variety of basic cutting techniques.

8 Use and understand specific tools, techniques and products required for basic haircutting.

9 Recognise adverse results and deal with them effectively.

10 Provide aftercare and product advice.

Introduction

What is it?

These are the fundamental cutting skills that form the foundation of all cutting techniques.

What are the basic cutting techniques?

One length above or below the shoulders; uniform/round layering; and long graduation and short graduation.

Are these techniques difficult to learn?

No, not at all. Surprisingly, with practice and by following a few simple rules, cutting hair is not as difficult as you might think.

The foundation of a great hairstyle – the cut

Until the 1960s, the hair 'cut' was not nearly as important to the style as the way it was 'dressed'. The sole purpose of cutting hair was to make it shorter, so that it could be set or dressed into the chosen look. At the time, the cut didn't matter as hairdressers built their reputation on their dressing and setting skills. Amazingly, hair cutting was actually considered a relatively unimportant skill for a ladies' hairdresser. Not any more...

Vidal Sassoon showed that by focusing on the cut, it was possible to create looks and shapes that needed little or no setting or drying. The art of the haircut was born. For the first time in history, your hairstyle was not dependent on your being able to afford a weekly trip to the salon. Hair fashion was open to everyone and it meant that a new and exciting look was possible with every six-weekly appointment. This revolutionised hairdressing and transformed it into the exciting and creative industry that leads fashions, generates huge incomes and turns hairdressers into household names and celebrities.

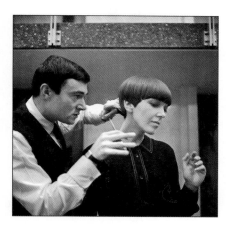

Vidal Sasson cutting Mary Quant's hair

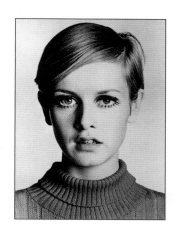

Twiggy

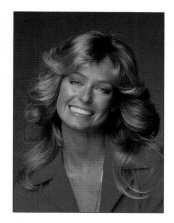

Farrah Fawcett

You are a part of that industry! The cutting techniques developed by Sassoon and countless other inspirational hairdressers are there for you to learn. And you can take these skills, build on them, develop them and take creative cutting to new and exciting places!

And it starts here, with the basics.

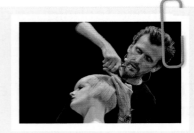

Case study
Start at the beginning

'Everything begins with the Classics. The Sassoon precision technique relies on a geometric approach to cutting and colouring that has been continually refined over the course of the company's 50-plus-year history. It is this geometric method, which, with a series of modernist principles applied to hair, allows their team to create cuts and colours of timeless understated simplicity or avant-garde complexity.'

'The ABC method is about the Rules of Freedom: know the rules, and then how and when to break them. It is a comprehensive technical system to create unlimited hair cutting and colouring possibilities.'

'Without mastery of technique, you cannot hope to control hair or develop a style of work that is so crucial to individual success.'

Mark Hayes, Sassoon International Creative Director

Hair cutting – the fundamentals

The cut is the foundation of all hairstyles and the basic cutting techniques are the foundation of all haircuts. Once you've mastered these techniques, you can combine them, add others and create amazing looks, shapes and styles.

There are two key principles in haircutting and they apply to all the techniques you will ever use, from basic one-length cutting to scissor-over-comb and slide cutting:

> hair travel
> detail and precision.

The first principle – hair travel

Understanding the principle of hair travel is key to hair cutting, and once you grasp this, the rest is easy.

Hair travel – hair always travels to the longest point!

What does it mean?

Hair will always want to fall in the direction it grows naturally, but you can change or at least influence this direction by using this basic principle and make it go the way you want it to.

What is the longest point?

It is where the hair of a particular section or area is longest. It can be on the outside perimeter line or a longer layer within the haircut. When the longest point is on the outside perimeter it's called length, and when it's on the inside of the haircut, it is called weight.

Keywords

Section: the piece or area of hair to be cut.

Sectioning falls into two categories:

- Sectioning off: parts of the head or areas of the hair that are separated from other areas, usually with clips, to enable you to work on a specific area without other hair getting in the way. These sections can be any size, but should be uniform as a general rule.

- Cutting section: the individual amount of hair to be held in the fingers and cut. These sections should be slightly shorter than your index finger, and generally no thicker than two fingers' width.

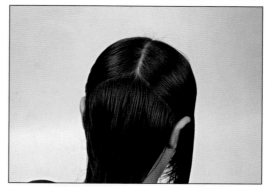

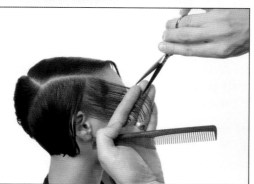

How does this affect a haircut?

When you cut a hairstyle, what you are actually doing is creating various points of length and weight that make the hair behave in a certain way. It's this control of movement and direction that enables you to manipulate the way the hair lays and creates shape and movement.

> Length: Cut a fringe straight across on straight hair and it will lie in a straight line. Cut it so that it's shorter on the left and it will fall to the right because it's longer.

> Weight: Cut a fringe straight across on straight hair and it will lie in a straight line. 'Layer' the left side and, even though the length is the same, the layered side will be 'lighter' so the hair will fall to the 'heavier' right side.

The stronger the natural growth direction, the more weight or length you will need to change or control it.

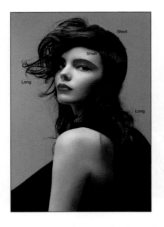

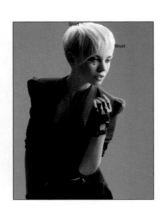

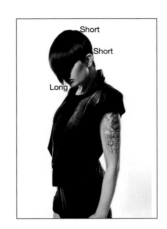

Look at these hairstyles, where we've noted the long and short points on various sections, and you can see how the principle works.

By understanding this principle, you will be able to work with the natural growth patterns to control and direct the hair into the style you want to create.

Keywords

Challenging growth patterns

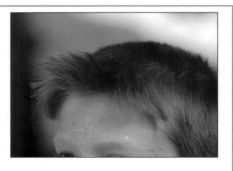

- **Cowlick**: a small section of hair that sticks up or grows in a different direction to the rest of the hair. Cowlicks are usually found on the front hairline, where they can make cutting fringes and controlling the hair difficult. They can also be found at the nape or anywhere on the head. Cowlicks can frequently be countered by using weight, although often it's easier to work with them and incorporate them into the style.

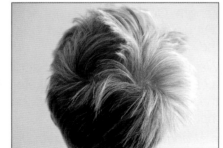

- **Double crown**: unruly or crown with two growth patterns. On most people, the hair at the crown grows in a semicircular pattern, radiating out from one single point. For clients with a double crown, they either have a growth pattern that does not follow a uniform direction, or they have two separate and often opposing patterns of growth. As with cowlicks, these can be controlled by weight, by leaving the hair longer in this area. Although it is not as easy as with cowlicks, double crowns can also be incorporated into the style and made into a feature.

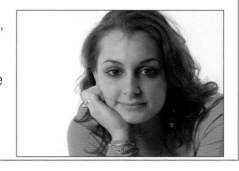

- **Widow's peak**: a pointed and prominent front hairline. When combed back, especially in men, a widow's peak can look great and can be a real feature of a hairstyle. For styles with a fringe, it can cause a problem, by stopping the hair from lying flat or causing it to part in the centre when combed forward. To deal with a widow's peak, you often need to leave the fringe heavier than you would normally, or cut it so that it's heavier in the centre. Geometric fringes also work well with widow's peaks, but it's usually advisable not to sweep all the hair over to one side, but to leave some softness.

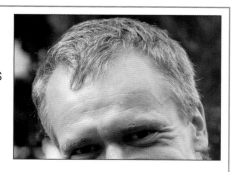

- **Recession line**: the point at the temples where the hairline recedes. Often a joint problem of a widow's peak, recession lines can be either the way the hair grows naturally or a result of male pattern baldness. The position of a parting on a client with deep recession lines is important. In the right place, it will disguise it; in the wrong place, it will accentuate it. Often, when cutting a style on a client with deep recession lines, you will put the parting slightly higher than normal. A full fringe can also disguise recession lines.

The second principle – detail and precision

The more attention you pay to detail and the more precisely you work, the better your cutting will be.

What does it mean?

It means exactly what it says: haircutting is a precision skill and you will never create good haircuts unless you work in a precise and detailed way.

How is it done?

It is done by always taking your time and concentrating; by learning to use your tools properly and looking at each client's hair individually; and, above all, by properly mastering the basic cutting techniques.

How will it affect a haircut?

It will mean the difference between a good haircut and an okay or bad one; between hair falling into its style or needing to be forced into place. This will be the difference between your clients returning to you or going elsewhere.

Basic cutting – looks

There are only three types of haircut: one length, layers and graduation. All haircuts and hairstyles are either one or a combination of these three haircuts. This is why they are called the basics.

> One length: cutting the outside perimeter of the hair as it lies.

> Layers: cutting sections of hair in lengths within the perimeter.

> Graduation: cutting hair so that it becomes gradually longer or shorter.

One length

This relates to the perimeter length or lengths of the hair, with it all being cut in a blunt line, without any layers or graduation. All of the hair will be combed in the direction it grows and cut to the same length. One-length haircuts will often have various or varying perimeter lengths, like a shorter fringe or a curved back baseline. In each of these areas, all of the hair is cut to the same line.

Keywords

Elasticity: hair's ability to stretch

All hair has a certain amount of elasticity. Hair in good condition has strong elasticity; it will be firm, hard to stretch and will instantly spring back. Hair in poor condition will stretch easily and take time to return to shape. As you cut hair using tension, it's important to factor in the elasticity of the hair when cutting.

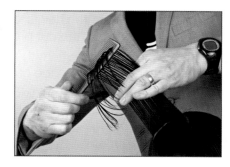

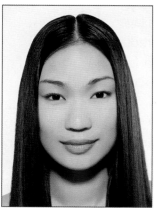

Baseline: the perimeter or outside length

This is the exterior length of the haircut. The baseline usually refers to the length at the back of the haircut, but the length at the sides and the fringe are also baselines. You can also have a baseline that is shorter than the natural hairline and inside the haircut.

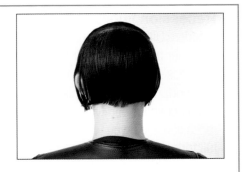

Layers

As the name implies, layers are sections of hair cut to lie on each other. Hair is pulled vertically from the scalp and cut so that, when released, it falls in sections of different lengths. Layers are used to add a further dimension of shape inside the perimeter line, reduce the hair's overall weight and give the hairstyle texture and volume.

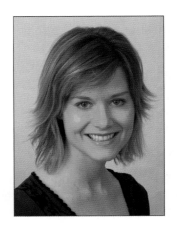

Graduation

With graduation, each section of hair is incrementally longer or shorter than the previous one. The difference in length from one section to the next continues by the same margin throughout the graduated area. The result is a blend, a gradual change from short to long or long to short. There are two types of graduation:

> Graduation: where the hair is longer on the outside and gets gradually shorter as the cut progresses up the head.

> Reverse graduation: where the hair is shorter on the outside and gets gradually longer as the cut progresses up the head.

Graduation can be used both within the haircut and on the perimeter line.

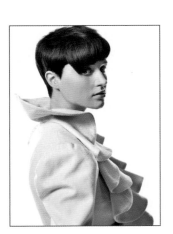

With these three cuts, you will be able to create the five looks you need for Unit GH12:

> one length
> uniform layer
> short graduation
> long graduation
> one look with a fringe.

Activity As all haircuts are made up of one or more of these techniques, start to look at the haircuts of your friends and family and see if you can figure out which techniques were used.

Basic cutting techniques

As your career progresses, you will learn many different ways of cutting hair, but the ones you will use most often are called the basic cutting techniques.

These skills are not only needed to complete this unit, they will form the foundation for all of your hair cutting.

Club-cutting: cutting hair held in the fingers

A term not heard much outside the classroom, club cutting is the most common cutting technique used in creating a wide range of looks, most commonly in layering. The hair is held taut between the index and the middle finger and cut in a straight line.

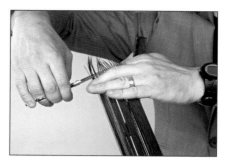
Club-cutting

Scissor-over-comb: cutting hair through the comb

Scissor-over-comb cutting is a technique used mainly on short layering and short graduation. It requires the hair to be supported by the comb while being cut. Differing from other techniques, the hair is usually cut while in continual motion.

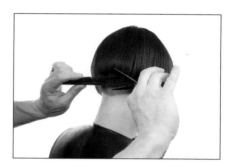
Scissor-over-comb

Free-hand: cutting hair without holding it in your fingers or in the comb

Free-hand cutting is a skill that is mainly used to cut exterior perimeter lines. Often it is used to finish fringes or hairlines and requires a steady hand.

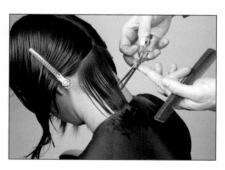
Free-hand

Pointing: using the ends of the scissors to cut small pieces of hair

Often called chipping in or texturising, pointing is the technique of removing small amounts of hair from the ends of a section, to remove some of the weight, to soften a hard line or to add texture. This can be done either while held in the fingers or freehand.

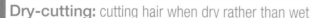

Keyword

Dry-cutting: cutting hair when dry rather than wet

Unless it's for finishing, as a general rule, hair should be cut wet, as this helps the hair to stick together and shows its natural fall, enabling you to cut it with more precision. If you cut hair dry, it can feel coarser and can become static and flyaway. Avoid over-combing hair when dry-cutting, and note that the hair may have been dried or styled and is not falling in its natural way. Not weighed down with water, dry hair clippings can also fly around more, so extra care should be taken to ensure that clients are well protected.

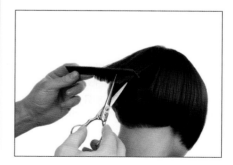
Pointing

Tools

Out of all the hairdressing services you learn, cutting requires the least amount of tools, and it's this that makes hairdressing such a portable skill. With only a pair of scissors and a comb, you can work just about anywhere! When working in a salon though, as well as these items, you'll find a few other things useful.

You will need:

> a pair of professional hairdressing scissors
> a cutting comb
> sectioning clips
> a water spray
> a neck brush
> thinning scissors (optional).

Scissors

Designed to be used for cutting hair, hairdressing scissors are very different from everyday household scissors. Thin-bladed and light-weight, hairdressing scissors are pointed and extremely sharp. Some hairdressing scissors have two different blades: one that has very fine serrations and the other that has a clean, sharp edge. The serrated edge helps to hold the hair in place, so that the sharp edge can cut it cleanly. Higher-quality scissors will have two extremely sharp, hand-finished blades. There are many different sizes and styles of hairdressing scissors on the market, mostly made from high-quality stainless steel. Hairdressing scissors can be very expensive and are usually the most expensive item in any hairdresser's tool kit.

Standard shape scissors

Traditionally shaped, geometric scissors, with removable little finger rest. Some scissors have an insert in the upper handle that helps the scissors fit tighter to the third (ring) finger.

Higher-quality scissors will be handcrafted and made of exceptional quality cobalt steel, which is light, but strong and durable, so the scissors stay sharp for longer.

Left-handed scissors

Left-handed scissors are the mirror opposite of right-handed versions. This enables left-handed people to cut hair with the scissors in the right position. (If a left-handed person uses right-handed scissors, they will be the wrong way round. The stationary blade will be at the back instead of the front.)

Ergonomic scissors

Ergonomic scissors have offset handles that are moulded to fit the hand. These scissors also have a hand-tightened screw that enables the hairdresser to finely adjust the cutting tension to their own style.

Top Tip

When you are learning, it's advisable not to spend too much on scissors, as you will most likely drop them a few times, which can damage them. You should invest in a fairly good pair though, as the quality will affect your ability to work and the finish of your haircuts. Once you have gained confidence in using scissors, you should invest in higher-quality scissors.

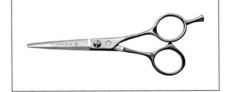

Contour 2-55

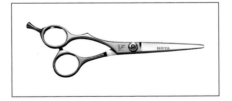

Utsumi Lefty 5.5

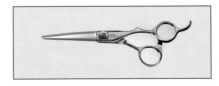

Utsumi Jyo SF-50

Keyword

Tension: the tightness with which hair is held when cutting

Holding the hair firmly and with even tension is important, as it helps to ensure that the hair is cut evenly. If you hold the hair between your fingers with loose or uneven tension, the line you cut will be uneven.

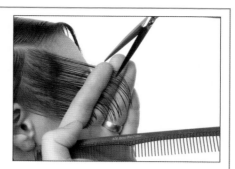

Traditional thinning scissors

These scissors have one 'toothed' blade and one cutting blade. The hair is cut between the teeth, so the more teeth thinning scissors have, the less hair they will cut.

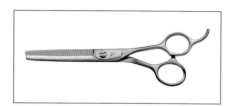

Utsumi U&U NS-30C

High-tech thinning scissors

There are many different types of thinning scissors on the market that enable hairdressers to refine and detail their haircut with exceptional precision.

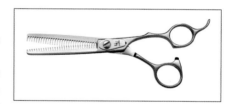

Utsumi U&U WT-60

Length of scissors

Scissor length is measured from the end of the handle to the point, with the blades accounting for roughly half the overall length. Scissors are often still measured in imperial lengths (inches) and this can make it confusing when buying scissors, so it's always best to buy them in person, to make sure you get the right size for you. There is no best size for scissors; some hairdressers use long scissors up to 17 cm (7 inches), while others prefer much shorter scissors of 11 cm (4.5 inches). There are hairdressers that use different-sized scissors for different work: longer ones for cutting bob lines and scissor-over-combing, and shorter ones for layering and texturising. Most, however, will use one pair for all cutting work. The length of scissor you use should be down to what you feel comfortable with.

Care of scissors

It is important to look after your scissors. Scissors should always be kept in a scissor case or box when not in use and never left loose in your tool bag. Keep them clean and occasionally use a little oil to keep them moving freely. Hairdressing scissors may have fine serrations and are delicately balanced, so only ever use a specialist company to sharpen or service your scissors.

Holding and using your scissors

Hairdressing scissors are held differently to normal scissors and it's vitally important that you learn how to hold them correctly, so that using them becomes comfortable and second nature.

Top Tip

To find the length of scissors that's right for you, try out the scissors of other hairdressers in your salon or class and see what feels right. But remember, always ask first!

Most normal household scissors are held between the thumb and index or middle finger, with the cutting action generated by opening and closing the hand so that both blades open and close.

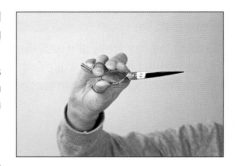

Control of the blades is crucial for precision hair cutting, so this method doesn't work for cutting hair. The scissors need to be held in a certain way to ensure that only one blade moves and you maintain a steady cutting edge.

Holding your scissors

Hold the scissors with the screw facing you. Place your thumb in the bottom handle. You only need to use the tip of your thumb, about level with the bottom of your thumbnail.

Place your third (ring) finger into the upper handle, again, not too far in, just past your first knuckle. The tips of your index and middle fingers rest on the top of the scissors. Your little finger stays free.

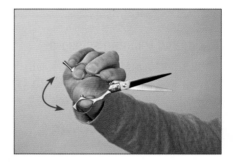

Using your scissors

The skill in using hairdressing scissors is to keep the bottom blade still while the upper blade moves up and down to cut the hair. This is achieved by sole use of your thumb to generate the cutting action.

Holding the scissors horizontally, move your thumb up and down to open and close the blades, while keeping your fingers and the lower blade still. Practise this as often as you can until it becomes comfortable.

> **Activity** When first learning to use your scissors, hold the bottom blade still with the tip of a finger from your other hand, and practise using only your thumb to open and close the blades.

Cutting comb

Cutting combs are straight, with uniform-length teeth, and are usually 16 to 18 cm long. The comb is divided into two halves: one with fine, narrow teeth and the other with wider-spaced, thicker teeth. The tooth on each end of the comb is tapered into a point that helps with sectioning, and some combs also have units of measurement on the back edge.

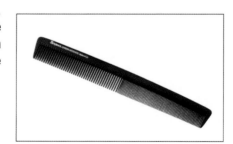

Using your cutting comb

The cutting comb has three specific functions when cutting hair:

> sectioning

> combing through

> creating tension.

Sectioning

The ends of the comb are used to take sections of hair that are to be cut. Use your cutting comb like a pencil, to 'draw' the section that you want to take before picking it up and combing it through.

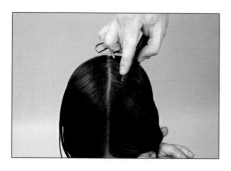
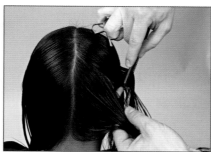

Combing through

The wide-toothed end of the comb is used to comb through the hair and each individual section, to remove knots and to ensure that all the hair is going in the same direction.

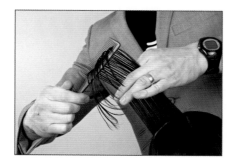

Creating tension

In order to cut hair cleanly, it is important that all the hair is held evenly and is taut. The fine-toothed end of the comb helps pull all the hair of the section tight and clean, so that it can be cut evenly.

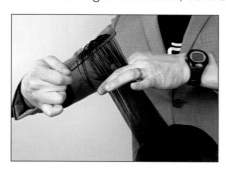

Activity Hold your comb in the middle and practise flipping it around, backwards and forwards, so that the fine-toothed and the wide-toothed ends are uppermost alternately.

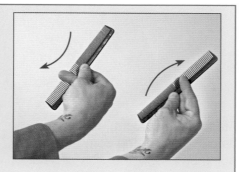

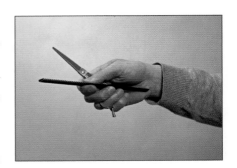

Using your scissors and comb together

This is not easy and it takes practice. In time, though, it will become second nature, almost as if your scissors are part of you.

If you are right-handed, you will hold your scissors and comb in your right hand and the section of hair between the index and forefingers of your left hand. If you are left-handed, it will be the other way round.

Taking a section

With the scissors on your third (ring) finger, hold them in the palm of your hand, making sure the blades are closed. You will probably need to let the handle slide further down your finger. Hold the comb between your thumb and index and forefingers. This enables you to take a section without the scissors getting in the way.

Holding the section

Hold the section of hair to be cut between the index and forefingers of your other hand. Keep your fingers straight – don't bend or cross them.

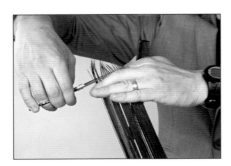

Combing through

Continuing to hold the scissors and comb in this way, comb the section through until it is tangle-free and all the hair is straight. You'll need to use the fine-toothed end of the comb to get good tension, so if you have taken the section and combed it through using the wide teeth, turn the comb round and comb through again.

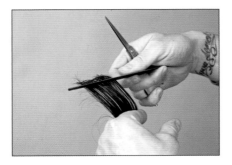

Cutting the section

When you have combed so that all the hair is straight, and you are holding it at the place where it's to be cut, transfer the comb to your other hand and hold it between your thumb and the side of your hand so that it's out of the way of where you are cutting. Bring your scissors to the cutting position by putting your thumb in the lower handle and moving the upper handle nearer to the tip of your finger. Cut the hair using just your thumb.

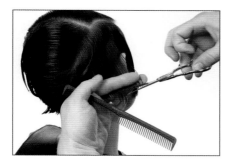

> **Activity** Practise holding your scissors and comb together, flipping or turning your comb, and moving your scissors from the holding to the cutting position.
>
> Also practise taking, combing through and holding sections of hair, using a block, or on a friend or colleague. If you can 'pull' a section of hair by holding it between your two fingers, then you've got it!

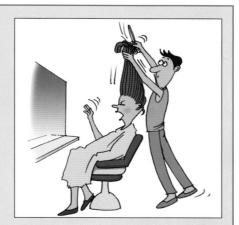

Top Tip

If you drop some of the section, lose the tension or cross your fingers while holding the hair, you must start again. If you cut the hair, it will not be straight and you will have to cut it again anyway.

Preparation

Safety first!

Hairdressing scissors are both sharp and pointed and can easily cause injury. Accidentally cutting or stabbing yourself or someone else is very easy to do, so you must take great care with your scissors at all times.

> When not in use, scissors should always be stored securely in a pouch or case.

> Never leave your scissors lying around on trolleys or counters.

> When carrying scissors, carry them safely within your hand.

> Make a note of any moles on your client's hairline and take care when cutting round the ears.

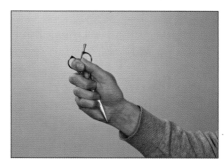

> Most of all, when cutting, make sure you stay focused on what you are doing, so you don't cut yourself or your client.

The correct position

It's important that both you and your client are in the correct positions while working to ensure the best result and to avoid injury. If your client is slouched or not sitting straight, it can affect the haircut and result in it being uneven. Also, if you are not standing correctly, it will be hard for you to cut the hair well and you could even end up injuring your back or hurting yourself.

The client

> The chair should be directly in front of and facing the styling mirror straight on.
> The client should be sitting up straight with their back against the backrest of the chair.
> Their feet should be flat on the ground or on a footrest. Do not allow their legs to 'dangle' if possible as this can cause pressure on the lower back.
> Their legs should always be uncrossed.
> Ensure they are comfortable throughout the haircut.

You

> Make sure you are wearing appropriate and supportive footwear.
> Make sure that the space around the chair is clear and uncluttered.
> Use the chair's height adjustment to raise or lower the client so that you don't need to over-stretch or bend down. Continually adjust the height during the haircut as you work on different areas.
> Stand straight, keep your weight evenly distributed on both feet and don't slouch your shoulders.
> Don't over-reach; always shift your standing position so that you are as close as possible and parallel to the section you are cutting.

Good preparation will make the task of cutting hair easier for you and will therefore enable you to produce the best possible result.

The client

> Ensure the client is gowned to protect their clothes.
> The client's hair should be shampooed to remove any grease, dirt or product build-up, and should have been conditioned if needed.
> Ensure the hair is towel-dried so that there is no dripping water.
> The hair should be combed through and tangle-free. (You may need to gently towel-dry again after combing through.)
> A towel or a cutting collar should be placed around the client's shoulders. (You may also place a strip of cotton wool inside the client's collar, to stop hair falling down their neck.)

Top Tip

When working on long hair or a very short client, rather than bending down, get the client to stand up when cutting the back length. This is so much easier and will help you do a better job.

> Make sure the client is sitting in the correct position and is comfortable.

> Ensure that any earrings are removed and that other jewellery is safely out of the way.

> Always ask if the client has any allergies to certain products, and check the scalp for abrasions or sores.

You

> Ensure that your hands are clean.

> You may need to wear an apron or protective gown if the hair has recently been coloured.

> Make sure that none of your jewellery will get in the way while you are working.

> Make sure that you have all the right tools and that they are clean and fit for purpose.

> Keep your working area as tidy as possible while carrying out your work.

> Make sure that you know how to work safely, with the correct posture, and that you are wearing clothes and shoes suitable for the service you are carrying out.

Choosing the hairstyle and deciding the techniques and methods to use

During the consultation process covered in Unit G7, we have seen how head and face shape, look and lifestyle should be taken into account when choosing the client's hairstyle. We have also seen how the hair's length, density, condition and texture can limit or influence the style options. These and other factors would have been considered, leading you to the final look and style decision.

Your skill as a hairdresser is then to decide the cutting techniques and methods you will need to deliver that chosen look. Whether you choose to use short graduation or layering, or to cut a graduated or one-length outline, has as much to do with the thickness, growth patterns and condition of the hair as it has with the style you are looking to create.

Some styles obviously dictate a particular technique or way of cutting to achieve the desired result. In other cases, different techniques or methods can be used to achieve the same overall result, but make it better suited to the client's individual hair.

For example:

> When cutting a chin-length bob on a client with thin, fine hair, using the finer side of the comb and more tension will give a thicker baseline.

> When cutting the same style on a client with very thick, heavy hair, you may decide to add some long layers to reduce the weight.

> Another client having the same hairstyle may have a difficult nape hairline, which grows upwards and will stop the bob sitting

correctly. In this case, you may decide to leave the hair longer, so the extra weight will counteract the hairline.

So it's important that during the consultation process you also think about how you will cut each area of the haircut to achieve the style being discussed. There's no point in agreeing a style if it's not technically possible to achieve it.

Basic cutting techniques

One length step by step – above or below the shoulders

Cutting the perimeter of the hair to a uniform length.

1 Section the hair into four sections, taking your first parting from the forehead, though the crown, and continuing to the nape. Split each section into two, starting from the crown, and continue to just behind the ears. Part the hair front and back by parting from the crown to the top of the ears, and section the back into two equal halves. At the back, take a section approximately 2 to 3 cm wide on each side, from the centre parting to the outside hairline, following the curve of the head. Use sectioning clips to secure the hair if needed.

2 With the head tilted forwards, comb the hair down and cut one side to the required length, following the curved line of the section.

3 For hair longer than the shoulders, comb the hair down in its natural position and cut the hair by using your fingers to hold it securely (a). Do not bend your fingers outwards, but keep them horizontal to avoid graduation.

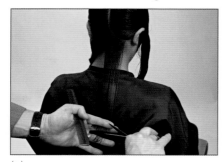

(a)

4 For hair shorter than the shoulders, cut it directly on the skin. Ensure that the hair is lying in its natural position and hold it firmly against the skin with your fingers when cutting. If you force it against the direction in which it grows, once you've cut it, it will return to its natural position and the line will be uneven or graduated.

5 Cut all the way to the outside hairline, ensuring that the hair is combed straight down and not forwards.

6 Cut the other side in the same way and, once complete, stop and check for symmetry.

7 Take another section up the back of the head, making sure that you can see and follow the guideline. Cut to the same length using the previous method.

8 Continue to work in this way, bringing sections down to the guideline (b). Slightly reduce the tension as you work up the head, to avoid creating graduation.

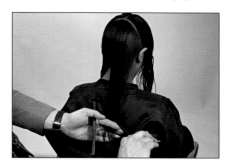

(b)

9 Continue to comb the hair into place to check the length and balance.

10 Once the back has been completed, with the head in the natural position, find the natural parting and use it to section the top into two halves.

11 At the side, take a section of approximately 2 to 3 cm above the ear, from the front hairline to behind the ear (so that it contains some of the previously cut hair (c)). Use sectioning clips if you need to.

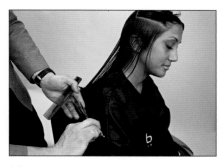

(c)

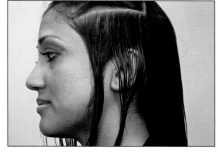

(d)

12 Using the previously cut hair as a guide, cut the hair to the same length in the same manner as before. It's really important to allow for the ear. If you pull the hair down over the ear and cut it, when released it will be shorter. You can overcome this by holding the hair loosely in your comb or in your fingers, allowing the hair to bulge out over the ear (d). Alternatively, you can over-direct the hair that falls over the ear backwards, so that it's slightly longer.

13 If you are unable to cut the hair on the skin, cut it between your fingers, but cut it dead flat and as close to the skin as possible, keeping your fingers horizontal (not bending them outwards) to avoid graduation (e).

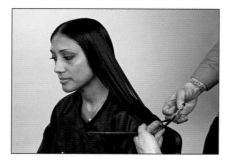

(e)

14 Continue to work up the head until you reach the parting. Lean the head away from you to check the line and remove any loose hairs or graduation. Ensure that the line and length are correct before moving on to the other side.

15 Begin working on the opposite side, taking great care to ensure that the first section matches that on the first side. Work up the head as before.

16 Check as before.

17 Comb or brush the hair and allow it to fall in its natural position. Comb it into place and check for any stray hairs.

18 Use scissors or clippers to remove unwanted hair from below the hairline if needed.

19 Brush down, apply styling products, dry and shape.

20 Once finished, comb the hair into place and check. Pay close attention to the sides and how the hair lies over the ears. Hold the hair in your comb and cut to remove any stray hairs or areas of graduation.

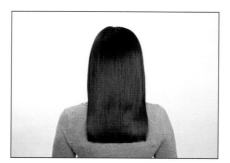

Keywords

Guideline: the first section you cut that you then follow

Whether it's layering, cutting length or the point at which you start your graduation, the first section you cut is the guideline. You then use this as a reference point when cutting follow-on sections.

Checking (cross checking): going over sections you have cut to make sure they are even and correct

Checking your haircut is a fundamental part of hair cutting. Checking is usually done by holding sections in the opposite way to how they were cut: if you cut layers in vertical (front to back) sections, you would check it horizontally (left to right), and vice versa. You also check by using your hands to 'feel' if the hair is the same, and look in the mirror to visually check the length and balance. You should also check with the client that they are happy with the progress of the haircut.

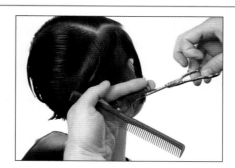

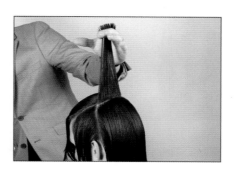

Uniform (round) layer step by step

Cutting hair at uniform length to create an even, layered haircut.

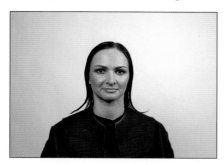

1. Take a section on the top of the head from the front hairline to the crown.
2. Starting at the crown, lift the section vertically at a 90° angle from the head and cut to the desired length (a).

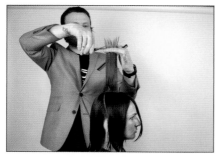

(a)

3 Continue forwards, increasing the length towards the front. As this is the haircut's guideline, check that it is correct before continuing to the next section.

4 Again, starting at the crown, take a section on the side of the head, using the top section as a guide.

5 Continue towards the front hairline, following the guide.

6 Continue working in this way (b), taking sections further down the side of the head until all the hair on the side has been cut. Depending on the required length of the side, you may need to either increase or decrease the angle.

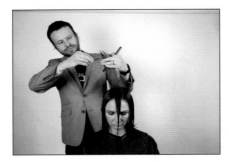

(b)

7 Cross check by using horizontal sections.

8 Repeat on the other side of the head (c).

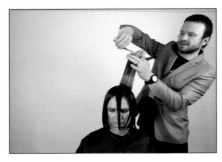

(c)

9 Once complete, compare both sides and review the overall shape.

10 Begin work on the back by taking a section from the crown to the nape. Lift the section vertically at a 90° angle and cut to the desired length, following the natural shape of the head (d).

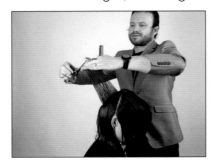

(d)

11 Using the cut section as a guide, continue from the centre to the side of the head in vertical sections.

12 Once completed, use the same method on the other side.

13 Cross check horizontally (e) and blend the side and back sections.

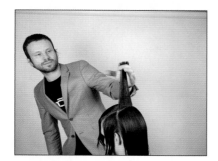

(e)

14 Begin work on the perimeter, cutting the back to the length you require (f). Use vertical sections to reduce weight and use pointing to personalise and finish.

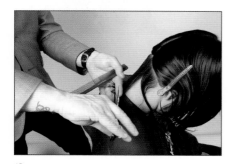

(f)

15 Use the same method on the sides and fringe, taking into account natural growth patterns and the styling of the finished look.

16 Review the shape, the weight, the way the hair is falling and do a final cross check.

17 Use scissors or clippers to remove unwanted hair from below the hairline.

18 Brush down, apply styling products and dry into shape.

19 Once complete, review the look and use pointing to soften and refine.

20 Apply finishing products.

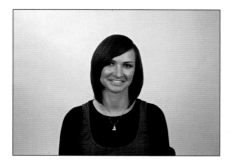

Elevation: lifting the hair away from the head

When you cut hair, specifically layers, you lift up the hair from the head and this is called elevation. You also elevate the hair when graduating.

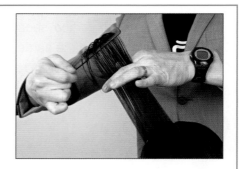

Angle: the angle or direction at which you hold a section for cutting.

For basic layering, the hair should be held at 90° from the head – that is, held straight and vertical. Increasing or reducing the angle at which you hold the hair is called over-direction, and this will change the length and weight of the section.

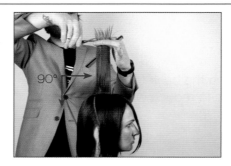

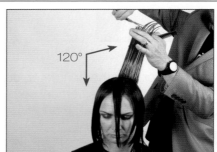

Short graduation step by step

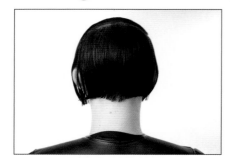

1 Separate the side area of the head in a section from the temple, right round the head, to a point that crosses slightly above and continues towards the lowest point of the nape on the opposite side. Comb all the other hair out of the way and secure using section clips if needed.

2 At the front hairline, take a diagonal section from the temple down. Pulling the section forward, approximately the width of your finger, cut the hair to the required length at a 45° angle, following the head shape (a).

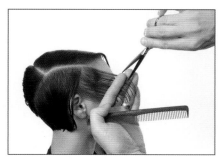

(a)

3   Using the previous section as a guide, take a following section above and behind the first. Again, comb it slightly forward, making sure you hold and cut the hair at the exact same angle, and with the same tension as the previous section (b).

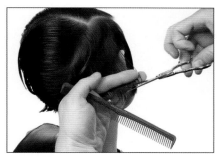

(b)

4   Continue to take sections at the same angle and following the same line as you work back and round the head. To produce even graduation, it is very important that your sections are cut at the same angle and with the same level of tension.

5   Once you have reached a point just past the occipital bone, stop, comb the hair down and check the graduation is even, with no bumps or lines.

6   Begin working on the opposite side. Make sure you take a section that mirrors the one you took on the first side. Again, take a section from the temple down, pulling it forward and holding it at the same 45° angle and at the same tension as before (c).

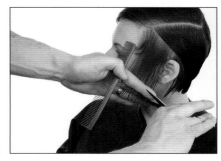

(c)

7   Work, as before, to just past the occipital bone on the far side, until you run out of hair.

8   Comb both sides down and check for balance.

9 After cutting both sides, you will have created an area of weight from the crown to the occipital bone that you may want to reduce. If so, take a horizontal section across the back at the point of graduation.

10 Reduce the weight (by rounding off the corner) and use this as a guide, continuing to take horizontal sections up to the crown, making sure that you follow the head shape (d). Continually comb the hair down to check the shape.

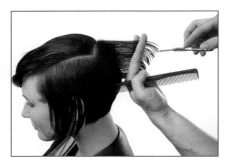

(d)

11 Once you have reached the crown, begin to work across the top, pulling the hair back to your crown line until no further hair reaches the line.

12 On the top of the head, place the parting in the hair where it is to fall. Take a vertical section and follow the line of your previously cut side graduation so that the hair is continually being pulled further away from the head (e).

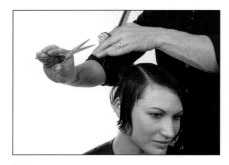

(e)

13 Continue to take vertical sections to the parting towards the crown until all the hair has been cut.

14 Comb the hair down and into place, and check for balance and evenness by cross checking the graduation. Remove any lines or areas of excess weight using scissor-over-comb.

15 Use scissors or clippers to remove unwanted hair from below the hairline (f).

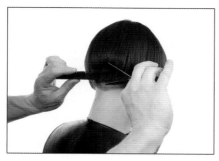

(f)

16 Brush down, apply styling products and dry into shape.

17 Once complete, review the look and use pointing or scissor-over-combing to soften and refine (g).

18 Apply finishing products.

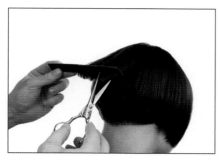

(g)

Long graduation step by step

1 Take a section 2 to 3 cm wide around the front hairline, from ear to ear. Starting in the centre, cut the fringe to the required length (a).

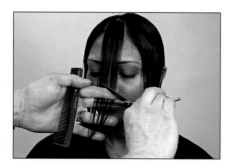

(a)

2 Hold the hair straight down and cut the fringe so that it's slightly curved, using the eyebrows as a guideline.

3 With the fringe as your guide, take a section on the side of the head, holding it forward and slightly downwards, and cut it so that it's gradually getting longer from the fringe (b).

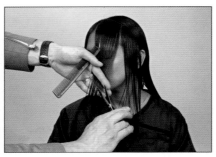

(b)

4 Continue to follow this line until you reach the bottom of this section. The angle at which you hold the hair decides the degree of graduation.

5 Repeat on the opposite side, ensuring that you keep the cutting angle the same (c).

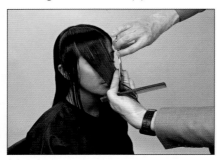

(c)

6 Once complete, check for symmetry and balance.

7 Take a further section around the hairline, behind the first, comb the hair to the guideline and cut as before.

8 Continue to work in this manner, bringing all the hair to the front guideline until you get to the crown. Lifting the hair up as you cut the sections towards the crown will increase the amount of graduation and make the haircut lighter.

9 Section the back of the head in two and take a side section 2 to 3 cm wide, from the temple to the nape. Comb the hair directly forward and continue the line of the previously cut front sections.

10 Continue to bring sections forward, ensuring that they are held at the same angle, until you reach the centre (d).

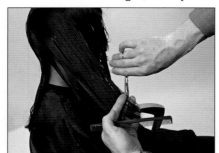

(d)

11 Repeat on the opposite side and, once complete, check for symmetry and balance (e).

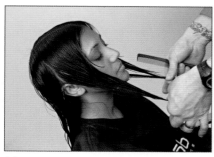

(e)

12 Without combing the hair back away from the face, move on to cutting the back baseline. Take a section on each side, from the centre to the outside hairline, following the curve of the head. Use sectioning clips to secure the hair if needed.

13 Comb the hair down and cut it to the desired length (f). You may wish to cut the back baseline in a curve rather than straight across, in keeping with the graduated front line. Cut the hair either in your fingers or by holding it flat with your fingers or comb.

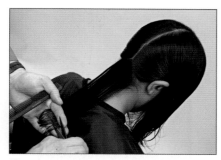

(f)

14 Check that both sides are even before bringing down further sections to cut to the guideline. Continue until all the hair has been cut.

15 Comb the hair into place and check the perimeter to ensure symmetry and balance.

16 Personalise the fringe and front sections by reducing weight or pointing to soften and feather if needed.

17 Brush down, apply styling products, dry and shape.

18 Use pointing to finish before applying finishing products.

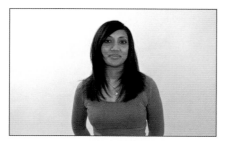

Finishing off

When you have finished your haircut, you have checked it thoroughly and you are happy, always take time to brush down the client carefully.

> Gently ruffle the hair to shake out any loose clippings.
> Using a soft (neck) brush, gently brush the client's face, ears and neck.
> Taking care not to let hair fall down the client's neck, remove the towel or cutting collar and shake off.
> Brush the neck area again before replacing the towel and/or the collar.
> You may want to give the hair a rinse at the backwash to remove all the loose hair.

Advise the client on how you will style and finish their hair, and the products you will use.

Housekeeping

Once you have finished your haircut, help keep the salon clean and safe by:

> cleaning the workstation and sweeping up as soon as possible
> putting hair clippings, dirty towels and gowns in the appropriate bin
> cleaning and sterilising tools, ready for the next client.

Aftercare advice

As most clients will style their hair at home between visits to the salon, it's essential that you advise the client on how to style and maintain their hair. Once you have created your haircut, take time to advise the client on how to maintain the haircut and how to recreate the look at home.

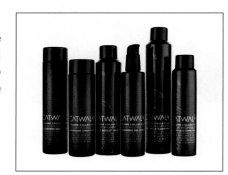

Advise them on:

> the best shampoo and conditioner to use to maintain the condition
> products and styling aids, and how and when they are to be applied
> how to dry and style the look, what tools and appliances to use and how to use them for the best results
> possible ways the style could be enhanced next time, with colour, perming or a conditioning treatment
> when they should book an appointment for a follow-up haircut to keep their hair looking good.

Finally, before they leave let the client know that if they have any problems with the haircut, or if they discover, for example, that the fringe or the back is a bit too long, they can always come back to have it adjusted. Clients are often embarrassed about coming back if there is something that they are not altogether happy with, and sometimes they will even go elsewhere. So always make sure they know that it's part of the service and that there is never a problem in coming back to have the cut adjusted slightly.

Case study
No compromise

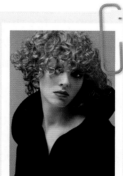

'The key to good hairdressing is not to compromise; always do your best. Never think "that'll do" or "that's good enough" if it isn't. Don't settle for a haircut that's more or less even, or scissor over combing that's just about smooth. If the blow-dry is not going the way you want it to, wet it down and start again.'

'If you can't do something, whatever you do, don't avoid doing it. Ask someone to show you and practise until you master it. And not just when you're training but throughout your career. Not only will you learn what you don't know, you will get better and better and your clients will respect and trust you.'

'By compromising and settling for work that's less than your best, not only will your haircuts never be as good as they could be, neither will you.'

Stephen Mackinder, International Educator, Mackinder Hair, Copenhagen, Denmark

Over the following pages we'll cover the fundamental areas of perming that you'll need to know for NVQ level 2 Unit GH14. Plus we'll show you the broad spectrum of exciting looks, styles and textures that can be created by perming.

In this chapter you will learn to:

> **understand perming products and how they work**
> **prepare for perming and neutralising**
> **perm and neutralise hair**
> **provide aftercare advice.**

You will be assessed against your knowledge and ability to:

1   Understand your salon's processes and procedures with regard to perming services.

2   Understand your legal and health and safety responsibilities when carrying out these services.

3   Understand your personal obligations to other team members and know when and from whom you should seek advice and assistance.

4   Maintain effective and safe methods of working and carry out perming in commercially viable time.

5   Consult with clients and consider key factors when deciding on the perming service to suit their individual needs.

6   Communicate effectively with clients using positive listening skills, body language and verbal communication.

7   Understand products and tools required for perming.

8   Test and assess the hair and prepare it and the client for perming services.

9   Carry out various perming techniques, process and neutralise.

10   Recognise adverse results and deal with them effectively.

11   Provide aftercare and product advice.

Introduction

What is it?

A perm is an abbreviated term for 'permanent waving', the process of permanently adding curl to the hair.

How is it done?

Rollers are put in the hair and chemicals are used to break down and re-form the structure of the hair.

Is it really permanent?

It can be. Some perms will drop out and soften over time, but the stronger the solution and the tighter the curl, the longer it will last, with some staying in the hair until they are cut out.

What's the difference between perming and straightening?

Nothing, except that with perming, straight hair is wrapped around to form curls. Straightening, or relaxing, as it's also called, is the process of removing or loosening natural curl. While the application method is different, the chemical process is the same.

What does this chapter cover?

This chapter covers perming and neutralising, from an explanation of how they work, to product selection and winding methods, as well as the perming process from start to finish – all that you need to know for the NVQ Level 2 Unit GH14.

Does it also cover straightening and relaxing?

No. While it covers the basic principle of changing the structure of the hair, perming concentrates on creating curl.

Creative curling – the fantastic and versatile perm

Permanently curling hair was first seen in salons in the early twentieth century. Clients were attached to huge machines that used a mixture of chemicals and electricity to break down the internal bonds of hair. It wasn't until the late 1930s that cold-wave lotion was invented, making perming not only more widely available, but considerably more comfortable and safer!

The impact perming has had on hairdressing can easily be put on a par with the Vidal Sassoon cutting revolution of the 1960s. Not only did it mean that women with straight hair could now have hairstyles with waves and curls; it also meant that by perming body and curl into the hair, dressing and setting became much easier. Hairstyles would last much longer and it made it much easier for women to do their hair themselves.

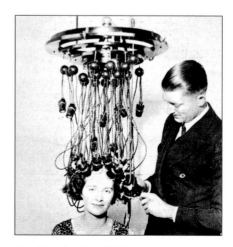

Perming in the 1920s

Perming soon became the most frequent technical service performed by salons, with the vast majority of women having a perm every 6 to 8 weeks. Perming remained a mainstay of salon business until straight hair became the fashion in the mid 1990s and the number of salon perms decreased.

And now the curl is back...

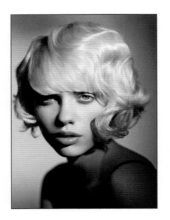
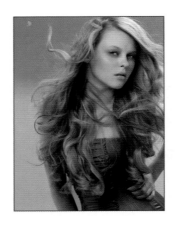
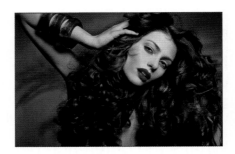

Waves, curls and volume are becoming ever more visible in fashion collections and on the catwalks.

Not that the perm ever completely disappeared, far from it. While the popularity of the curl may have waned for a time at hairdressing's fashionable end, the perm remained a bread-and-butter service for the vast majority of hair salons. Plus the vogue for straight hair saw a huge increase in relaxing and straightening.

Versatility – the key to the perm's continued success

Today, perming is one of the most versatile services you can offer as a hairdresser. More than simply about producing a curl to aid the styling process, modern perms enable you add direction, volume, waves and curls of every conceivable shape and size, to create a vast array of looks, styles and shapes. Modern perms are also far gentler and on the hair than their predecessors.

The looks shown here have all used perming to help create the look.

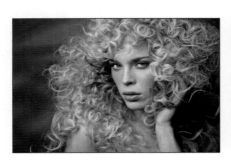
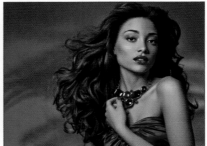

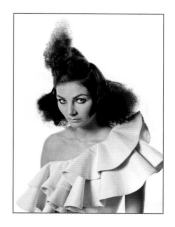
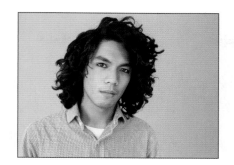
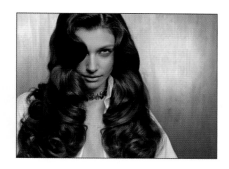

The science of perming

One of the chemical bonds that gives hair its strength and shape is the disulphide bond. While there are fewer disulphide bonds than hydrogen bonds, they are not so easily broken. Hydrogen bonds are weak and easily broken by water; they are re-formed when the hair is dried. The greater number of hydrogen bonds means that they are able to overpower the disulphide bonds and reshape and change the hair by blow-drying. Once wet, however, the hydrogen bonds will be broken and the hair will return to its original, natural shape and texture.

Although fewer in number, the disulphide bonds can't be changed so easily, so the hair will always return to its natural shape and texture. Perming breaks down and neutralising re-forms the disulphide bonds, 'permanently' changing the natural shape and structure of the hair.

The perm lotion swells the hair, opening the cuticle and enabling it to get to the hair's cortex, where the disulphide bonds are. The perm lotion then breaks these links. It doesn't break all of them, just a proportion – up to around a third (the more that are broken, the stronger the result).

Once enough of the bonds have been broken, the process is stopped by using water to rinse the perm lotion out of the hair. The disulphide bonds are then re-formed in their new position by using neutraliser. The hydrogen peroxide in the neutraliser acts as an oxidising agent and re-forms the bonds. (As it's an oxidising process, the disulphide bonds would in fact eventually re-form naturally. The neutraliser simply speeds up the process and re-forms the bonds in one go.)

1 Wet, straight hair is wrapped around a perm rod (perm roller).
2 Perm lotion is applied that swells the hair, opening the cuticle.
3 The perm lotion enters the cortex and begins to break down the disulphide bonds.
4 Once the desired bend has been achieved, the lotion is rinsed out with water.
5 After blotting out excess water, neutraliser is applied to oxidise and re-form the disulphide bonds in the new position.

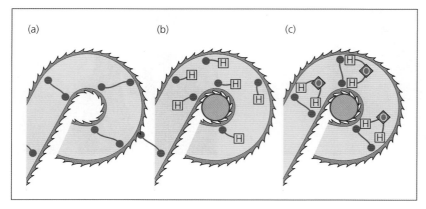

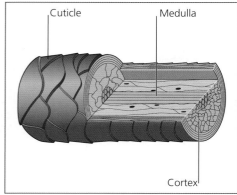

(a) Disulphate bonds (b) Reduction: breaking disulphate bonds
(c) Oxidation: forming new disulphate bonds

Perming doesn't affect the way the hydrogen bonds function – you can still blow-dry or set the hair as you would have done before. Once wet, however, the hair will return to the way the hair was permed.

Types of perms

Early cold perms were very harsh and often damaged the hair. Today's modern perms use a range of gentler chemicals that are more controllable and deliver much more consistent and reliable results.

Alkaline perms

Alkaline perms often contain ammonium thioglycolate, or a similar chemical, which has a high alkaline pH of 8 to 9.5. It's the strong alkaline that causes the hair to swell, enabling the lotion to get to the cortex, where it breaks down the disulphide bonds. Their strength means that alkaline perms break down more of the disulphide bonds than other perms, usually 20 to 30 per cent, which makes the results stronger and longer-lasting.

The strength of alkaline perms and their high pH value, however, means that they do cause hair damage. The cuticle can become rough and uneven, and the hair's natural moisture can be reduced, leaving the hair feeling dry and looking dull.

Acid perms

These have a far weaker pH strength of 4.5 to 6.5, on the acid side of the pH scale – hence their name. The principal ingredient is glyceryl monothioglycolate. Being fairly weak, acid perms require heat to help swell the hair, to open the cuticle and allow the lotion into the cortex. Heat is usually generated by using a plastic cap and placing the client under an accelerator or dryer.

Acid perms break down fewer of the disulphide bonds, meaning the results are softer, but they cause much less hair damage. For this reason, acid perms are often used on dry hair, hair that has previously

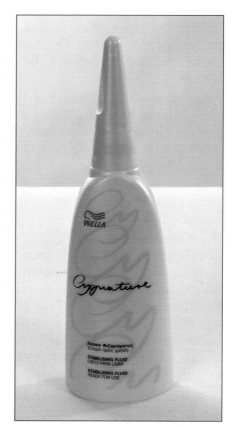

been chemically processed, or for styles that only require a small amount of body or curl.

Unlike alkaline perms, acid perm lotion needs to be mixed just prior to application, as this activates the chemicals. Once mixed, the lotion has to be used and it cannot be saved for use at a later date.

Exothermic perms

A fairly recent innovation in perming, exothermic perms, roughly speaking, are acid perms that generate their own heat. When mixed, the chemicals in the perm make the lotion warm, which helps the perm to enter the hair and the perm to process. Some of these perms have a set duration of time that the heat will last, effectively stopping the processing once that time has elapsed.

The main feature of exothermic perms is their ability to produce the results of an acid perm without the need for an accelerator or dryer.

Preparation – the key to successful perming

To get the right result, you've got to get your preparations spot on. Get it wrong and you could end up with a poor result, an injured client or even a lawsuit.

To ensure you do get it right, always follow these three simple rules:

1 **Test** – test the client's skin for sensitivity and test the hair for compatibility and condition.
2 **Select** – choose a product that suits the client's hair and desired hairstyle.
3 **Protect** – ensure the skin and clothes of both you and your client are protected.

Test

There are a number of tests that need to be carried out to ensure that a perm is suitable for the client and their hair.

First, you need to enquire into the client's history, to find out if they have previously had a perm and if they've ever had a reaction to perm lotion. You should also ask if they have any product or other allergies, skin disorders, or if they have any medical conditions that could interfere with or be affected by the perming process. Don't just think about how the perm lotion may affect the skin or the scalp. If the client has an injured neck, for example, they may not be able to sit at the backwash for the length of time it takes to neutralise.

Sensitivity testing

What is it?

Sensitivity tests (sometimes referred to as patch, skin or hypersensitivity tests) are used to check if a client will have an allergic reaction to the chemicals in the perm lotion.

How is it done?

Generally, a small amount of the perm lotion to be used is applied to a clean patch of skin behind the ear or in the fold of the arm. (If it's an acid perm, you will have to use the mixed solution.)

How long does it take?

The test takes moments, but it can take up to 24 hours for a reaction, after which time, if there's no reaction, the client can receive their colour treatment.

What reactions can occur?

Redness, itching, inflammation or general local soreness and discomfort may occur. If the client experiences any of these reactions, the product should not be used. You may decide to retest using a different type of perm lotion, as the chemicals vary between acid and alkaline perms.

Do I have to carry out a sensitivity test for all perm services?

Yes, especially if it's a new client or you are using a new product they've not had before.

Do I have to carry out a sensitivity test each time the client has a perm?

As a rule, yes, you should. While it might not be practical, clients can develop allergic reactions over time, and for this reason, some manufacturers recommend testing prior to each use, or at least periodic testing.

Note:

> Testing requirements may vary from product to product, so make sure you check the instructions.

> Always ask the client if they have any medical conditions or have been advised that they should not have a perm.

> Never take a client's word that they have been tested – they might be lying.

If in doubt, always seek advice from a more senior colleague or the manufacturer.

Pre-test curl and incompatibility test

What is it?

It's a test carried out to see how the hair reacts to the perm lotion and the result it produces.

When is it used?

It is used any time that you are unsure of the result the particular lotion will produce on the hair, or if you are concerned that the lotion may react with the hair or products that have been used previously.

How is it done?

There are two ways: you can either snip off a small piece of hair or you can perm one small section of the hair. In each case, you need to

---

Top Tip

If you're testing acid or exothermic perms, where you have to mix the lotion, you can often take a small amount out of each bottle and mix it in a tint bowl to test. Or you can use some of the lotion that is being used on another client. But if you are using leftover lotion, make sure that it's fresh and hasn't gone past its productive stage. If in doubt, use fresh lotion.

carry out the entire perming process just as you would when perming the client's hair.

> If you are concerned about how the hair will react to the perm lotion, or that it might have an adverse affect on the hair or its condition, you should remove a small section of hair for testing.

> If you want to check the strength or durability of a perm, you may want to test a small section (one roller) on the head. This can be done at the nape of the neck or around the occipital bone (anywhere that it won't be noticed). Remember, though, if you are curl-testing on the head, you should carry out a sensitivity test first.

How long does it take?

If you are testing for compatibility, you will know as soon as the process is finished. If the hair has reacted to chemicals in the hair, this will be apparent straightaway. If you are testing to see the result, you will need to review the result in a week or so, to see how the curl has lasted.

Do I have to carry out a pre-test curl or incompatibility test for all perm services?

No. You only need to carry out either test if you think that the hair may react to the lotion or you want to test the result.

> **Activity** Practise carrying out sensitivity tests and test curls on friends and colleagues. Pre-test curls can be fiddly, so practise until you can do them quickly and easily.

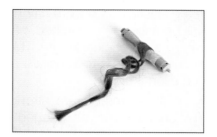

Top Tip

If you are going to snip off a section of hair, make sure that it represents the hair you need to test. If you are testing for reaction with another product already on the hair, make sure that the section you test has enough of the product. Likewise, if you are testing for damage, make sure that the section you choose represents the most damaged hair. Also, as with sensitivity testing, you may not need to mix a full bottle of perm lotion.

Porosity and condition testing

What is it?

This tests how absorbent the hair is, how stretchy it is and the hair's general condition.

Why is it done?

For perming, it's really important to assess the porosity of the hair, as this will affect how quickly the perm is absorbed and how quickly it will process. It's also very important to assess the condition of the hair so that you can choose the right perm lotion.

When should you carry out the test?

You must assess the condition of every client's hair prior to any chemical process; this can be done during your consultation.

How is the test carried out?

Testing the condition is generally done visually and by touch.

> If the hair is overly porous, it will feel rough and coarse when you rub strands with the ends of your fingers. Also, it will remain heavy and saturated, even after towel-drying.

> If the elasticity is poor, a hair held near the root and near the tip will be easily overstretched, have little or no tension, and won't return to its original length. This will also determine if the hair is brittle. If it snaps too easily, it could be a sign of damage to the hair's inner cortex.

Any of these results are strong indicators of damaged hair. The condition can also be gauged by its general texture, sheen and tendency to tangle, which is a sign of damaged cuticle.

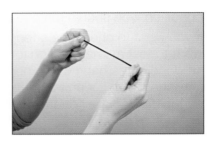

How do I decide if the hair is too damaged to proceed with the service?

Consider the additional damage that is likely to be caused by perming before proceeding, and always take the most cautious approach.

What should I do if the hair is too damaged to proceed?

Recommend that your client books a professional in-salon conditioning treatment, and advise on intensive home hair care to rehabilitate the condition.

Test curl

What is it?

This is a test carried out to see if the perm has processed to the desired point.

When is it carried out?

All perms need to be tested before neutralising. When you carry out the test depends on the hair, the perm you have used and the result you want. Soft perms and perms on dry or damaged hair will need to be checked sooner than those aiming for a firm result on strong, virgin hair. Follow the manufacturer's instructions on testing, but always check sooner rather than later. Checking will not affect the processing of the perm, so it doesn't matter how often you check.

How do you check a test curl?

Select a roller, unfasten the elastic and unwind the hair, without pulling it so that the hair is loose. You often don't need to completely remove the roller, just unwind it a couple of turns so you can see how the hair falls. You are looking for well-formed curls or waves that reflect the shape and size of the roller. If the perm is ready, the hair will form a good, firm 'S' shape.

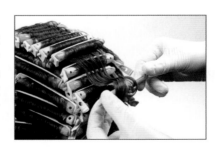

Do you only check one place?

No, it's always advisable to check various places around the head, as they often process at different speeds, especially if there are variations in temperature. If you are using heat, always check the front of the head and both sides, as clients often lean on one side or lean forward to read a magazine!

What if the hair is not processing?

There are a number of reasons that this could be happening.

> If it's not processing all over the head:

> you may need to add or increase heat
> you may need to add more perm lotion if the hair is thick or particularly strong.
> If it's not processing in certain areas:
>> check how the client was sitting, as they may have been leaning closer to the accelerator on one side; if so, reduce or remove the heat from the side that's processing well, while keeping it on the areas that need it (if it's only one small section, you could use a hairdryer)
>> check that the hair is wet with lotion and reapply if you think it's needed.

Testing perms is a knack that needs to be learned. While the instructions will give you guidelines, it's your skill that has to decide when to rinse off the perm lotion so that you will achieve the result you want. Rinse it off too soon and it will be too loose and may drop out, meaning that you'll have to do it again. Leave it too long and the perm can be too tight and you can seriously damage the hair. As with everything in the salon, if you are unsure, ask. There is no embarrassment in asking someone with more experience for a second opinion.

Note: Always ask for help and advice if you need help reading a result or deciding how you should proceed.

Select

There are three elements to the selection process for perming:
> the perm lotion
> the rollers
> the winding method.

Advice on how to select the right lotion and the right-sized rollers is set out here, while winding methods are covered later in the chapter.

Choosing the right perm

There are many factors involved in getting the right result in perming, but the selection of the lotion is crucial. Too weak and the perm won't take or won't last; too strong and you will seriously damage the hair and could injure the client.

The key to choosing the right perm is knowing your products. The best way to get to know your products is by watching and learning. During your training, you will be introduced to various perming products and be given an insight into how they work and the results they produce, but this is no substitute for experience. Through using the products regularly, the technicians in your salon will know the characteristics of the perms in the salon and will be able to use this knowledge and experience to select the best product and perming method for the desired look on each individual client. Don't expect this knowledge to come quickly; it takes time and the best way to acquire it is to watch and to ask.

The table should give you some starting guidelines, but remember, each client will be different, so always read the instructions and ask for advice if you are unsure.

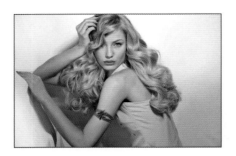
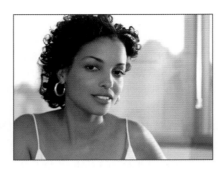
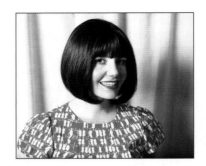

Style	Hair type	Roller size	Lotion
Soft, loose, wash-and-wear curls	Good-condition, shoulder-length, virgin hair	Large	Alkaline
Short, tight curls for setting/ blow-drying	Previously permed and coloured, dry hair	Small	Acid/exothermic
Add volume to a fine-hair bob	Some highlights	Medium	Acid/exothermic
Add volume to a thick-/coarse-hair bob	Fairly good-condition, natural hair	Small/medium	Alkaline
Fringe part perm to control direction	Coloured, but fairly good condition	Medium/large	Acid/exothermic

Choosing the right perm

Choosing the right perm rollers

There are quite a lot of things to consider when deciding on the size of rollers you will use when perming.

Style

What hairstyle are you trying to create? Do you need different amounts of curl or do you need to control direction?

Hair type

Is the hair fine, thick, in good or bad condition? Fine hair will need a larger roller than thick hair to achieve the same result. Also, dry hair will take quicker and stronger than virgin hair, so will also need larger rollers.

Result

Do you want to create body, waves or curls? The smaller the roller, the tighter the curl, so consider the shape and size of the curl you want to achieve.

Finishing

Is the hairstyle to be blow-dried, set or left to dry? If the style is to be blow-dried or set, it will need to be firmer than if it's to be left to dry naturally, as blow-drying will stretch out the perm.

> **Activity** First, learn the various characteristics of the perm lotions used in your salon. Then pick two hairstyles that could be achieved by perming and write down the lotions and the size of rollers you think would be used to achieve that result on a work colleague's or friend's hair. Ask your salon's perming technician or educator to check your suggestions, to see how well you have done.

Size of rollers

As well as the lotion you use, the size of roller will determine if the perm will be soft or tight. There is a rule of thumb that will help you decide the size of roller to use.

> **To create body** – the hair should not go round the roller more than one and a half to two times.

> **To create body and soft curls** – the hair should go round the roller two to three times.

> **To create strong curl** – the hair should go round the roller three times or more.

It is of course possible to create a stronger or weaker curl on the same roller size by using a stronger or weaker perm lotion, but this a good general guide to selecting rollers.

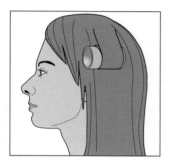
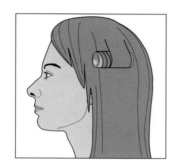
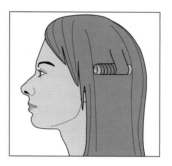

Protect

Perming products generally won't stain or harm the skin, but you should avoid skin contact where possible. They can damage fabrics and furnishings, and, as they tend not to smell too nice, it's important to ensure that you, your client and nearby surfaces are properly protected.

Whenever you carry out perming services it's important that you follow the guidelines set out below.

Your client

You should ensure that your client:

> is wearing a gown that covers their clothes

> has removed any collars or high-necked clothing, or that these are turned down and adequately covered

> has had barrier cream applied to the skin around the hairline (avoiding the hair) and on the ears

> is correctly positioned and comfortable.

You

You should:

> wear gloves

> wear an apron or gown

> ensure that your sleeves, hair and jewellery are out of the way and won't interfere with your work.

Your working area

> The gown should cover the chair (if possible) or the chair should have a protective back cover.

> You should use a mobile trolley, to keep the rollers and papers close to where you are working.

> Wipe up any spills as soon as possible.

Tools and equipment

Tail comb

A comb with one end tapered into a point. (For perming, you should not use metal combs (unless they are stainless steel), as they may react with the perm lotion.)

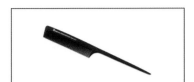

Perm rollers

Often called rods or perm curlers, standard perm rollers come in various sizes that are colour-coded. Perm rollers are usually fitted with an elastic fastener (sometimes called a perm rubber) that secures the hair around the roller and keeps it in place. Medium and large rollers are usually hollow, with holes helping the lotion to reach all the hair. There are also spiral and flexible, foam-covered rollers.

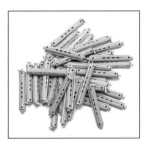

End papers

'Wet-strength' end papers are used to ensure that the ends of the hair are straight and smooth around the roller. There are various sizes and brands of end paper, and some can be washed and reused. End papers are either used dry, straight from the packet, or are dipped in water before use. If the hair is long and/or strong, the end papers can be dipped in perm lotion.

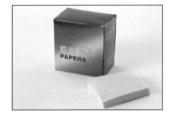

Strips or plastic pins

Thin plastic strips or pins placed between the elastic and the hair to stop the elastic marking the hair.

Water spray

To keep the hair damp and make it easier to wind.

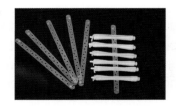

Barrier cream

As its name implies, barrier cream forms a barrier that stops the lotion coming into contact with the skin and is used to protect skin around the hairline. Do not get barrier cream on the hair, as it will also stop the perm lotion penetrating the hair shaft.

Cotton wool

Used in a strip around the hairline to absorb any perm lotion that runs off the scalp. This can be dampened down to dilute any lotion that comes into contact with the skin.

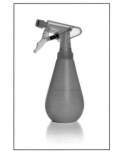
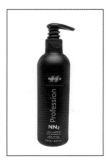

Gloves

Protective gloves for your hands should be used during all perm services. The current health and safety recommendation is for talc-free, non-latex (nitrile) or vinyl gloves to be used for salon work.

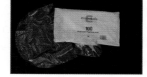

Gowns

Dark-coloured gowns are used to protect your clothes and the client's.

Plastic caps

Used to aid processing by retaining the heat from the head. It's important to check the perm instructions to see if caps can be used or not.

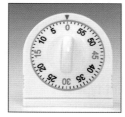

Timer

Used to remind you when processing needs checking or is complete.

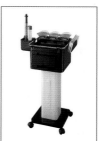

Trolley

Mobile workstation used to place roller trays, end papers, clips, lotions and other tools used during perming. Trolleys should be sturdy, with wheels (castors) free from hair.

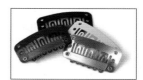

Clips

Larger, 'grab' clips are used to keep large sections of hair out of the way. Pin-curl clips can be used instead of rollers for creating small, flat or directional curls. (Only stainless steel or plastic pin-curl clips should be used in perming.)

Bowl and sponge

Used to apply neutraliser.

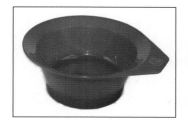 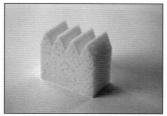

Client record card

Used to record all technical services the client has and other relevant information (see next page).

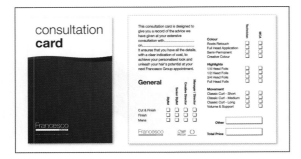

Accelerators

What are they?

Accelerators are used to speed up the processing time of some perm applications.

How do they work?

Mainly used with acid perms, they use heat to assist and speed up the processing.

Are there different types?

Yes. Some use straightforward heat; others use infrared; while others also use a fan to produce 'hot air'. A hood dryer or a hairdryer can be used to accelerate processing times.

Are they easy to use?

Generally, yes, although as some require product and application information to be entered, it's important to be trained on how to use and position each machine individually.

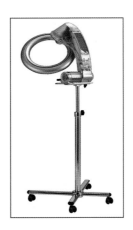

Do I need to use an accelerator with all perm services?

No. Acid perms often require heat, but exothermic perms usually don't. They are useful for speeding up processing times, or for targeting specific areas of the head in order to create an even result. You should always check the instructions to see if heat can be used to help processing. Also, if the salon is warm you may not need any additional heat.

Dryers

Although not as comfortable, hood dryers can also be used in the same way to speed up the processing of perms.

Getting started

Before you start perming, it's important that the hair is prepared for the process. You should also make sure that you have all the right tools and equipment ready. You don't want to have to keep stopping to go and get something you've forgotten; worse still, you don't want to forget something that will affect the result or the client's safety.

> **Activity** When you see an accelerator or dryer being used with a perm, ask why it's being used and by how much it will speed up the processing. Also, learn how to position it properly and how it should be stored when not in use.

Pre-perm preparations

As hair products and conditioners can form a barrier that can interfere with the absorption of the perm lotion, it's important that the hair shaft is as clean as possible.

Pre-perm shampoos

You should always shampoo the hair before a perm with a pre-perm shampoo, as these are designed to remove product residue and leave the hair clean. Also, they do not contain any additives, such as colour protectors or conditioning agents that can be left on the hair. Some pre-perm shampoos do contain agents that help to balance the pH.

You should never use conditioner before perming, as this will coat the hair shaft and stop the perm lotion getting into the hair.

Pre-perm treatments

What are they?

Pre-perm treatments are designed to be used prior to a technical service like a perm.

What do they do?

They even out the porosity of the hair. If the hair has highlights or has been permed or coloured previously, the porosity will vary between the hair that has been treated and the hair that hasn't. This means that the perm lotion will be absorbed at different rates, so some hair will process faster. Pre-perm treatments reduce the porosity of the damaged/dry hair, so that all the hair absorbs the lotion in the same way.

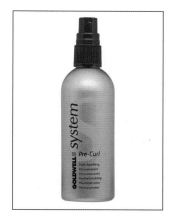

Do you need to use them before all perms?

Technically, yes, as the porosity of everyone's hair will vary. In reality, no. If the condition of the hair is fairly uniform, it won't make much of a difference.

How do I know when to use one?

During your technical and product training, you will learn what pre-perm treatments your salon uses and when they tend to be used. Always read the product's usage directions and, if you're unsure, ask your salon's educator.

Pre-damping

What is it?

Pre-damping is when you put perm lotion onto the hair before you begin winding.

Why do you pre-damp?

Pre-damping is a way of giving the perm a head start, so that the lotion can begin to swell the hair and start the process. As you only add a small amount to the wet hair, the lotion is diluted and won't fully process the hair; it will just start the process so that when the lotion is applied it is absorbed quicker.

When would you pre-damp?

You usually only need to pre-damp on long or very strong hair. For long hair, which can become very thickly rolled around a roller, you may want to dip the end paper in perm lotion as you wind. This will help ensure that the perm lotion gets through to the ends of the hair.

Can you pre-damp with all perms?

No. You generally only pre-damp with alkaline perms, although it is possible with some acid perms. Always read the instructions.

When would I decide to pre-damp?

With experience, you'll learn the hair and the styles with which pre-damping would help. It's particularly advisable to pre-damp long hair, to make sure the perm lotion penetrates the hair. If you do pre-damp, you need to know roughly how long you'll take to wind the head, as, even diluted, you don't want to leave lotion on the hair for too long. For this reason, while you are training and until you can perm proficiently, it's best not to pre-damp unless advised to do so.

Winding techniques

There are many ways that hair can be permed to achieve various different and exciting results. As you progress in your career, you will get an opportunity to learn many different winding techniques, but for Unit GH14 we will focus on the three basic methods:

> nine-section winding
> brickwork winding
> directional winding.

These three methods will form the basis of all your future perming skills and, properly learned, will allow you to create a wide range of looks and styles.

Also, as it's the principal way individual rollers are wound into the hair, the following step-by-step process uses the technique that achieves maximum root lift without drag or over-directing the roots. The aim is to have the roller resting on the roots of the hair and not on the scalp of the section parting. Once you have perfected this method, you can explore other rolling methods to achieve different degrees of lift or movement.

Winding step by step

The key to a good perm is consistent and evenly wound rollers. Always ensure that your sections are even and that you have the right amount of hair for the size of roller.

1 Divide the hair into sections appropriate to the style of wind you have chosen. Each section should be no wider than the roller you will use.

2 Comb through the section you will work on, so it's smooth.

3 Using a tail comb, take a small section across the main section, approximately the thickness of the roller.

4 Comb this section 90° from the head, so it is smooth and straight.

5 Without pinching it together, hold the very ends of the hair between your thumb and index finger (a).

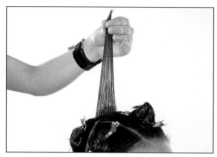

(a)

6 With your other hand, take an end paper and, without loosening the tension, place it around or over the hair (b).

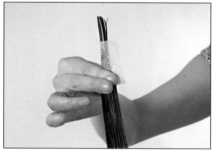

(b)

7 Take a perm roller and place it on the end paper, in front of the hair (c).

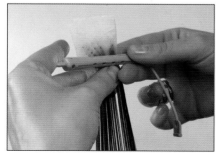

(c)

8 Holding the roller between your thumb and index finger of both hands, pin the hair firmly against the roller.

9 Slide the roller and the end paper up until they are just past the ends of the hair.

10 Roll the roller towards you, holding the paper and the hair tightly onto the roller.

11 Turn the roller down the hair, keeping the ends smooth and flat (d).

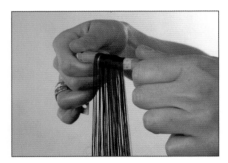

(d)

12 Use the end of your tail comb to pass round between the hair and the roller (e), following the direction of the hair to ensure that the ends are in the right direction.

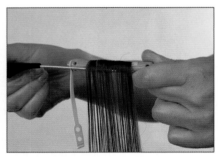

(e)

13 Roll the roller down the hair, keeping the hair straight and the tension even, so that the hair is spread evenly across the width of the roller.

14 Roll the roller down so that it sits on top of the section's roots (f). If the hair is too bunched on the roller, you may need to remove it and take a smaller section.

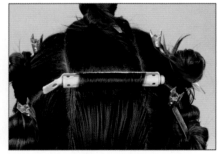

(f)

15 Fasten with the elastic, ensuring that the tension on the roots is taut, but not overly tight. (If the skin of the scalp is raised or 'white', it is too tight.)

16 Insert a plastic strip or pin under the elastic and push it down under the elastic of each following roller.

17 Always ask the client if the rollers are comfortable. Loosen slightly any that are too tight.

Preparation

What to consider for your perm

> Movement or curl required.
> Condition of the hair – hair with some damage may require a gentler lotion and reduced processing time.
> Texture of the hair – coarse, strong hair may require stronger lotion and smaller rollers.
> Hair length – longer hair may require pre-damping.
> Hair density – finer hair may require larger rollers and a gentler lotion.

The client

> All clients having a perm must have had their hair and skin properly analysed and tested.
> Protect the client's clothes with gowns, capes and towels.
> The hair should be shampooed with the appropriate product. Conditioners should not be used, as they will coat the hair and prevent the perm lotion from penetrating into the hair.
> Pre-treatments should be applied if required.
> Ensure that any earrings are removed and that other jewellery is safely out of the way
> Ensure that the client is seated comfortably and that you are able to carry out the service.

You

> Ensure that your hands are clean.
> Review the client record card and consult with the client, taking into account that the hairstyle may change after perming. (For further details, see Unit G7.)
> Decide on the winding method, rod size, perm lotion and processing method, and if you need to pre-damp.
> Ensure that you have read and understood the product instructions.
> Make sure that none of your jewellery will get in the way while you are working.
> Protect your clothes with an apron and your hands with gloves.
> Make sure that you have all the right tools and rollers, and that they are clean and fit for purpose.
> Set out tools and rollers on a trolley.
> Section the hair evenly, as this will help to create an even result.

> Keep your working area as tidy as possible while carrying out your work.

> Make sure that you know how to work safely, with the correct posture, and that you are wearing clothes and shoes suitable for the service you are carrying out.

Note: Most salons will use older or special towels for perming, as they can become stained or smelly. Make sure you always use the appropriate towels.

Nine-section perm step by step

1 Ensure that the hair is clean and that any pre-perm treatment needed has been applied.

2 Section the hair into nine sections.

> Part the hair from recession line (temple) to the nape on each side of the head, ensuring that each panel is the same width.

> Section the centre panel at the crown, and secure the hair from the crown to the front in a clip.

> Section the back of the central panel in two, just above the occipital bone, and secure the two sections with clips.

> Divide the two side panels into three, following the guidelines of the central section, and secure with clips.

> Once completed, you should have nine sections (a). These should be wound in order, as they are numbered in the diagram.

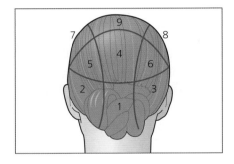

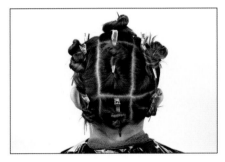

(a)

3 Starting at the top of section one, take a section approximately the same size but slightly narrower than the roller. Ensure that all the other hair is clipped out of the way.

4 Wind the roller towards you, into the hair, with even tension, until it rests on the roots (its base), and then fasten.

5 Place the end of a strip or pin under the elastic (b).

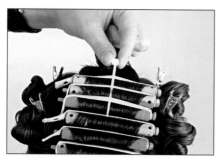

(b)

6 Continue down the section, keeping the sections even and pushing the strip under each elastic. You may need to reduce the size of the roller as the hair gets shorter, to ensure that the curl remains uniform.

7 Once finished, begin work on the next section and repeat until the entire back is completed (c).

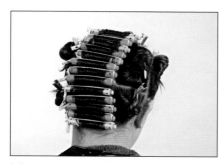

(c)

8 Begin work on the sides, working from the top of each section, down to the top of the ears (d).

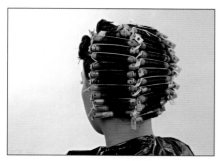

(d)

9 Finally, wind the top section, working forward from the crown (e).

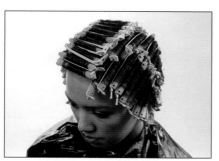

(e)

10 Check that the client is comfortable before applying barrier cream and cotton wool around the hairline (f).

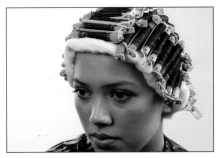

(f)

11 Apply the perm lotion according to the manufacturer's instructions (g). Ensure that each roller is completely wet with perm lotion, but not overly saturated so that it drips.

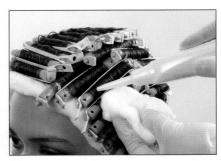

(g)

12 Replace the cotton wool if it becomes saturated.

13 Place a plastic cap over the entire head (h), use heat or leave uncovered, according to the processing instructions.

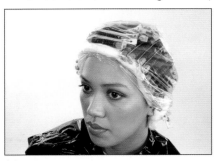 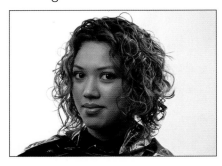

(h)

Brickwork perm step by step

1 Ensure that the hair is clean and that any pre-perm treatment needed has been applied.

2 Comb all the hair back from the face. Standing behind the client, take a section in the centre on the front hairline (a). The section should be approximately the same size but slightly narrower than the roller.

3 Wind the roller towards you, into the hair, with even tension, until it rests on the roots (its base), and then fasten.

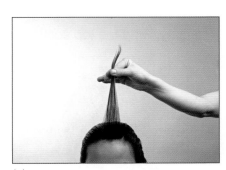

(a)

4 Place the end of a strip or pin under the elastic (b).

5 Using the centre of the first roller as a guide, part the hair and take a section of the same size from the part that's down. Wind the roller in as before, keeping it 90° from the head and keeping the tension even.

6 Take a mirror section on the other side of the part and roll as before.

7 Next, following the line on the first roller at the front of the head, take a section across the centre.

8 Again, make a parting behind the centre of the previous roller and take a section to the side of the centre.

9 Repeat on the other side and continue this line down both sides of the head, until you run out of hair.

10 Place plastic strips or pins under the elastics and push them down so that they go under the next parallel roller.

11 Continue working in this method backwards, keeping the sections uniform (c). You may need to reduce the size of the roller as you approach the nape, to ensure that the curl remains uniform.

12 Check that the client is comfortable before applying barrier cream and cotton wool around the hairline.

13 Apply the perm lotion according to the manufacturer's instructions. Ensure each roller is completely wet with perm lotion, but not overly saturated so that it drips.

14 Replace the cotton wool if it becomes saturated.

15 Place a plastic cap over the entire head (d), use heat or leave uncovered, according to the processing instructions.

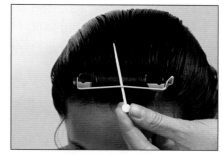

(b)

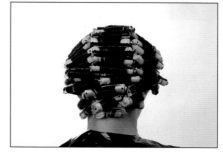

(c)

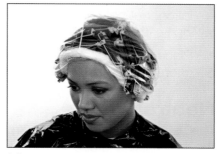

(d)

Directional perm step by step

1 Ensure that the hair is clean and that any pre-perm treatment needed has been applied.

2 Decide the direction that you want the hair to be permed and section the hair in roller-width sections that follow this direction. If you need to, section off the hair so you can work cleanly.

3 Starting at the panel nearest the front, take a section that follows the direction of the section, approximately the same size but slightly narrower than the roller (a).

4 Holding the hair at 90° from the head, wind the roller towards you, into the hair, with even tension, until it rests on the roots (its base), and then fasten.

5 Place the end of a strip or pin under the elastic.

6 Continue down the section, keeping the sections even and pushing the strip under each elastic. You may need to reduce the size of the roller as the hair gets shorter, to ensure that the curl remains uniform.

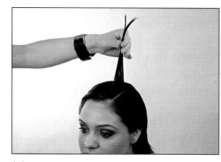

(a)

7   Once the top/front section is finished (b), begin work on the side sections until they are both completed.

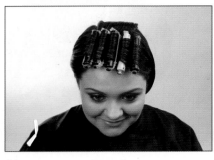
(b)

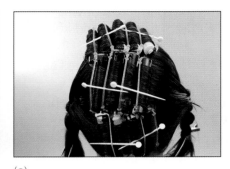
(c)

8   Begin work on the back, from the crown down to the nape (c). Either work in three vertical panels or in a brickwork pattern, placing plastic strips or pins under the elastics as you go.

9   Check that the client is comfortable before applying barrier cream and cotton wool around the hairline.

10 Apply the perm lotion according to the manufacturer's instructions. Ensure that each roller is completely wet with perm lotion, but not overly saturated so that it drips.

11 Replace the cotton wool if it becomes saturated.

12 Place a plastic cap over the entire head (d), use heat or leave uncovered, according to the processing instructions.

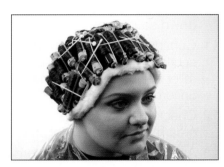
(d)

Neutralising

This is a crucial stage of perming, when you 'set' your perm. If the neutralising stage is not carried out properly, all the winding and preparation will have been for nothing. The hair will need to be re-permed, which will not only be bad for the hair, it will be an inconvenience for the client and a financial loss for the salon. When training, you will probably have to neutralise for other hairdressers in your salon, and you won't be popular with either the client or the stylist if the perm fails due to your poor neutralising. You definitely won't get a tip! So make sure you concentrate when you neutralise, regardless of how many times you have done it before.

Read the instructions!

Not all perms are neutralised in the same way, so make sure that you read the specific instructions for the perm you are using.

Basic neutralising

While the details may vary from product to product, usually neutralising requires the hair to be rinsed to remove the perm lotion, the hair to be towel-dried (blotted) to remove excess water, and the neutraliser applied to re-form the disulphide bonds before the rollers are removed. Finally, the hair is conditioned and the pH balance restored if needed.

Prepping for neutralising

> Once the perm has processed, take the client over to the shampoo area. (Perms should only be neutralised at a backwash basin. Front-wash basins should not be used.)
> Ensure that you are wearing a protective apron and gloves.
> Recline the client before removing the cotton wool or cap.
> Make sure that the gown and towel are secure and that the client is covered and protected.
> Make sure that all the rollers are in the basin before commencing rinsing.

Rinsing

> Set a timer for the duration of time the rollers are to be rinsed.
> Adjust the water so that it's warm but not hot. During perming, the scalp may become sensitive, so the water should be slightly cooler than for a usual shampoo. Check that the temperature is comfortable for the client.
> Ensure that you thoroughly soak *all* the rollers, so that the perming process is stopped over the entire head.
> Take care when rinsing, especially the front hairline, as water can splash off the rollers. Use your hand to shield and stop the water running onto the client's face. If the rollers at the nape are hard to get to, get the client to sit up and back as far as possible. Again, use your hand to stop the water running down the client's neck.

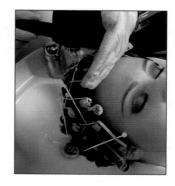

> After the initial rinse, begin to methodically rinse the entire head. Working from the front, slowly rinse the rollers across the entire head, from left to right and back again, gradually moving down the head until you reach the nape.
> Continually repeat this process until the time has elapsed.

Blotting

> Once the rinsing is complete, place a dry towel over the rollers and gently press to absorb the water.
> Never rub the rollers, as this will disturb the hair.
> Once the hair has stopped dripping, blot the front hairline. Then, while supporting the client's head in the towel, sit them upright.
> Blot the rollers at the nape of the neck.
> With the client in this position, check that the towel and gown have not become wet. If they have, change them.
> Continue to blot the rollers, using a new dry towel if necessary.
> Using the towel, go over each roller, gently squeezing it to remove the water.

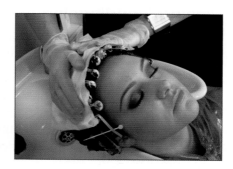

> Once complete, check the rollers to make sure none have come loose or unwound. If they have, replace or re-tighten them. (If you are unable to do this, ask someone else to help you.)

Applying the neutraliser

> Different neutralisers are applied in different ways, so make sure that you apply the neutraliser according to the product instructions.

> Recline the client at the basin. You may also want to put a strip of cotton wool round the front hairline to stop drips.

> For bottle applications, gently squeeze the bottle, applying the neutraliser slowly, starting at the front and working rhythmically back and downwards until you have covered all the rollers. (Don't squeeze the bottle too hard initially or you risk running out of neutraliser before you get to the back.) Once you have reached the nape, begin the process again until all the rollers have been covered and soaked. You may need to apply a second application when the rollers are removed. If so, make sure you have saved enough to do so.

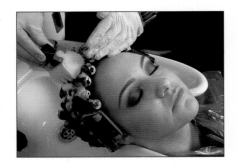

> For sponge applications, pour the neutraliser into a bowl and soak some into a sponge. Begin at the front, using the sponge to push the neutraliser into the hair. Ensure that you cover the entire roller. (The neutraliser will usually foam up.) Again, work down and back until you have covered all the rollers and then repeat. You may need to apply a second application when the rollers are removed. If so, make sure you have saved enough to do so.

> Check the neck and hairline for drips.

> Set the timer for the required processing time.

Removing the rollers and applying more neutraliser

> Once the processing time is up, starting at the nape, gently remove the rollers.

> Do not pull or stretch the hair. Unwind gently and let the hair fall off the roller.

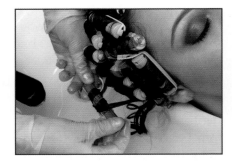

> Once all the rollers are removed, apply the second neutraliser if needed. Apply gently, supporting the curls.

> Gently loosen so that the hair is not weighed down or flat to the head.

> Check the neck and hairline for drips.

> Set the timer for the required processing time.

Rinsing, conditioning and readjusting the pH

> Once the processing time is up, after checking the temperature, gently rinse the hair to remove the neutraliser.

> Do not pull or stretch the hair.

> Once thoroughly rinsed, gently squeeze to remove excess water.

> Apply an anti-oxidant (post-perm) conditioner or product recommended by the manufacturer. Anti-oxidant conditioners help to restore the natural pH level of the hair to 4.5 to 5.5, as this has probably been altered by the acid or alkaline perm lotion.

Top Tip

While the second neutraliser is on, use the time to rinse and dry the rollers and discard the end papers. This way, the basin will be clear and ready for the next client. Check the elastics on the rollers as you go, and put to one side any that need replacing.

> Finally rinse the hair again, taking care not to stretch or pull the hair.

> Gently towel-dry the hair and return the client to the styling station. Avoid letting the client sit with a towel on their head, as this can flatten the perm.

> Check the scalp and hairline for sores or reactions to the chemicals.

> Check and change wet or damp gowns and apply any special leave-in post-perm product.

After neutralising, the perm is still weak, as many of the disulphide bonds may not have re-formed. They will slowly re-form and strengthen over time, so it's important to treat the perm as gently as possible during and straight after the neutralising process.

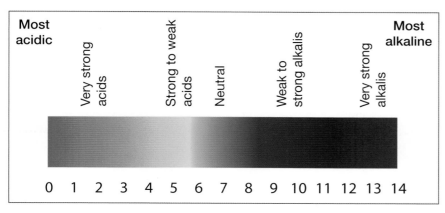

pH scale

Perming problems

Review your perm to check that it's even and that you have achieved the desired result. If not, you may need to take corrective action or at least make a note on the client record card for next time.

Note: Seek the advice of a senior team member or manager if you are unsure of how to deal with something that happens during or after the perming process. *Never ignore or try to hide a problem and always be honest.*

The scalp is tender

Reason

> The rollers were wound too tight.
> Too much or too high heat was used to process the perm.
> The perm was over-processed.

What to do

If the client's scalp is tender, you need to ensure that this is not a reaction to the perming. Always seek the advice of your manager and/or first aider before proceeding.

Next time

> Wind looser.
> Don't use or reduce the heat.
> Take care with processing times.

The hair is broken

Reason

> The rollers were wound too tight.
> The perm was over-processed.
> The elastic on the roller was too tight and rested on the hair.
> The lotion was too strong for the hair.

What to do

Even if only a small amount of hair is broken and it may not be noticed, you should still advise the client and consult your manager to decide the course of action. There may be need for corrective action or reconstructive treatments.

Next time

> Wind the rollers looser.
> Take care with processing times.
> Ensure you use plastic strips or pins.
> If you think it was the perm lotion, carry out a pre-test curl.

The hair is dry and frizzy

Reason

> The perm was over-processed.
> The rollers used were too small.
> The perm lotion was too strong.

What to do

> Apply a restructuring conditioning treatment.
> Trim the ends to reduce the frizz.

Next time

> Take care with processing times.
> Use larger rollers.
> Use a weaker lotion.
> If you think it was the perm lotion, carry out a pre-test curl.

The curl is too loose

Reason

> The hair was not properly cleansed.
> The perm was not processed properly before neutralising.

> The neutralising wasn't carried out properly.
> The perm lotion was too weak.
> The rollers were too large.
> The roller sections were too large.

What to do

> Re-perm the hair if the condition allows.
> If not, explain to the client and arrange for them to return at a later date.

Next time

> Make a note of the reason and readdress the problem.
> If you think it was the perm lotion, carry out a pre-test curl.

The curl is too loose in one area

Reason

> This area was not processed properly before neutralising.
> This area wasn't neutralised properly.
> The rollers in this area were too large.
> The roller sections were too large.

What to do

> Re-perm this section of the hair if the condition allows.
> If not, explain to the client and arrange for them to return at a later date.

Next time

Make a note of the reason and readdress the problem.

The hair colour has lightened or changed

Reason

> The hair was porous and the peroxide in the neutraliser has lifted the colour.
> The perm lotion has reacted to a chemical.

What to do

> Ask for advice from a manager.
> Apply a toner either straightaway or after a week or so, when the hair has recovered.

Next time

> Ensure you carry out an incompatibility test.
> Avoid perming until the hair is in better condition.

Fish-hook ends

Reason
The ends of the hair were not smoothly around the roller.

What to do
Trim off where needed.

Next time
Take extra care when winding.

Finishing up

As well as being unsightly, dirty bowls, tools and part-used perm lotions and neutralisers left lying around can damage clothes and surfaces, and may even cause injury if they come into contact with skin or are ingested. They can also contaminate other products, so it's important to dispose of unused perm products and clean tools as soon as possible after use.

> Clean up any spills or dropped papers or rollers.

> Tidy the perm tray and put it away.

> Discard part-used lotions, cotton wool, and so on in the correct bin, noting that some of the packaging may be recyclable.

> Rinse perm rollers and discard used papers. Dry the rollers and put them away.

> Advise the relevant person of any stock that needs reordering.

Aftercare

Perms damage the hair and are not cheap, so it's important to advise your client on how to look after their perm.

Especially when they are new, perms can lose some of their strength and curl if they are overly stretched or straightened with brushes or styling tools, or by using heavy conditioners or styling products. For this reason, make sure that you advise your client on what to do and what not to do to take the best care of their perm.

The better care they take of their hair, the better it will look and the better it will last. Also, the better the condition, the more additional services, such as colour, they can have, and the sooner they can have another perm!

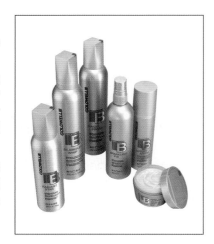

> Recommend shampoo and conditioning products that will help to repair any damage and keep the perm looking good.

> Advise them on how to look after their perm so that they don't cause it to drop or damage the hair, and what other services they should avoid.

> Show them how to style their hair and what products to use.

> Give the client advice on and show them how to use styling products and tools to get the best results.

> Inform the client how best to protect their hair from damage by heated stylers or other electrical tools, to maintain condition and keep their perm looking good.

> Let the client know how sunlight, swimming and other lifestyle activities can affect the condition and how the hair could be protected.

> Suggest additional services, such as treatments that will improve the look or their ability to maintain the style.

> Advise them when they should come back for a trim or if they need to come back for a treatment.

> Advise the client on how long they should expect their perm to last.

Finally, before they leave let the client know that if they have any problems with the perm, they can always come back to have it adjusted. Clients are often embarrassed about coming back if there is something that they are not altogether happy with, and sometimes they will even go elsewhere. So always make sure they know that it's part of the service and included in the price!

For the record...

It's important that you maintain accurate and up-to-date client records. It ensures that you can repeat the same perm if the client wishes, and provides a valuable record of the processes and chemical treatments the client has had, which is all important information that should be considered when deciding on future technical services or treatments.

It's also important to record the details of the service just in case there are any future problems that may lead to legal action. If your client has an adverse reaction to the perm and decides to sue your salon, you need to be able to prove that you carried out all the required tests, asked the appropriate questions and did everything possible to avoid a reaction. Even if the client has not told the truth or did not give you the correct information at the time, if you fail to make proper records, you will not be able to prove that you weren't at fault.

Always record the following:

> results of sensitivity or other tests

> any relevant information learned during the consultation, as it may be of importance to a future service

> date of the service

> pre-treatments and preparations

> perm service details – winding method, rod size, pre-damp, and so on

> perm lotion used – be sure to note the product name clearly

> processing – time and method

> neutralising – time and method

> personnel – who carried out the winding, lotion application and neutralising

> shampoo, conditioning and treatment products used, how they were applied and any processing information
> result – if the perm was good and if you achieved the desired result, and if the client was happy
> notes on the hairstyle
> retail products purchased
> any information that would be useful for next time.

Case study
A great career choice

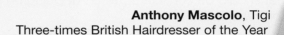

'Hairdressing is a wonderful career. It offers so many opportunities and is all about making people look good and feel good. I believe that to achieve the utmost in hairdressing you must never stop learning and sharing your ideas; it is fundamental to retaining motivation and continuing on your own hairdressing journey. I believe in sharing everything that we do – as soon as we do it! In giving others our new ideas, we are constantly pushed to improve our own work. Being part of a team is what keeps my ideas fresh and helps me to learn new techniques and create new collections – even after so many years of being in this wonderful profession.'

Anthony Mascolo, Tigi
Three-times British Hairdresser of the Year

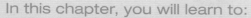

In this chapter, you will learn to:

> **cut men's hair to achieve a variety of looks**
> **cut beards and moustaches to maintain their shape**
> **dry and finish men's hair**
> **plan, agree with clients and create patterns in hair**
> **provide aftercare.**

You will be assessed against your knowledge and ability to:

1   Understand your salon's processes and procedures with regard to promoting products and services.

2   Understand your legal and health and safety responsibilities when carrying out these services.

3   Understand your personal obligations to other team members and know when and from whom you should seek advice and assistance.

4   Maintain effective and safe methods of working and carry out services in commercially viable time.

5   Consult with male clients, consider key factors and decide looks and styles that suit their individual needs.

6   Communicate effectively with male clients, using positive listening skills, body language and verbal communication.

7   Cut, dry and style men's hair, using a variety of basic cutting, drying and styling techniques.

8   Cut and shape beards and other facial hair.

9   Use and understand specific male-orientated tools, techniques and products.

10 Recognise adverse results and deal with them effectively.

11 Provide aftercare and product advice.

Introduction

What is it?

Men's hairdressing, often referred to as barbering, covers the skills and services you'll need to learn to work on male clients.

What's the difference between men and women's hairdressing?

While some barbering skills such as clipper-cutting and scissor-over-comb are occasionally used in women's hairdressing, they're more often used in men's. Other techniques like shaving and cutting facial hair are obviously only used in men's hairdressing.

Are these the only differences?

As far as technique is concerned, yes, but there are differences in hairstyles, the products used and sometimes in the way you work.

If I plan to work only in women's hairdressing, do I still need to learn about men's hairdressing?

Yes. First, you need to cover men's hairdressing to get your NVQ qualification. Second, you never know where your career will take you, and learning these skills will make you a better all-round hairdresser.

What does this chapter cover?

The cutting elements of Units GB3 and GB5 are covered, plus the styling and dressing covered in Unit GB5, as well as clipper use and patterning from Unit AH21. Additionally, this section explores the cutting and shaping of facial hair from Unit GB4.

Men's hairdressing – the misconceptions

There are two myths about men's hairdressing that seem to contradict each other: it's easy and that it's difficult!

It's a misconception that cutting men's hair is easier than cutting women's hair. You need the same level of skill and technical expertise for men's hair as you do to cut women's. It is true that cutting a five-point graduated bob is far more technically difficult than a short-layer cut, but many of today's male styles are just as complex as those for women. In fact, in some cases, even cutting simple styles on short, thinning or coarse and unruly men's hair requires a greater level of skill to get it looking good.

It's also a misconception that male-specific techniques and services, such as beard trimming, shaving and razor use, are extremely difficult. They are not at all. They are no more difficult to learn than any other skill you need to master to become a hairdresser.

These two misconceptions have led to men's hairdressing having a strange and unique position in the UK hair industry. A man's haircut is generally 25 to 30 per cent cheaper than a woman's. At the same time, there are very few places that offer shaving and male grooming services, and those that do charge a premium for them!

This situation is slowly changing. The high level of skill required in men's hairdressing is becoming more appreciated, and the cost gap between men's and women's haircuts is narrowing. Plus, an ever-increasing number of salons and barber's shops are training their staff to offer shaving and other male-specific services.

> Today, the world of men's hairdressing is just as creative, exciting, vibrant and financially rewarding as women's.

> Today, image-conscious men spend huge amounts on looking good, and a large proportion of that is spent on haircuts and hair products.

> Today, top salons and celebrity hairdressers produce amazing men's work, and use traditional barbering techniques to create exciting and innovative looks on women.

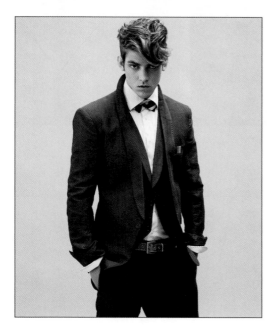

His and hers

In today's society, the boundaries between men and women are not so much fuzzy as impossible to define. Sexual equality means that in our modern society, men's and women's lifestyles are almost universally interchangeable. Women work as builders and mechanics, while men stay at home, keep house and bring up the children. Men learn to bake and do yoga, while women go to football matches and drink pints! In fashion, too, there is little difference between the genders. There are few hair and clothes fashions that are not sported by both men and women.

There are exceptions though. There are looks and styles that are strictly male and some that are strictly female. More importantly, there are nuances – subtle differences in the way that men and women dress – that define the genders. And it's these differences, more than anything else, that separate a man's haircut from a woman's.

Some of the differences between men's and women's cuts are obvious, while others are not so clear. Overleaf are some examples that show you some of the differences in men's and women's hairdressing. These are not definite rules, as many of the features can be found in either gender's haircuts. They are more general guidelines that, especially if combined, will help you to see the differences in shape, detail and finish that define men's and women's hair.

Activity

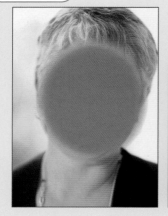 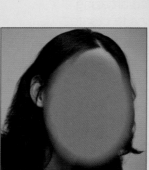 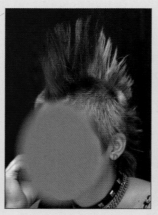 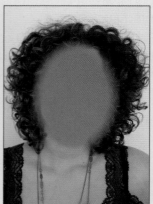

Look at the images above and see if you can decide which is a man's cut and which is a woman's.

The answers are on the next page. So how did you do?

Perimeter

> Men: The perimeter of a man's haircut is often well defined, with clean, strong lines.

> Women: The exterior lines of women's hairstyles are often shattered, rounded, tapered or soft.

Necklines

> Men: The back of men's hairlines tends to follow the natural growth shape and direction, as most men don't style the back of their hair.

> Women: Short haircuts for women will have a tailored and shaped hairline.

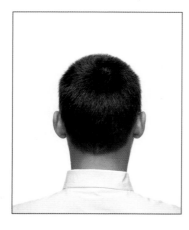 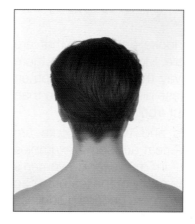

Length

> Men: Men's hair is generally shorter. Short, mid-length and long hairstyles for men will be shorter than similar styles on women.

> Women: A short haircut for a woman, even a crop, will rarely be as short as a man's crop, and there are few men who will have hair longer than their shoulders, whereas women and girls often have hair of that length.

Volume

> Men: Generally men's hairstyles do not have much volume. If they do, it's usually only in one key area.

> Women: Volume is more important in women's styles and tends to be overall and balanced.

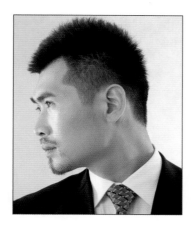 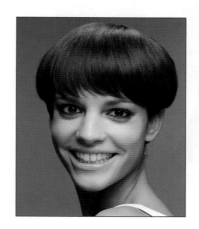

Activity

Activity answers

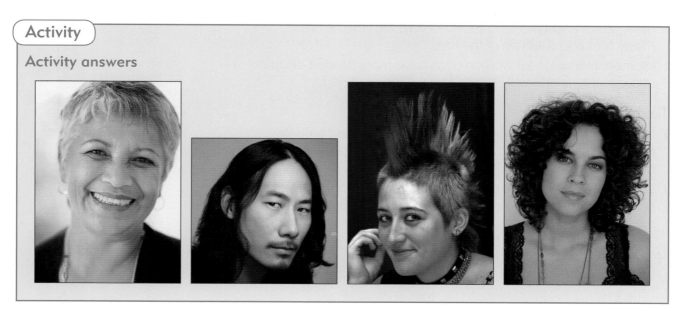

Shape

> Men: While it may be accentuated in some areas, the shape of men's hairstyles tends to follow the natural head shape.

> Women: Women can wear hairstyles with more accentuated and stronger head and anti-head shapes.

Sides

> Men: Men's haircuts will use sideburns to add feature to a haircut or to accentuate the face shape.

> Women: While length around the ear is used to add softness, women's haircuts do not accentuate hair that grows on the face.

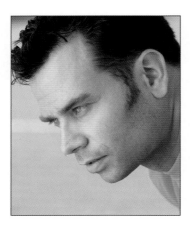 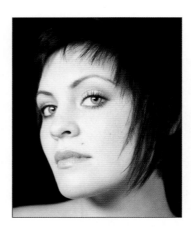

Direction

> Men: Men's hairstyles tend to work more with the natural movement and direction of the hair.

> Women: Hairstyles for women often have more defined direction and one that is artificially created by cutting or styling.

Texture

> Men: Very few men's styles are universally sleek and smooth. Most men's looks rely on natural or unstructured texture and movement.

> Women: Many women's styles have a uniform, smooth, sleek finish. Even messy styles will still retain an air of polish.

Colour

> Men: Hair colour in men is rarely all over, but tends to be specific to an area or spot application. Generally, bleaches and lighter colours are used to add highlights and feature to a haircut.

> Women: Women's hair colouring tends to have either a natural finish or is an all-over, strong, rich or vibrant colour, to give a style brightness, sheen and vitality.

Communication and language

As well as subtle differences in hairstyles, there is also a difference in the language used in men's and women's hairdressing. Most hairdressing terms are generic, but there are some that tend to relate to one gender more than another. For example, a female client would be keen to have a conditioner if you told her it would make her hair 'silky-smooth, soft and bouncy'. A male client is more likely to respond to 'shiny' or 'manageable'.

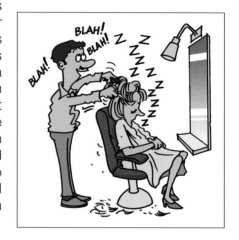

It may sound obvious, but there are also differences in how you talk to male and female clients – not so much in the way you address them, but in the topics of conversation you choose and even whether you talk at all! Again, there are no set rules, but while some clients will enjoy a good natter while they're having their hair done, others will want to sit quietly and read a magazine. Part of your skill as a hairdresser is to know not only when a client wants to talk and when they don't, but also to be able to talk about and discuss subjects that they would be interested in. Most male clients are not going to be interested in talking about shopping and make-up! This doesn't mean you need to know about football teams or which spin-bowler should be taken on the next Ashes tour, but you do have to be prepared to listen and take an interest. Remember, this is their time, and as well as making them look good, listening and taking an interest in them will make them feel good too!

Tools

Most of the tools you use in men's hairdressing will be the same as those used in women's hairdressing: scissors, combs, brushes, dryers, and so on. (Details of these can be found in Units GH12 and GH10.)

There are some tools, however, that you will use more often or will find useful in men's hairdressing. Most of the tools can be used on both wet and dry hair.

Large comb

This is a larger version of a cutting comb, with broader, thicker teeth, used for scissor-over-comb cutting, where the hair is to be cut short, with a light, loose finish.

Cut-throat razor

This is an open-bladed razor with either a sharp edge or replaceable blades. It is used for face and hairline shaving and razor cutting.

Shaper razor

This is a covered, hand-held razor, used for thinning, shaping and razor cutting. It can be used on wet or dry hair.

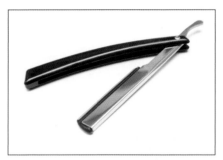
Cut-throat razor

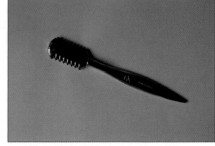
Shaper razor

Clippers

Corded or cordless, electrically powered clippers are used for general clipper-cutting and edging. A toothed upper blade passes side to side across a stationary lower blade, clipping off hair that goes between the teeth. Most have adjustable blades and guards of various lengths, for cutting hair at uniform lengths. They can be used on damp or dry hair; the hair should not be saturated.

Clippers should be checked before each use to see that the blades are level (parallel) and should be adjusted if not. Most clippers have a small screw that holds the blades in place, and this can be undone to allow for the blades to be realigned. This screw can also be undone to remove the blade for cleaning or to replace it when worn. Always check the manufacturer's cleaning and maintenance instructions.

Clipper guards

These are tapered plastic attachments that fit over the blades of the clippers and restrict the length of hair that can be cut. Clipper guards are measured either by number (the higher the number, the longer the hair) or in actual length (millimetres).

Always make sure that you are using the right guard for the clipper and that it is properly attached before you start work.

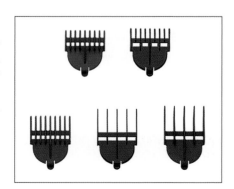

Trimmers

Similar to clippers, trimmers are usually cordless and smaller, with a narrower cutting head. These are used for edging and finishing, but can also be used for trimming eyebrow, ear and nose hair. They are generally used on dry hair, but can be used on damp hair. Trimmers are levelled, clean and maintained in much the same way as clippers.

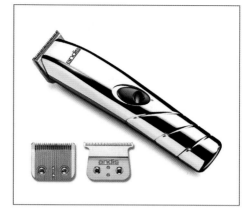

Shaving tools

There are also tools specifically used for shaving services, such as soaps, shaving brushes, strops and skin products. As shaving is covered in the next level of hairdressing, these are not covered in this book.

Note: Make sure that clippers and trimmers are cleaned and maintained. Use clipper oil to keep the blades working smoothly and use a small brush (usually supplied with the clippers) to brush and clean off hair between clients. Always follow the manufacturer's instructions on cleaning and replacing blades. Never use clippers with damaged wires or that are not in good working order.

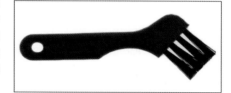

Products

As with tools, most hair products, such as colours, perms, shampoos, conditioners and styling products, can be used for both men and women. Today, though, there is an ever-increasing number of male-specific styling ranges on the market from professional hair product companies. As well as having male-orientated packaging and fragrances, male-specific products are designed to work with male hairstyles and finishes and/or particular male hair issues, such as thinning.

While there are no set rules, below are some general differences between men's and women's products.

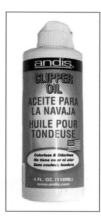

Shampoos

As well as having fragrances more appealing to men, male-orientated shampoos often have stronger detergents. This is because men often don't wash their hair every day or work in dusty, dirty environments. Also, it helps to remove the build-up of the waxy, stronger male styling products.

Conditioners

Conditioning products designed for use by men are generally lighter than those for women. This is mainly because men's hair, being short, with less chemical processes and less likely to have heat damage from dryers and stylers, usually needs less damage repair.

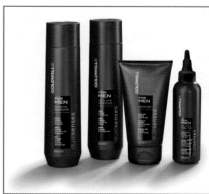

Styling products

Women tend to use products as a styling aid, using them together with brushes, dryers and stylers to create their look. Men tend not to, instead using the product itself to form and shape the look. This is why men's ranges have more waxes, moulding and styling pastes. In addition, gels and mousses will often be stronger than their counterparts for women, to enable men to create the look they want without the use of a dryer.

Consultation pointers for male clients

The consultation process for male clients is the same as that for female clients. (In-depth details of this process can be found in Unit G7.) That said, when carrying out a consultation on a male client, there are a few particular things that you should pay more attention to.

Thinning hair and receding hairlines

Men can start to lose their hair from as young as 17 and can be very sensitive about it. Most male hair loss is caused by male pattern baldness (androgenic alopecia) and affects the hair in three ways.

> Receding front hairline: the hair stops growing on the front hairline, often more so at the temples, slowly receding towards the crown, increasing the size of the forehead.

> Balding crown: the hair around the crown thins or stops growing, resulting in a bald patch. The size of this patch can continue to grow or it can reach a certain size and then stop increasing.

> Thinning: the overall amount of hair reduces, so that the hair becomes thinner. This can happen over the entire head or be concentrated in particular areas.

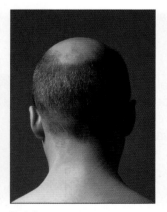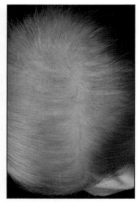

Receding front hairline   Balding crown   Thinning hair

Men with male pattern baldness will lose hair in one or more of these ways. The condition is hereditary and, while there are many remedies on the market that may ease or slow hair loss and may even encourage some growth, there is currently no cure. There are medical procedures where clumps of hair follicles are transplanted into the bald areas, as well as other specialised treatments that are available.

(Other causes of hair loss are covered in Unit G7, which looks at conditions and infections of the hair, skin and scalp.)

Your principal role as a hairdresser will be to help create looks and styles on your male clients that disguise or compensate for hair loss. It's important that you assess the amount of hair loss and the client's feelings about it during the consultation process. Some clients will be unconcerned about their hair loss, while others will be very self-conscious about it. This will have a bearing on the way you discuss style options with the client and the look you eventually decide on.

Sometimes these consultations can be difficult and uncomfortable. You may have a client who has been wearing a style that they believe is disguising their hair loss, when in fact it is actually drawing attention to it. In these cases, you need to be very tactful in pointing out the flaws in their current style and suggesting how a different approach might be a better option. Often, in these cases, pictures and examples of men who have made the same style choices can help. It is important never to rush the client in these situations; give them time to make up their own mind about how to proceed. It may be necessary to approach the change in stages, rather than in one dramatic step. Remember, you are the professional; they are looking to you for advice and guidance.

Styling and aftercare

When deciding on a hairstyle, it's important to bear in mind the amount of aftercare your male client is prepared or likely to do. As men generally don't use dryers and stylers to create their looks at home, you need to ensure that they will be able to recreate the look themselves.

You can get a good idea about the amount of time a male client is likely to spend on his hair just by looking at him. If his overall look is well put together, with attention to detail, he spends time on his appearance. If the opposite is true, he'll be looking for a style that's quick and easy to manage.

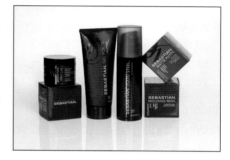

Ask what the client does after they wash their hair, and what products they use, as this will be a key factor in the time they spend on their hair. All of this will enable you to make a decision on the style to suit the client.

Lifestyle

As in all consultations, it's important to pay attention to lifestyle. There are still rules about dress code that men have to follow that women don't, so you need to take into account the work they do. Plus, many of the sports and activities more often enjoyed by men may influence their chosen style.

> Do they work in a dirty environment, meaning that their hair needs to be washed hard every day?

> Do they have a job with rules about hair length or style?

> Do they do sports where long hair would be a hindrance, such as swimming?

> Do they have a hobby or a pastime, like playing in a band, where they need their hairstyle to be versatile?

Note: While women also have facial piercings, they might not be so obvious on a male client and could be hidden by a beard or sideburns. Take extra care when dealing with male customers and check if they have any piercings that might get in the way of your work, as these may have to be removed.

Preparation

Safety first!

Hairdressing scissors are both sharp and pointed and can easily cause injury, and cut-throat razors and their blades are particularly dangerous. It's easy to accidentally cut or stab yourself or someone else with either of these items, so always take great care when using and storing them.

Scissors

> When not in use, scissors should always be securely stored in a pouch or case.
> Never leave your scissors lying around on trolleys or counters.
> When carrying scissors, carry them safely within your hand.
> Make a note of any moles on your client's hairline and take care when cutting round the ears.
> Most of all, when cutting, make sure you stay focused on what you are doing, so you don't cut yourself or the client.

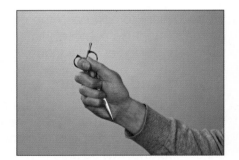

Razors

> When not in use, razors should always be secured closed.
> Never leave razors open or leave blades lying around.
> Use a new or sterilised razor for each client.
> Be careful about any moles or lumps on the skin when shaving the neck.
> Always use water or a shaving agent when using a razor on the skin.
> Dispose of used razors correctly. Never throw them in the bin!
> If your salon uses disposable razor blades, it should have a sharp objects bin to comply with health and safety regulations. It will usually be a small, solid, yellow box that has instructions on how it should be disposed of once full. You should not use disposable blades unless there is a system in place to deal with them once they are finished with.

Good preparation will make the task of cutting hair easier for you and will therefore enable you to produce the best possible result.

Activity Practise asking male friends and family about their work and lifestyle. Each time, make a list of the things that would influence their haircut and why. If you can, carry this out in class or with a fellow trainee. Compare results and see if you come up with the same things.

The client

> Ensure that the client is gowned to protect their clothes.
> The client's hair should be shampooed to remove any grease, dirt or product build-up, and should have been conditioned if needed.
> Ensure that the hair is towel-dried so that there is no dripping water.
> The hair should be combed through and tangle-free, to make it easier to take sections and work. (You may need to gently towel-dry again after combing through.)
> A towel or a cutting collar should be placed round the client's shoulders. (You may also place a strip of cotton wool inside the client's collar to stop hair falling down their neck.)
> Make sure the client is sitting upright and is comfortable.
> Ensure that any earrings are removed and that other jewellery is safely out of the way.
> Always ask if the client has any allergies to certain products and check the scalp for abrasions or sores.

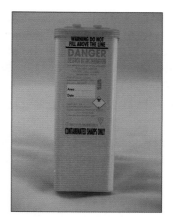

You

> Ensure that your hands are clean.
> You may need to wear an apron or protective gown if the hair has been coloured recently.
> Make sure that none of your jewellery will get in the way while you are working.
> Make sure that you have all the right tools and that they are clean and fit for purpose.
> Make sure that you know how to work safely, with the correct posture, and that you are wearing clothes and shoes suitable for the service you are carrying out.

Male-specific hairdressing techniques

Generally, men's and women's hairdressing uses the same techniques and skills. There are a few, however, that tend to be either more commonly or exclusively used on men. To pass the NVQ Level 2 in men's hairdressing, you will need to know about the following techniques.

Thinning – removing volume and thickness from hair

Although widely used in women's hairdressing, thinning is a technique associated with cutting men's hair. Thinning hair is used to reduce the amount of hair without changing the shape of the style. It is used to reduce bulk and give more control to thick, wiry hair.

Thinning hair is done either by using thinning scissors (see the scissor section on page 236) or manually by using normal scissors. Thinning scissors have a toothed blade that cuts generally 30 to 40 per cent of the hair of a section. Usually when thinning, hair is cut approximately 2 cm or more from the scalp. (If you cut hair any shorter it can actually add volume, by the shorter hairs sticking up and holding up the longer hairs.) Thinning scissors can also be used to soften a heavy fringe or hairline.

If you are using standard scissors to thin hair, this is done in one of two ways:

> Pointing – using the end of the scissors to chip out hair, either at the ends or in the mid-lengths of a section.

> Weaving – using the point of the scissors to weave out hair from a section and cut it to a short length.

Always take care when thinning hair not to cut too thin. Continually check the look and fall of the hair as you work.

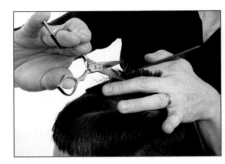

Pointing

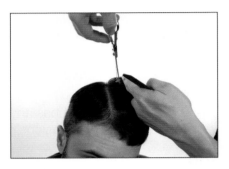

Weaving

Cut hair using basic barbering techniques – using a razor to clean the neck and finish the haircut step by step

1 Make sure your razor has a new blade or has been sterilised.

2 Do not open your razor until you are ready to work.

3 Place an additional towel on the shoulder of the client (to use to clean the blade). Also, have clean, damp cotton wool to hand, in case you nick the skin.

4 Use cotton wool to moisten the neck with warm water. **Note**: Some salons don't wet the neck, instead opting either to use talc or to shave the neck dry. Using water or a shaving soap solution will make the process easier and more comfortable for the client. You should always check your salon's working practice guidelines.

5 Beginning at the edge of the haircut, stretch and hold the skin taut with one hand, and, with the other hand, hold the razor at 30 to 45° to the skin, gently sliding the blade across the surface of the skin in short, smooth motions (a).

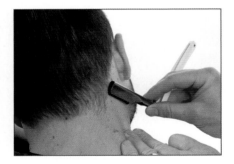

(a)

6 Wipe the blade clean on the towel after each section.

7 Continue working down the neck, re-moistening the skin as necessary (b).

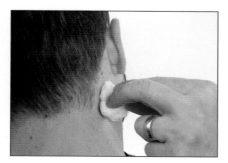

(b)

8 Take care to avoid catching any moles or bumps in the skin.

9 Once complete, close your razor and put it down in a safe place.

10 Clean the neck with moist, cold cotton wool before dabbing it dry.

11 Apply a post-shave cream or balm (c).

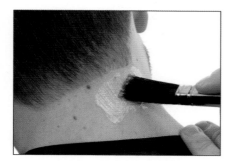

(c)

12 Sterilise or carefully dispose of disposable razor blades.

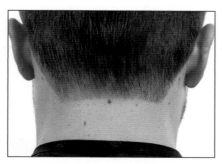

Note: If you cut the skin:

> for small nicks and scratches, apply pressure with damp cotton wool and hold until the bleeding stops

> apply antiseptic cream and a plaster if needed

> for deeper cuts and wounds, immediately apply pressure and call for assistance

> follow the instructions of the first aider.

Always involve your salon's first aider and enter the incident in the accident book.

Clipper use – cutting and edging hair with clippers

Clippers work in the same fashion as hedge trimmers, in that one set of teeth slides across the top of another, slicing off any hair that falls between them. Clippers are also different from scissors in that once they are turned on, they continue cutting until they are turned off. So you must always be aware where the clippers are when you are using them, as it's very easy to cut off more than you want to!

Clippers can be adjusted or used with guards to cut hair at different lengths. Most clippers have a lever that lets you vary the distance between the blades on the unit itself, varying the length form short to very short. The removable guards keep the clipper blades a set distance away from the scalp, so that the hair is all cut to a uniform length. You may have heard crop haircuts being referred to by number, with a number one being the shortest and number four being a fairly long crop. This relates to the size number of the guard. While not all clippers have numbered guards, in men's hairdressing, many hairdressers and clients still use this method to explain or determine the length the client would like. For example, number one at the back, number two at the sides and number four on top would be a haircut that was very short at the back, slightly longer at the sides and with a longish crop on the top.

Here are some cropped haircuts showing the approximate length relevant to each number.

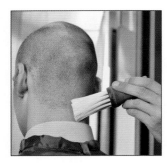

Number one

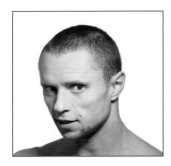

Number two

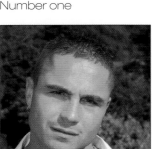

Number three

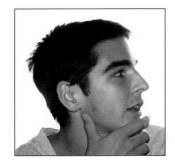

Number four

Clippers are used to cut universal-length crops, cutting scissor-over-comb and for edging.

Cut hair using basic barbering techniques – creating and finishing men's hair using clippers step by step

1 Make sure that the clippers are clean and in good working order. If they are cordless, make sure that they are charged.

2 Check that the cut-length adjustment is at the correct setting or that you have attached the correct guard for the length.

3 Remember that, unlike scissors, clippers will cut continually, so always ensure that you are in control of the cutting edge.

Universal crop and general hair cutting with clippers

1 Working with a guard, begin at the hairline and move the clippers up the head, through the hair and out in a smooth, arching motion (a).

2 When working without a guard, use your comb to control the cutting length (b). Work in the same manner, ensuring that he clippers are in continual motion. This enables you to compensate for unevenness in the head shape.

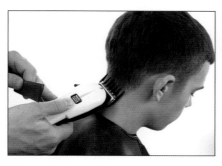

(a)

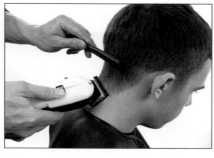

(b)

3 Work up and around the head until the desired length is achieved.

Edging and finishing – square and rounded hard lines

1 Turn the clippers over and use the blade edge to cut sharp lines, noting that this will remove all the hair through to the scalp. Take care not to press, as it may cut the skin.

2 For straight lines, start in the centre and work outwards, keeping the line straight to the edge of the hairline (c).

3 For curved lines, pick a point on the outside hairline, approximately level with the bottom of the ears. Starting in the centre, work in a soft round curve, from the base of the nape up to this point on either side (d).

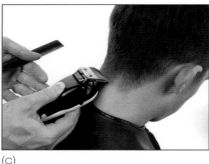
(c)

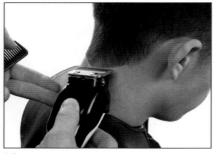
(d)

4 Keep lines uniform and even, and check for balance.

5 Without a guard and on the shortest setting, working from below, shave up to the pre-cut line to remove all straggly hairs.

Edging and finishing – tapered, blended and faded lines

1 Working without a guard, work up from below to the hairline, removing all straggly hairs.

2 Place the fine end of a comb in at the hairline as a guard and work the clippers up and onto it (e).

3 As you move further up into the haircut, slowly increase the length of the hair by moving the comb away from the head (f).

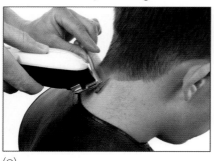
(e)

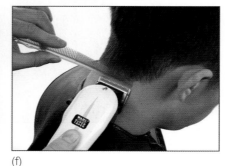
(f)

4 Begin to use the thick end of the comb to further increase the length.

Haircut and outline shapes

Today, most haircut and outline shapes are unisex, so the techniques and looks you create on men's hair will also be used on women's hair. As some shapes are more often found in men's hairdressing, they feature in Unit GB3 of the NVQ Level 2. These looks and shapes are as follows.

Outline shape – the overall shape of the perimeter of the haircut

> Natural – a shape that follows or uses the natural growth patterns of the hair. Natural outline shapes vary in length, but they are cut so that the hair falls naturally.

> Created – the hair is cut into a specific shape, overriding the natural growth patterns. Created shapes also vary in length, but tend to have straight lines and a more tailored, symmetrical appearance.

> ## Top Tip
>
> Listen to the sound of your clippers before you use them. They should vibrate lightly and give off a low, smooth hum. If they are noisy or are vibrating a lot, they may need oil, cleaning or the blades readjusting. The blades may even be damaged, so check thoroughly before use. You may want to check them on your arm hair.

> Tapered – a tapered shape, as its name implies, gets gradually shorter from a longer upper part of the haircut, tapering out towards the outline. Tapered haircuts are generally short.

Neckline shape – the way the haircut is finished at the back of the head at the nape

> Tapered – the hair is cut to 'fade', so that there is little or no defined line. Tapered necklines are short and often follow the natural growth patterns, but are usually tidied and refined for neatness. Tapered lines are created using clippers or scissor-over-comb.

> Square – the baseline at the back of the haircut is cut across in a straight line, with all the hair below the line removed to make it more defined. Square lines ignore the natural growth patterns at the nape and create their own strong line. Square lines can be cropped short or longer, but they are always uniform. Square lines are created using clipper-edging or freehand scissor-cutting.

> Rounded – rounded or curved nape-line shapes are softer than the harsh, square lines and more structured than the tapered line. Curving up from the centre, the rounded line also has all the hair below it removed and can be close-cropped or longer. Square lines are created using clipper-edging or freehand scissor-cutting.

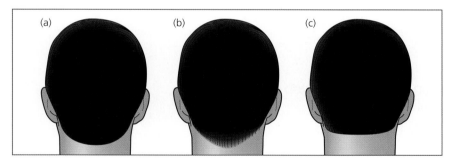

Neckline shapes: (a) Rounded; (b) Tapered; (c) Square

What to consider before starting your haircut

> Look and lifestyle – how will the haircut match the client's lifestyle, in both look and manageability?

> Hair density – how will you take into account the hair's thickness? Is there any male pattern baldness and how will you deal with it?

> Hair texture – what is the texture of the hair and what cutting techniques and products will best suit it?

> Head shape – how will the haircut match or counter the client's head and face shape?

> Growth patterns – how does the hair grow in different areas and what will you do to work with or counteract these patterns?

> Condition – how will the condition and elasticity affect the way you will cut the hair?

> Jewellery – will any piercings, earrings or necklaces get in the way of your work, and should these be removed for safety?

> Scalp and skin health – are there any cuts or bruises that you need to avoid, and are the scalp and skin healthy and free from infection?

Basic men's cutting techniques – uniform (round) layer step by step

Creating a stylish short men's haircut by combining layering and scissor-over-comb techniques.

1 Section off the top of the head, from the recession line on each side of the front hairline to the crown.

2 Within this panel, take a vertical section from the crown to the front hairline. Lift the section vertically at a 90° angle from the head and cut to the desired length from the crown forwards (a).

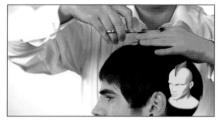

(a)

3 Starting at the crown, take a section across the main top section and cut both sides to match the guideline (b).

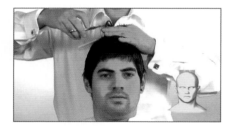

(b)

4 Continue towards the front hairline. Once complete, cross check the section for accuracy.

5 Move onto the front right panel. Take a section from the top down the side. Hold at a 90° angle and, following the curve of the head, use the previously cut top section as a guide (c).

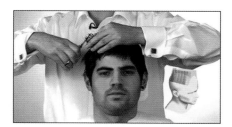

(c)

6 Continue working in this way, taking sections back along the side of the head until you reach the crown.

7 Cross check by using horizontal sections.

8 Repeat on the other side of the head.

9 Once complete, compare both sides and review the overall shape.

10 Begin work on the back and, as with the sides, take a section from the crown down and follow the angle of the head and the guideline. Work from the centre forwards on both sides until you reach the previously cut front sections (d).

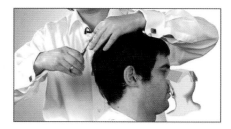

(d)

11 Once complete, cross check the upper part of the haircut for accuracy and balance.

12 **Scissor-over-combing:** Beginning on the lower right side, take a large toothed comb to allow the hair to move freely in the comb (e). Note: the thickness of the teeth will determine the length of the hair.

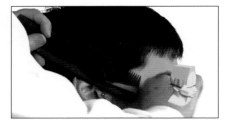

(e)

13 Placing your comb in at the hairline, begin working upwards, aiming for the guideline of the previously cut upper side section. Work in small sections at a time, ensuring both the scissors and comb are kept in constant motion to avoid cutting 'steps'.

14 Continually go over each small section until the hair is even and blended with the upper section.

15 Begin to work backwards around the head, continuing to blend the sections with the upper and recently cut lower side sections.

16 Once you have reached the back of the head, begin work on the other side of the head, cutting the hair in the same fashion.

17 With both sides complete, starting at the nape, work up the back towards the previously cut crown area, blending together the two side sections (f).

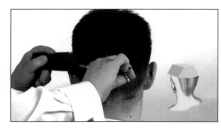

(f)

18 Once complete, review the shape, the weight, the way the hair is falling and do a final cross check.

19 Finally, use pointing to texturise the hair cut and trim and tidy the hairline (g).

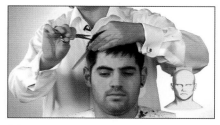

(g)

20 Brush down, apply styling products and dry into shape.

21 When dry, review the look and use pointing to soften and refine.

22 Apply finishing products.

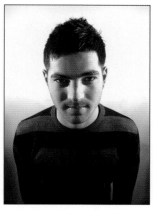

Basic men's cutting techniques – graduation and scissor-over-comb step by step

Creating a modern man's haircut using graduation and scissor-over-comb.

1 Beginning at the side of the head, take a horizontal section from the front hairline to the top of the ear. Comb the rest of the hair cleanly out of the way (use sectioning clips if needed) (a).

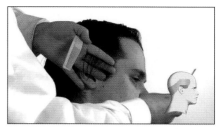

(a)

2 Cut the hair between the fingers close to the head.

3 Bring a finger-width section down from above and cut to the same line, ensuring you hold the hair at the same elevation.

4 Continue working up the head to just below the recession line.

5 Take a section from just behind the ear, diagonally across the back of the head to just below the occipital bone (b).

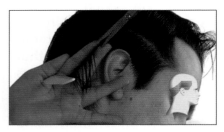

(b)

6 Using the previously cut hair as a guide, take finger-sized sections from this larger section and continue to cut the hair in the fingers following the section line.

7 Continue to take sections through this panel, ensuring you cut the hair at the same level of elevation. Comb the hair flat to check your graduation is even.

8 Now that a guide from front to back has been established, working from the front hairline, bring sections down to this line. Continue cutting, working back around the head.

9 As you work around the back, follow the diagonal line, working towards the opposite side of the nape (c).

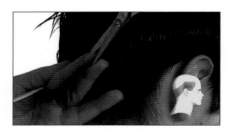

(c)

10 Continue around the side and back of the head, bringing hair down to this line until you reach the top section (level with the recession line). Check continuously for balance and smooth graduation.

11 Now begin on the opposite side, working in the same way. Check your new guideline to make sure it's even with the first (d).

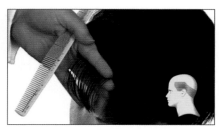

(d)

12 Work as before, first cutting above the ear, then creating the back guideline before continuing to cut the sides and back, working across to the opposite side of the nape as before. Continually stop to check the balance and line of the graduation.

13 Once the sides are complete, take a vertical section from the crown to the front hairline. Lift the section at a 90° angle from the head and cut to the desired length from the front to the crown (e).

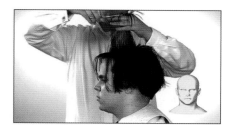

(e)

14 Starting in front of the crown, take a section across the main top section and cut both sides following the guideline.

15 Continue towards the front hairline following until the top section. Once complete, check the section for accuracy.

16 Use the same method to cut the crown area.

17 Blend the sides by starting at the crown and bringing all the hair up at a 90° angle from each side until there is no more hair (f).

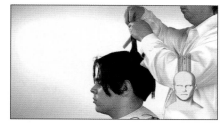

(f)

18 Refine the back section by holding the hair horizontally to smooth out the graduation and remove the corner of weight.

19 Check that the graduation is uniform throughout the sides and back and that the haircut is balanced.

20 **Cutting the fringe:** If the fringe is too long for the client, take a 2 cm deep section from the parting across the front hairline and clip away the rest of the hair. Pull down and cut between the fingers using the eyebrows as a guide.

21 Blend the end of the section with the side graduation (g).

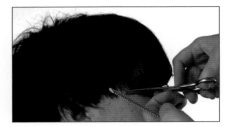

(g)

22 Bring the remainder of the hair down to this line and cut to the same length, elevating the final few sections to reduce the weight.

23 Refine the outside line. Hold down the ear and cut the perimeter line following the hairline and use scissors or clippers to tidy the neck and sideburns (h).

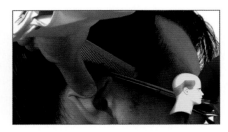

(h)

24 Finally, use pointing to texturise the haircut.

25 Brush down, apply styling products and dry into shape.

26 Once dry, review the look and use pointing to soften and refine.

27 Apply finishing products.

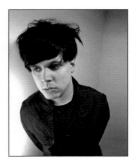

Finishing off

When you have finished your haircut, you have checked it thoroughly and you are happy, always take time to brush down the client carefully.

> Gently ruffle the hair to shake out any loose clippings.

> Using a soft (neck) brush, gently brush the client's face and ears and neck.

> Taking care not to let hair fall down the client's neck, remove the towel or cutting collar and shake off.

> Brush the neck area again before replacing the towel and/or the collar.

> You may want to give the hair a rinse at the backwash to remove all the loose hair.

Advise the client on how you will style and finish their hair and the products you will use.

Housekeeping

Once you have finished your haircut, help to keep the salon clean and safe by:

> cleaning the workstation and sweeping up as soon as possible

> putting hair clippings, dirty towels and gowns in the appropriate bin

> cleaning and sterilising tools ready for the next client.

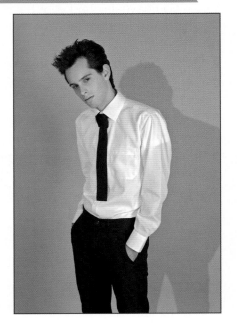

Introduction

What is it?

This is how to dry and finish men's hair after a haircut.

What's the difference between drying and finishing men's and women's hair?

As far as tools and preparations are concerned, there is no difference. You will use many of the same tools and techniques covered in Unit GH10. The main difference is the looks and textures you use to finish men's hair.

There isn't much to it, is there?

A common misconception is that men's hair needs little or no finishing. In fact, it does. There is not a great deal more to learn than what's covered in Unit GH10, but what there is, is very important to know.

Although many men's haircuts have a casual feel, that doesn't mean that they are unfinished. Many young hairdressers make the mistake of thinking that men's hair doesn't need to be dried and finished with the same care and attention as women's hair; it does.

Finishing men's hair is a skill that's not to be underestimated. Casual looks don't mean a casual approach. Often, it's quite hard to get a style to 'look' as though it's unstyled and dishevelled.

The main difference between finishing men's and women's hair is texture. The finish on women's hair concentrates on shine, smoothness and movement. With men's hair, texture and shape are the primary goals.

When finishing men's hair, there are some key points to remember.

> Avoid creating overall volume and root lift. Height and volume are usually concentrated in one specific area, like the fringe.

> Don't 'roll' the hair when drying, as this will create bend. Keep the ends straight and flat.

> Keep the sides and the back of the haircut flat to the head.

> Work with the dryer on a slow setting, so that the hair is not blown around too much.

> Work with the hair's growth patterns, allowing it to fall naturally.

> Use round brushes to straighten and smooth hair, but, unlike with women's hair, don't lift or roll.

> Use flat paddle brushes to push hair around the head into shape, to add more polish and finish than finger-drying.

> Constantly look at the shape, and if it's beginning to get too 'big', damp it down and start again.

> Only use product to enhance the finish and texture, not to create it.

Tools

The tools you need to blow-dry and finish men's hair are exactly the same as you would use for women's. (See Unit GH10.) What you may find is that certain tools, like the vent brush and paddle brush, are used more often. Also, you will find that in finishing men's hair, you use your fingers a great deal.

Preparation

During the consultation process you will already have decided on the final finished look. Now you need to prepare the client and gather the correct tools and products to create the look.

What to consider before starting to blow-dry

> Look and lifestyle – how will the finished look match the client's lifestyle, in terms of both look and manageability?

> Hair density – how will you take into account the hair's thickness? Is there any male pattern baldness and how will you deal with it?

> Hair texture – what is the texture of the hair and what drying techniques and products will best suit it?

> Head shape – how will the haircut match or counter the head and face shape?

> Growth patterns – how does the hair grow in different areas and what will you do to work with or counteract these patterns?

> Condition – how will the condition and elasticity affect the way you will cut the hair?

> Jewellery – will any piercings, earrings or necklaces get in the way of your work, and should any of these be removed for safety?

> Scalp and skin health – are there any cuts or bruises that you need to avoid, and are the scalp and skin healthy and free from infection?

The client

> Ensure that the client is gowned to protect their clothes, and that there is a towel round their shoulders to absorb any dripping water.

> The client's hair should be shampooed to remove any grease, dirt or product build-up, and should have been conditioned if needed.

> Blot, squeeze and gently towel-dry the hair well, to remove excess water. Try not to rub the hair too much, as this will roughen the cuticle and make the hair harder to manage.

> The hair should be combed through and tangle-free. (You may need to gently blot the ends again after combing through.)

> Make sure that the client is sitting upright and is comfortable.

> Ensure that any earrings and facial piercings are removed and that other jewellery is safely out of the way.

> Always ask if the client has any allergies to certain products, and check the scalp for abrasions or sores.

You

> Ensure that your hands are clean.

> You may need to wear an apron or protective gown if the hair has been coloured recently.

> Make sure that none of your jewellery will get in the way while you are working.

> Make sure that you have all the right tools and that they are clean and fit for purpose.

> Make sure that you have selected the correct styling products for the client's hair type and the desired result.

> Make sure that you know how to work safely, with the correct posture, and that you are wearing clothes and shoes suitable for the service you are carrying out.

Styling products

Women tend to use products as a styling aid, using them together with brushes, dryers and stylers to create their look. Men tend not to, instead using the product itself to form and shape the look. This is why men's ranges have more waxes, moulding and styling pastes. In addition, gels and mousses will often be stronger than their counterparts for women, to enable men to create the look they want without the use of a dryer.

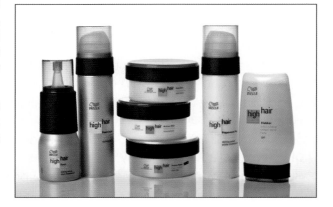

The styling products you use will depend on the client's hair and the result you are trying to achieve. Four simple factors should help you to decide on the best products for your chosen style:

> condition

> volume

> hold

> texture.

Condition

Consider the condition of the client's hair and how it will be affected by the styling methods you are planning to use.

> Will a leave-in conditioner make styling easier?

> Are you planning to use hot curling irons, straighteners or stylers? And, if so, should you use a heat protector?

Volume

Consider the type of hair, the thickness and the amount of volume your style should have.

> Does the style require any root lift in key areas? If so, how much, and would a mousse or spray gel be best?

> If you want to keep the hair flat and smooth, will you need a frizz or volume reducer?

Hold

Think about the hair type, length and condition, and how it will hold the style. Also, consider how much movement the style should have and how long the client needs the style to last.

> Is the hair soft or fine, and will it need a gel or wax to hold the style?

> Are you dramatically changing the direction or texture of the hair, and, if so, do you need a gel or moulding paste to keep it in place?

> Is the hair heavy, do you need to use a mousse or styling lotion to stop the weight pulling out the style?

> Will you need a hairspray to hold the finished look and help to protect against moisture?

Texture

Finally, think about the texture of the hair and the finished style. Think about whether you need to change the texture of the hair, and what texture you want the look to have.

> Do you need to control frizz, curl or flyaway hair?

> Will you need to create or accentuate detail, using gel, moulding paste or styling spray?

> Will you need a wax or pomade to break up and add texture to the ends?

You should also bear in mind how you plan to style the hair – finger-drying or using a brush – as some products work better with certain styling methods.

Note: Be careful when using waxes and moulding pastes during styling, as they can make the hair heavy and greasy. Use these types of products at the end and use them sparingly, adding a little at a time until the desired look is achieved.

Finger-dry men's hair step by step

Finishing a man's haircut using the fingers.

1 Ensure that the client is gowned, with a towel round their shoulders, and that the hair is cleansed and conditioned. Towel-dry the hair to remove excess water and add styling products.

2 With the dryer on slow and on a low heat, begin to push the hair round the head to remove the excess moisture, taking care not to lift the hair where you want it to remain flat (a). Check that the heat of the dryer is okay for the client.

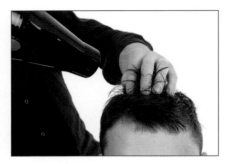

(a)

3 Following your hands with the dryer, push the hair backwards, keeping it flat against the sides of the head.

4 Continue working towards the nape, pushing the hair from side to side, keeping it flat to the head (b).

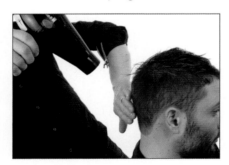

(b)

5 Move up the sides, gently beginning to lift the hair slightly away from the head, so that the airflow gets to the roots (c).

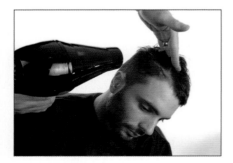

(c)

6 Do the same at the back of the head above the occipital bone, to create a light anti-head shape, taking care not to lift the hair too much.

7 From the front, lift the hair so that the airflow gets into the roots and pull the hair gently forward. As you release, allow the dryer to blow the hair up, to give a little more height and movement.

8 At the front of the hair, over-accentuate the lift. Hold the hair up and forward while drying the roots. Keep your hands and the airflow moving through the hair.

9 To add texture on the top of the head, grasp a handful of hair, heat with the dryer and hold until cool. Release and loosen with the dryer and your fingers.

10 Continue through the top.

11 Use the dryer to blow through the hair to loosen the style (d).

12 Use a wax or moulding paste to smooth the sides and the back.

13 Finally, use your fingertips to scrunch product onto the top of the hair and pull out tendrils (e).

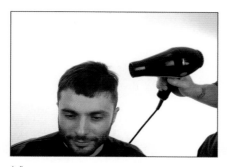

(d)

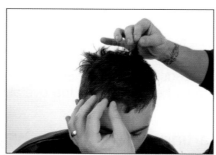

(e)

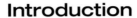

Introduction

What is it?

It's removing hair to create individual designs.

How is it done?

Usually with clippers – hair is shaved off so the skin of the scalp shows through the hair.

How long does it last?

Around two weeks, depending on how dark the hair is and how fast it grows. Once the hair starts to grow back, the pattern will begin to disappear.

Creating designs in cropped hair is a great way of individualising your haircut and showing your artistic flair. Patterns in hair can be as simple as 'tram-lines' – parallel lines that run down the sides of the head – or more intricate designs with swirls. Some talented hairdressers can create amazing, intricate pictures and wording.

Preparation

In order to create patterns, the hair needs to be short enough to make the design visible. The hair should be clean, with the overall haircut complete and finished.

What to consider before starting

> Design – what pattern are you going to create? Discuss the options with the client and consider their look and lifestyle. Use a pen and paper if needed to draw the design you are going to create. Never start a design unless you know what you are going to do!

> Head shape, scalp and hairlines – look at the shape of the head and how the hair grows around the hairline. Also look for any bald patches or scars, as you may need to take these into account when deciding on a pattern. Make sure you check each side of the head if the pattern will be on both sides. Also check the scalp for any sores or abrasions.

> How to do it – what will you use to create the pattern? You may not be able to create fine detail with large clippers. If the clippers or trimmers are cordless, are they fully charged?

> Your ability – can you actually create the design? Don't try to create a design unless you know you can do it. Only suggest patterns and designs you are confident that you can create.

> Do you have enough time? Whatever you do, don't rush. Make sure you have ample time to do the work. If you rush, you're more likely to make a mistake!

The client

> Ensure that the client is gowned to protect their clothes, and that there is a towel or cutting collar around their shoulders.

> The client's hair should be clean, dry and free from product. It should also be short enough that the pattern will be visible.

> The perimeter of the haircut should be clean and neatly finished.

> Make sure the client is sitting upright and is comfortable.

> Take care to ensure that any earrings and facial piercings are removed and other jewellery is safely out of the way.

You

> Ensure your hands are clean.

> Make sure your jewellery will not get in the way while you are working.

> Make sure you have all the right tools and they are clean and fit for purpose.

> You should know how to work safely, with the correct posture. Wear clothes and shoes suitable for the service you are carrying out.

Cutting patterns in hair step by step

1 With the client sitting up straight, begin at the front hairline. Working horizontally towards the crown, slowly remove hair in a line approximately 3 to 4 mm wide (a). Create a loop so that the line drops down vertically, following the hairline (b) (c).

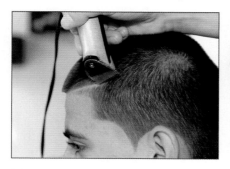 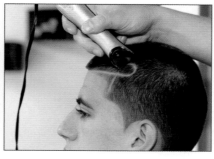 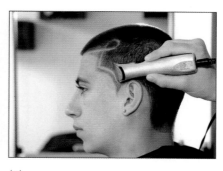

(a)   (b)   (c)

2 If the pattern is to be repeated on both sides, do the same on the other side of the head, checking continually for balance.

3 Follow the front perimeter, making sure the line stays the same distance from the hairline. Follow the hairline around the ear to the nape (d).

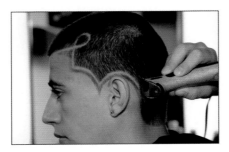

(d)

4 At the nape, create swirls and curves, ensuring that they mirror the size and shape of the previously created loop (e).

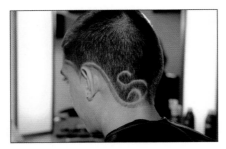

(e)

5 Using the ear as a guide, cut additional loops and curves on the side of the head, again making sure that the size and shape remains the same as those previously cut.

6 Check the pattern for balance.

7 Finally, clean and tidy the lines with scissors or a razor.

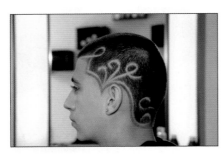

Activity Using a cropped block, start by practising cutting straight line patterns. Cut three lines on each side of the head so that they are evenly spaced and parallel.

Next, following on from the end of each straight line, cut three curved lines on each side, in to the back. Again, make sure they are evenly spaced and match those on the opposite side.

Finally, cut three circles on the top of the head. Cut one small one to start with, then cut two further circles around it, each evenly spaced around the first one.

Top Tip

Use a coin or your thumb as a size guide to keep the loops and curves even.

Introduction

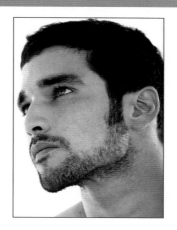

What is it?

This is the cutting and shaping of beards, sideburns and moustaches. It also includes clipping ear, nose and eyebrow hair.

How is it done?

A range of techniques are used to cut facial hair, including clipper-cutting, scissor-over-comb, clipper-over-comb and freehand cutting.

When is it done?

When cutting sideburns, it's carried out as part of the haircut. Beards, moustaches and other facial hair are usually cut after the haircut, so that the beard can be cut to match the hairstyle.

This is one of the hairdressing skills many hairdressers find difficult and avoid. In fact, they are fairly easy skills to master. Being coarse, you can't control the direction of facial hair as you can with scalp hair. As they are generally left as they grow, beards and moustaches are shaped and trimmed rather than cut and styled. It's an important difference, as it's closer to topiary (cutting hedges) than cutting hair!

When cutting beards and moustaches, you are cutting the hair to a visual shape. In other words, you are cutting it to 'look' even, rather than actually to be even, as you would in a haircut. For this reason, you tend to use more freehand and scissor-over-comb methods to cut the hair, instead of holding it in your fingers. Clippers are often used in trimming, as they enable the hair to be cut where it lies.

Most men won't comb their beards, so they will be left in the shape you cut them. The shape you cut depends on both the style of beard or moustache the client wants and the shape of their face. As well as a fashion statement, beards and moustaches are often used to create a stronger feature, such as to make the jawline more prominent, to hide a cleft lip or to distract from a prominent nose.

The best way to decide on the shape you are going to cut is to 'comb' the beard into various shapes by puffing it out or flattening it down. Use your hands and fingers to show how the beard would look if some of the hair was removed completely. Look at the shape of the face and see how the beard could be used enhance the face shape.

> A square beard will hide a weak or pointed chin.
> Sideburns and a goatee will elongate a round face.
> A beard trimmed shorter on the sides and longer at the chin will narrow a wide face.
> A beard fuller at the sides will widen a thin face.
> For smaller faces, keep the beard short and close to the outline of the face.

> Removing the beard from the neck, so that it stops at the jawline, can make the neck seem longer.
> Sideburns can be used to accentuate cheekbones.

When trimming beards or sideburns, you slowly reduce the amount of hair until you get the desired shape, so it's important to know the shape you are aiming to achieve and continually check how it's coming along. It's important to remember that a beard shape is three-dimensional, so you need to make sure you review it from all angles.

Key points to note when cutting facial hair

> It can take up to 15 minutes to carry out a beard trim, so make sure you have allowed sufficient time between clients.
> Beard trimming is best carried out with the client slightly reclined. The best type of chair is a reclining, sturdy barber-style chair, with an adjustable headrest. If your salon doesn't have one of these, you can use the backwash basin. You may need to move adjacent chairs to give yourself adequate room to work.
> As with cutting hair, work on both sides of the client to achieve balance.
> Facial hair is rarely combed or styled, so it remains in the shape in which you cut it.
> Where possible, it's best to cut the beard to follow the natural hairline of the face. Cutting within this line means that the client will have to shave this area to maintain the shape.
> Clippers are good for general beard cutting, but a smaller, narrower-bladed trimmer is often better for detail or for working on confined areas.
> Always check if the client has a scar or a mark that they are keen to keep covered and incorporate this into the shape.
> Sideburns, beards and moustaches can vary in density, so take into account the thickness of the beard throughout when deciding on the shape.
> Facial skin has more elasticity than the scalp, so you need to take care when using tension.
> Facial contours, skin folds or dents can affect the growth and how the beard lays.
> Beards, moustaches and sideburns often hide moles and spots that can be cut, so check carefully beforehand.
> Facial hair is generally finer than scalp hair, and cutting it too short can make it appear bald and patchy.

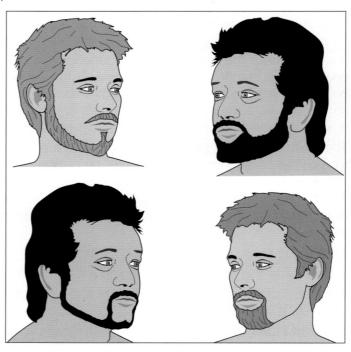

> Head shape and hairstyle should be considered when deciding on the shape and style of facial hair.

Preparation

> Discuss the shape and style of the beard with the client, and ensure that you have all the correct tools.

> Check for abrasions or skin conditions.

> The beard should be clean. If it is not, ask the client to wash their face or use facial wipes.

> If possible, recline the client, either in the chair or at the backwash basin.

> Ensure that the client's clothes are protected and that there is adequate protection to stop the clippings going down their neck.

> Cover the client's eyes with cotton wool pads or a towel (you must at least have them close their eyes).

> Your hands should be clean and your clothes protected.

> Make sure that you have all the required tools to hand and that they are clean and ready for use.

Cutting and shaping a beard step by step

1 Comb through the beard so that it's free from knots.

2 Using a large comb, 'pick out' the beard so that it's full.

3 Starting at the sides, and placing the comb in from underneath, use scissor-over-comb or scissor-over-clippers to begin to cut the shape (a) (b). Ensure that you blend the beard to the haircut.

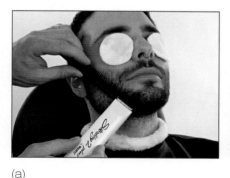
(a)

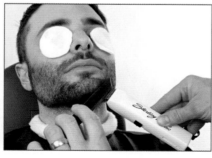
(b)

4 Work symmetrically towards the centre, cutting one side and then the same area on the other, continually checking for balance and shape. Continue until you have reached the chin (c).

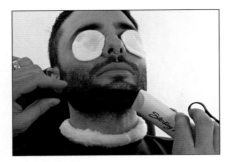

(c)

5 Cut each side of the moustache and then blend the two sides together.

6 Use the edge of the clippers or your scissors freehand to cut the length of the moustache, taking care to avoid the lip and nose (d).

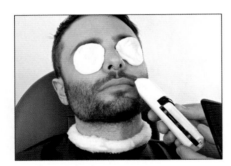

(d)

7 From the bottom of the neck, use the clippers to trim the hair under the chin (e). In most cases, this hair will be cut shorter or even removed altogether.

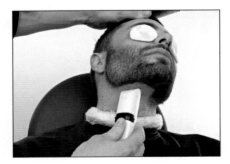

(e)

8 Use the clippers to remove any untidy hair on the cheeks or on the neck.

9 Check the beard from all sides and use cross checking, by holding the hair in the opposite way to how it was cut, where possible, to ensure that the beard is even.

10 Finally, use the edge of the clippers to sharpen or define any lines (f).

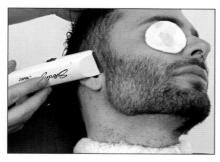

(f)

11 Use a neck brush to brush off the client's face and neck (g).

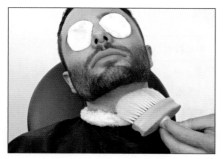 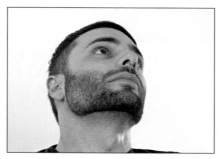

(g)

Note: As the client can't see what you are doing, stop occasionally so that they can see how the look is progressing.

Other facial hair

Ironically, as well as losing their hair to male pattern baldness, when men get older, their nose hair thickens and grows longer, as does the hair on their ears and eyebrows. Although not all salons offer these services, the trimming of nose, ear and eyebrow hair is still carried out in some salons, especially in traditional barber's and male grooming salons.

Eyebrows

Unlike women's eyebrows, with men you are only cutting the hair shorter, not shaping them. Use scissor-over-comb to cut long hairs and reduce bushiness.

Ear hair

Cutting ear hair requires care, as it's easy to nick the skin. Comb all the head hair well out of the way, so that you can clearly see the ear hair that needs to be cut. Most hairdressers find holding and stretching the ear makes trimming this hair easier. While freehand cutting with scissors can be used, a cut-throat razor is best. However, if you don't feel confident using a razor on the ear, clippers or trimmers can also be used.

Nose hair

Don't be embarrassed about cutting nose hair – it's really no big deal. When cutting nose hair, all you are doing is trimming off any long hair in

> **Top Tip**
>
> When cutting sideburns, it's important that you treat them as a beard and not as hair, and cut them in the same way as you would a beard. Generally, though, there is no need to recline the client when cutting sideburns, unless they're particularly long.

the nostrils. This is easiest if you put one finger on the end of the nose and push it upwards, so that it stretches open the nostril. Some hairdressers will use a special small, narrow nose-hair trimmer for this, while others will just use scissors. Care has to be taken when cutting nose hair, as it's easy to nick the skin. If you are using scissors, make sure you only use the very ends to slowly and gently nip away the hairs. For hygiene and etiquette, trimmers used for nose hair should not be used for anything else. If you use your scissors, make sure that cutting the nose hair is the last thing you do, and sterilise your scissors once you've finished.

All tools used to cut facial hair should be properly cleaned and sterilised before being used again.

Aftercare

As with all hair services, it's important to advise the client on when they next need to have their facial hair cut in order to maintain the look and shape. Clients should also be advised on how to keep their facial hair looking good between visits, and any home tools that they might find useful.

Finishing off

When you have finished your haircut, have checked it thoroughly and you are happy, always take time to brush down the client carefully.

> Gently ruffle the hair to shake out any loose clippings.
> Using a soft (neck) brush, gently brush the client's face, ears and neck.
> Taking care not to let hair fall down the client's neck, remove the towel or cutting collar and shake off.
> Brush the neck area again, before replacing the towel and/or the collar.
> You may want to give the hair a rinse at the backwash to remove all the loose hair.

Advise the client on how you will style and finish their hair, and the products you will use.

Housekeeping

Once you have finished your haircut, help to keep the salon clean and safe by:

> cleaning the workstation and sweeping up as soon as possible
> putting hair clippings, dirty towels and gowns in the appropriate bin
> cleaning and sterilising tools ready for the next client.

Aftercare advice

As most clients will style their hair at home between visits to the salon, it's essential that you advise the client on how to style and

Activity Look at the shape and styles of beards and moustaches on men you see and in pictures. Think about the shape, how they are cut, what areas are left long, and which are cut short or removed.

Also, practise cutting the nose, ear and eyebrow hair of friends and family. This will help you to improve the skill and to get over the embarrassment of doing it!

maintain their hair. Once you have created your haircut, take time to advise the client on how to maintain the haircut and how to recreate the look at home.

Advise them on:

> the best shampoo and conditioner to use to maintain the condition

> products and styling aids, and how and when they are to be applied

> how the style can be changed or altered to meet work, sports and social needs

> how to dry and style the look, what tools and appliances to use, and how to use them for the best results

> possible ways the style could be enhanced next time, with colour, perming or a conditioning treatment

> when they should book an appointment for a follow-up haircut to keep it looking good.

Finally, before they leave let the client know that if they have any problems with the haircut, or they discover, for example, that the fringe or the back is a bit too long, they can always come back to have it adjusted. Clients are often embarrassed about coming back if there is something that they are not altogether happy with, and sometimes they will even go elsewhere. So always make sure they know that it's part of the service and that there is never a problem in coming back to have the cut adjusted slightly.

Case study

The importance of training

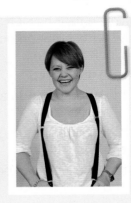

- To be creative and inspiring you sometimes have to break the rules.
- To be creative you have to understand the rules.
- But to break the rules you first have to learn them....

This is why the training you receive when you first become a hairdresser should not be rushed – it is your opportunity to learn all the techniques that will make you into the hairdresser you want to become.'

'What might be trendy and fashionable now may not be in a few years' time, and if you have not learnt your trade well it will be a very short-lived career. Think about when you visit a doctor – when they train, they first learn about the entire body and all fields of medicine. Only when they've done this do they choose their specialist area. It is the same with us hairdressers – learn everything first then decide if you want to concentrate on one area or not.'

'And remember if you're struggling to learn one thing in particular, it's all about practice, practice, practice! I can remember thinking that blow-drying was the hardest thing in the world and I would never get it. Now, my hairdryer feels like a natural part of my arm!!'

'Your basic training is your foundation to your career – the stronger the foundation, the better your career.'

Sally Brooks, Brooks+Brooks, London

Section 3
With the team

The teams that work in a salon have a direct impact on the business. This section takes in all the skills you will need to excel in your role as a proactive team player. Cultivating great relationships is the very foundation of a successful salon and a rewarding career, so this section begins with the communication skills you will need to make great professional relationships work for you. Hairdressing is an industry that encourages tireless self-improvement and also provides you with lots of opportunities to do just that; in 'With the team', we look at the ways in which you can manage your own career development and carve out a reputation as an outstanding team performer. Finally, we consider your role in growing the salon business and how that links directly to the breadth of customer service you offer.

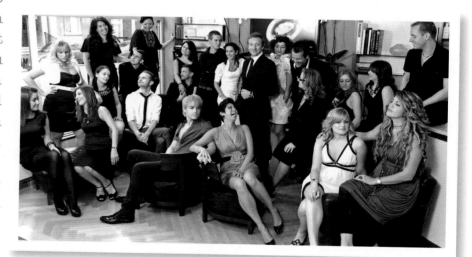

Chapter objectives for Unit G3

In this chapter, you will learn:

> **how to communicate well with staff and clients**
> **what a good attitude is**
> **how to perform to the best of your ability within your role**
> **how to manage your own work performance and work well with your colleagues to create a successful salon business.**

You will be assessed against your knowledge and ability to:

1 Understand your job role and responsibilities, and the standards of behaviour, productivity and conduct that your salon requires of you.

2 Deal with clients in a polite, efficient and positive way that promotes goodwill and trust.

3 Understand your role in helping your colleagues and creating a positive working atmosphere.

4 Assist your colleagues in a positive, polite and proactive way.

5 Seek and act on opportunities to learn and grow within the boundaries of your role.

6 Seek and act on ways to improve your performance, through help from your colleagues and other sources.

7 Regularly review your role and share information with your salon manager or supervisor that will help you manage your performance and output.

8 Monitor your own performance through reviews and feedback.

9 Use your time and skills in an appropriate, efficient and effective way.

10 Ask for help when you need it.

11 Understand how to resolve conflict.

Chapter objectives for Unit G8

In this chapter, you will learn:

> **how to manage your own work performance and work well with your colleagues to create a successful salon business.**

You will assessed against your knowledge and ability to:

1 Understand your job role and responsibilities and the

standards of behaviour, productivity and conduct that your salon requires of you.

2 Seek and act on ways to improve your performance through help from your colleagues and other sources.

3 Monitor your own performance through reviews and feedback.

4 Assist your colleagues in a positive, polite and proactive way.

5 Use your time and skills in an appropriate, efficient and effective way.

6 Understand how to resolve conflict.

Case study
Winning teams

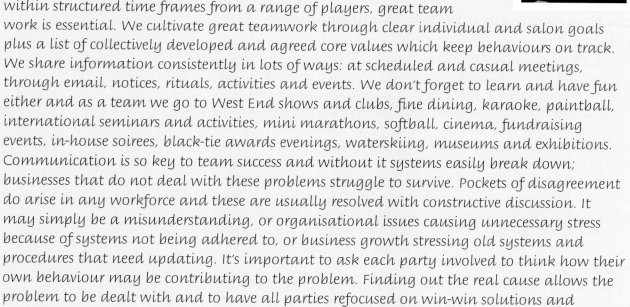

Michael Van Clarke has a premium salon in the heart of London's shopping district. He and his teams have won many awards in every aspect of hairdressing.

'Salons are a little bit like theatre and often just as entertaining for the clients. In this environment where high standards have to be delivered within structured time frames from a range of players, great team work is essential. We cultivate great teamwork through clear individual and salon goals plus a list of collectively developed and agreed core values which keep behaviours on track. We share information consistently in lots of ways: at scheduled and casual meetings, through email, notices, rituals, activities and events. We don't forget to learn and have fun either and as a team we go to West End shows and clubs, fine dining, karaoke, paintball, international seminars and activities, mini marathons, softball, cinema, fundraising events, in-house soirees, black-tie awards evenings, waterskiing, museums and exhibitions. Communication is so key to team success and without it systems easily break down; businesses that do not deal with these problems struggle to survive. Pockets of disagreement do arise in any workforce and these are usually resolved with constructive discussion. It may simply be a misunderstanding, or organisational issues causing unnecessary stress because of systems not being adhered to, or business growth stressing old systems and procedures that need updating. It's important to ask each party involved to think how their own behaviour may be contributing to the problem. Finding out the real cause allows the problem to be dealt with and to have all parties refocused on win-win solutions and positive goals.'

Michael Van Clarke, owner of Michael Van Clarke

Relationships at work and your performance

In this section we cover Unit G3 (Contribute to the development of effective working relationships) and Unit G8 (Develop and maintain your effectiveness at work), plus all the key information you need to manage working relationships and personal performance.

Hairdressing is a relationship-based business, so maximising your relationship with your clients and your team members will speed your success. Your attitude, conduct and communication can be a huge asset in your career, giving you access to opportunities and rewards that a poor approach could never achieve. The communication and body language skills you will learn from Units G7 and G17 will reinforce your commitment to building great relationships with your team and your clients. Applying some of the research and problem identification skills from Unit G18 will empower you to anticipate the needs of those around you, and will contribute to your reputation as a proactive, supportive and clear-thinking team player.

There is a huge difference between working *with* your colleagues and working alongside them – together you can achieve a great deal more than you can alone. It's essential to understand the part you play in contributing to a successful business, and the steps you can take personally towards growing in competence, skills and confidence in order to improve team performance.

How do you create effective relationships at work?

You need to take responsibility. Be your own ambassador. Invest the effort and time it takes to be skilled, confident and, above all, constant in your working life. Take the trouble to identify and read all of your salon policies and procedures, and learn the key roles and responsibilities of the team members you work with, so you know exactly who to turn to when you need help. The first step on the road to knowing how to contribute to working relationships is to understand the full scope of your own role and responsibilities within your salon or company, which can typically be found in your job description. Your job description should give your title, describe your role and list the main tasks contained within it. If you are unclear about your role or those of your teammates, ask your supervisor or salon manager for guidance.

Healthy, positive and happy working relationships contribute to the atmosphere in a salon. A good atmosphere is one where staff want to stay and clients want to return to again and again; a bad atmosphere will have a significant impact on staff and client turnover.

There are common characteristics in developing relationships of any kind. Whether it's a relationship with your client or your colleague, you will need to communicate well, conduct yourself appropriately and fulfil your obligations to the very best of your abilities.

Your communication

Effective communication is the bedrock of good relationships. You need to use both verbal and non-verbal communication (body language) to help you build trust, serve your clients, help your colleagues and generally remain a positive influence on the salon floor. This section covers the main communication tools that will assist you in developing effective relationships in the workplace.

Open questions

Open questions are those that require a more complex answer and are likely to deliver more information than a simple yes or no response. An example of an open question might be: 'What kind of beverage can I bring you today?' instead of: 'Would you like any refreshments?' Use open questions to uncover good information about how you can help your clients or colleagues. Once you have the information, don't forget to act on it!

Active listening

Maintaining comfortable eye contact, nodding attentively, asking relevant questions, leaning slightly towards the speaker, not inter-rupting or getting distracted are all ways in which you can show you are listening. Good listening skills are key to building trust and rapport quickly.

Tone of voice

Your tone of voice says a lot about you. The tone in which you speak rather than what you are saying can express everything from anger to stress. Don't speak too fast, use a high-pitched tone or mumble. Speak clearly and evenly, so that your communication has clarity and you project confidence and calm.

Spoken language

The words you use will help with clear communication. You should try to adjust the language you use to suit the person you are communicating with – for example, it's perfectly acceptable to talk about percentage peroxide and tint numbers with a colleague, but not with a client. In all your interactions, remain polite and respectful.

Summarising

Repeating back to your client or colleague the key points of your conversation will show that you have listened and will give them confidence that you have understood – for example, 'So you want me to prepare the equipment trolley and comb your client's hair through while you finish your last blow-dry. Is that right?'

Facial expression

Narrowing your eyes, pursing your lips and biting your bottom lip will have a negative impact on your colleagues and clients. Welcoming any interaction with a genuine smile, no matter how small, will show you to be warm, helpful and approachable.

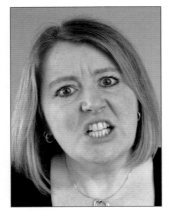 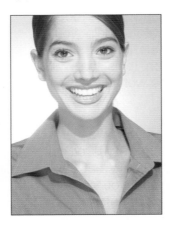

Be aware of your facial expression

Open body language

Body language has a lot to do with being 'available' to assist your colleagues and clients. Standing upright, with your shoulders back, hands held loosely in front or at your sides, and head held high will make you look available to help. Crossing your arms, looking down and turning your body away will give everyone the impression you are either unwilling or unable to help.

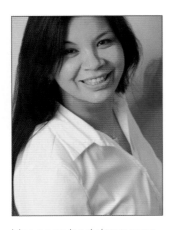 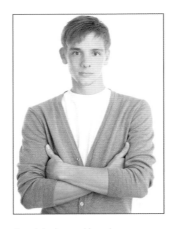

Use open body language

Avoid closed body language

Personal space

Standing too close to someone can feel too intimate or threatening. Respect the other person's space and keep a distance that is roughly arm's length – any further away and you are in danger of losing rapport. When you are conducting a service, keep distance and touch appropriate to the situation.

Note: If you are in any doubt about the correct way to communicate, simply ask your supervisor or salon manager for some coaching. Try to give them real examples of when you have been uncomfortable and role-play solutions with them.

Your behaviour

Behaviour can be contagious, so take the opportunity to 'spread' good behaviours by conducting yourself well and maintaining high standards. Remember that you are cultivating the 'brand of you', and think about the behaviours you want to be associated with. Take the time to find out your salon's guidelines on conduct, behaviour and appearance, so that you have a benchmark to work to. Here you can discover the key ways in which you can exhibit great workplace behaviour.

Don't be late

Lateness is a huge insult to your employer, your colleagues and your salon clients. Lateness has an impact on the service levels in your salon, which could result in clients not returning. Your lateness will also put your colleagues under added and unnecessary pressure. You are contractually obliged to be available and ready for work at a certain time, so make sure you stick to it. Pay attention to journey times, and if the weather, roadworks or public transport problems are likely to make you late, make sure you leave home earlier. Arrive at least 10 minutes before your start time so that you can at least remove your coat and prepare yourself for the day ahead. Remember, your start time is the time you are *available for work*, not the time you step in through the salon door.

Timekeeping

Every salon relies on the appointment structure to function efficiently. Think about the time allotted to tasks within your job description and work in a timely and efficient manner. Work with your colleagues to be flexible around their needs and those of the client. For example, if a client arrives late, you could reduce the time allotted for a shampoo and head massage by a few minutes to help the stylist to stay on track. Use the time you spend with your client in a positive way, and think about how you can match your salon's services and products to their needs – for example, if you do end up talking about holidays, you can tell the client about the 'sun protect' products available in the salon.

Time management has a lot to do with experience and planning. Ask more experienced colleagues for their advice on how long they believe services will take, and use the information to help you plan your day. You can check your list of appointments and use any downtime to prepare work trolleys or equipment for the service ahead.

Don't gossip

Gossiping about your colleagues and clients will erode trust and cause upset, so avoid it. Use the time you have with your client effectively, to build rapport or discuss their needs and desires and

Activity

Think about the ways in which your colleagues, friends, clients and family show that they value their relationship with you. Make a list of the things they do – for example, listen, help you learn, say supportive things.

Now make a list of behaviours you have observed and experienced in those you see regularly who do not make you feel valued – for example, not doing what they commit to, looking away when you speak.

the ways in which the salon can help with services and products. Gossiping about your colleagues is not an appropriate use of your time and energy. Use that time and energy to notice your colleagues' strengths – you never know, you might learn something!

Manners matter

Good manners are a simple and very effective way to promote positive working relationships. Remember to thank your colleagues. A word of thanks has even more impact if it's specific. Don't just say, 'Thanks!' say, 'Thanks for gowning Mrs Thomas for me. I was getting behind and it meant she wasn't sitting around in reception feeling forgotten.' So remember the what and the why when it comes to thanking others. Always be polite in all your conversations and particularly when asking for help from your colleagues. Good manners include good timing, so make judgements about the right moment to offer assistance to your colleagues or ask for their help.

Be appropriate

Behaving and communicating in a way that does not discriminate against or cause offence to others is important. Don't swear or make personal comments or comments of sexual nature; don't touch your colleagues or clients in an improper manner. If you find a team member's speech or behaviour offensive, speak to them about it clearly and concisely. Tell them why you find the behaviour or comment offensive and that it is not acceptable to you and must not be repeated.

Your attitude

A positive attitude to your job, your colleagues and your clients will be a great asset. Our state of mind has an enormous influence on the way we act and the way we are perceived, so a good attitude is essential. This section highlights ways that you can exhibit a good attitude towards your job role and your salon.

Keeping up appearances

Your salon may have a uniform or colour clothing policy – for example, all trainees should wear black and white. Adhere to your salon's policy and make sure your clothes are clean, ironed and appropriate for the weather and the type of work you are doing. Your hands will constantly be on view and in physical contact with the client; they are also your most valuable work tool, so treat them well. Pay attention to good hand hygiene (see Unit G20 for hand care information). Make sure your hair is cut, coloured and styled appropriately, so that you can be a good walking advertisement for your salon and your colleagues' skills.

Be customer-focused

You have 'internal customers', who are your colleagues, and 'external customers', who are your salon clients. They are all deserving of good customer service. Good customer service involves the following.

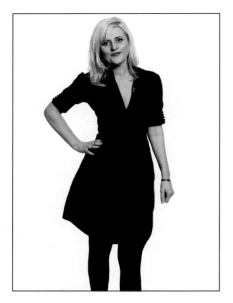

Your appearance matters – look the part

Being attentive to your customers' needs

From the client in the salon chair to the colleague standing behind it, pay attention and anticipate ways in which you can make their experience better or their job easier. Check that clients are comfortable and have everything they need. If the client raises any concerns that you cannot deal with directly, quickly connect them with a colleague who can help them. Be as sensitive to a client's body language as you are to your own. If you see your client flustered or fidgety, frowning or sighing, it's likely that they are upset or unsure about something, so use open questions to see how you can help. With colleagues, learn the correct way to assist them with pins, grips, sections, appliances, workstation cleaning, and so on. Make sure that you clearly understand when any kind of assistance is required, so that you help rather than hindering the flow of the salon service.

Protecting your customers' interests

Great customer focus means putting yourself in your client's shoes. For example, you should protect your client's clothing, with gowns and towels, just as you would protect your own, and treat your client's belongings as safely as you would treat your own, making sure they are returned at the right time. Consider ways in which you can help your colleagues by fulfilling all of the responsibilities in your job description to the very best of your abilities, and making certain that you offer your assistance in a timely and effective way.

Being available

There is always something to learn by observation on the salon floor, so don't linger on breaks or spend more time in the staff room than is absolutely necessary. A lot of good customer service is simply about making yourself available to help and being open to helping.

Be a team player

Speaking in a polite, friendly way towards your colleagues is a basic requirement of good salon etiquette. Remember to ask your colleagues for help and information whenever you need to, and if you experience any problems in carrying out your job, or you perceive any problems that might stop your colleagues from carrying out theirs, report the incident quickly to your salon manager or supervisor.

Be hungry to learn

The more you learn, the better hair professional you will be, so take every opportunity to broaden your knowledge and experience. Observing in the salon, reading trade magazines, participating in model nights and checking out the internet for hair-related sites are all good sources, and show that you have a positive attitude towards improving your performance.

How do you maintain your effectiveness at work?

The way you do your job and the way you practise and improve your skills combine to define your level of effectiveness. Great salons thrive on employees who actively seek out ways to 'go the extra mile'. This doesn't mean acting beyond your level of responsibility or doing things outside your job description; it simply means being the very best that you can be, consistently. So when your job description calls for providing clients with refreshments, great performance will make sure that it's laid out beautifully, with clean cups and saucers, and delivered with a smile in a timely manner. Being effective means that you make a difference, and as the demands of clients and the colleagues you work with change constantly, it means making sure that you remain effective by being flexible and equipping yourself with all the knowledge you need to do so.

Your performance

If you have a great attitude and good workplace conduct, you are already on your way to the kind of job performance that will get you noticed. Always remember that while you are creating the 'brand of you', you are also working as part of a salon team. What you do and how you do it makes a difference to everyone around you, every day. Your performance will have a direct impact on your colleagues, your clients, your salon and, of course, your career. Whether you choose to be a first-class salon-based stylist or an international session stylist for catwalk shows and photo shoots, be assured that performing to the best of your ability will bring you income, support and opportunities that will otherwise pass you by. The first steps required for great performance are as follows.

Identify your role and responsibilities

Your job should come with a clear contract of employment and a job description. The contract will define the main areas of your responsibility, and will clarify things like workplace address, working hours, holiday, salary and the salon's rules and regulations on conduct and behaviour. Employment contracts are in place to protect both you and your employer, and ideally they should be reviewed each time your role changes with the same employer. Your job description will show your job title, and will describe your role and each of the key tasks and responsibilities within it. It may go so far as describing the behaviours that a successful employee in that position should exhibit, such as good organisational skills or clear communication. It's important that while you fulfil all your responsibilities, you don't take on decision-making or responsibility beyond your job role and capabilities – doing so may result in problems for you and your salon. Your salon may take disciplinary action if you fail to fulfil your role or if you act beyond the limits of your responsibility. You should understand your salon's organisational structure – that is, the way that job roles interact and who reports to whom. Your salon will have experts who can help you – for example, colourist, receptionist, health and safety officer, education director, artistic director. If you are in any doubt as to which team member can help you in a particular situation – for example, if a client has a complaint – or if you are unclear about any task you have been given, you should ask your salon manager or supervisor for clarification. Every employee is important to the smooth and successful running of a salon business, so take pride in your role.

Set measurements for success

It's hard to stay motivated if you don't have a goal, so measuring yourself against certain success factors is important. It's also hard for

---

Stylist job description

> Must be in at least 15 minutes before starting work.
> Greet clients.
> Give a full, thorough consultation.
> Cut hair to a high standard within 45 minutes.
> Colour hair to a high standard.
> Be able to recommend products used.
> Be able to recommend treatments when needed.
> Answer phones and book appointments.
> Be able to achieve a complete restyle.
> Control a busy column.
> Help keep the salon clean and tidy to a high standard.
> No chewing gum at all.

Prerequisites

To be a Stylist the applicant must meet the following criteria:

> Be able to cut current trends with influence from the current collections.
> Be able to colour using advanced colour in combination with classic techniques.
> Be able to complete, to an excellent standard, a cut and blow dry in no more than 45 minutes.
> Be able to complete, to an excellent standard, a full set of foils in no more than 1 hour.
> Do classic hair up.
> Be able to open up, cash up and close the salon in the absence of a Manager.
> Regularly teach on model nights.

A clear job description
Courtesy of Falltricks

your salon to plan the number of staff they need to maintain and grow their business if everyone isn't pulling their weight. You will need to set your own goals with your employer, but here are some examples:

> Achieve NVQ Level 2 within a certain timeframe.
> Achieve a certain number of retail product sales per week.
> Achieve a 99 per cent attendance record over 6 months.
> Achieve a 99 per cent punctuality record over 6 months.
> Attend one model workshop per week.

Make sure that you understand the methods of measuring your goals. It might be your manager's records, your NVQ folder or your salon's computer system, but be clear, so that you can have confidence in the end result.

Your development

The hair industry is very active in continuous learning and most salons will encourage progress and development at every level. Don't leave your career development up to your employer; take an active role. Find out your salon's policy and procedures with regard to performance reviews and development plans. Make sure that you participate in all the formal and informal meetings and conversations that take place with regard to your progress, and use the information to plan your self-improvement. One-to-one feedback in the form of an appraisal is necessary to planning your future, but remember also that you have a whole team from whom you can seek assistance.

Good career development means the following things.

Being honest with yourself

We all have strengths and weaknesses – things that we are good at and areas where our skills and knowledge can be improved. Recognising your own strengths and weaknesses, either through self-assessment or through feedback from your team members and manager, is essential to your development. Think about your day-to-day job and the things you do with confidence – these things are likely to be your strengths. Now think about the things you routinely avoid, dislike or feel least confident with – these areas are likely to be your weaknesses.

Seek feedback

You don't have to wait for your formal appraisal or review meeting to get useful feedback – just ask! Remember to use open questions and make sure you ask all of your customers – both external and internal. Ask clients: 'How could your head massage have been improved?' Ask your colleagues: 'What can I do to assist you better?' Ask your manager or supervisor: 'What areas of my role do I need to improve on?' It's hard to hear criticism, even when it is constructive, so try not to react defensively. If you are unclear about the response, ask your customer to tell you more. Keep your tone even, your manner polite

Case study

Be the best you can be

Debbie G has worked for the industry's top names and delivers training to individual salons, salon groups, seminar audiences and shows around the UK and the world.

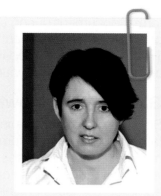

'I teach lots of young trainees for employers and the qualities that are common to the best of them are their energy, their enthusiasm and their mindset. Even the areas of hairdressing that they are not passionate about, they still approach with a good attitude. The more information a trainee takes in, then the more confident they will be as hairdressers. I teach a good mindset – I tell trainees, "If you think this is going to be boring, it will be. If you approach a lesson with 'I think I will get as much out of this as I can' then you will learn something valuable."'

'Being great at what you do takes practice, practice, practice. There are no shortcuts. Vidal Sassoon practised every line until it was perfect. David Beckham always stayed longer than the other lads in his training sessions when he was a kid. Backstage catwalk and photographic work stylists such as Guido Paulo and Eugene Souleiman practise the hair before every show and session, even if they've done something like it before because nothing is left to chance. Try and find your learner type – we all learn differently and it's important to know how you learn. Do you need to write information down? Are you better with lots of visual images around you? Do you need post-it notes around your home to remember things? To help techniques stick, think about why you did something, think about how you did something and then think about how you might do it differently. Every technique a trainee learns has depth and takes time to learn so I recommend lots of patience, but what you get out of hairdressing is far greater than those first hard years you put in. To be able to discuss a hair cut all night and love it is wonderful. We get to travel to amazing places and get paid for it. We get to change people through a haircut and colour and give them confidence or make them happy. It's fantastic.'

Debbie G, Debbie G training

and your body language neutral. Always summarise the key points, because if you've gone to the trouble to ask for feedback, you need to understand exactly what it is that you need to do more of, or need to do differently.

Getting involved with formal appraisals

Formal reviews will take place with your manager or supervisor, but may involve some input from your colleagues and even client feedback on your performance and progress. Typically, formal reviews are regular, but not frequent, perhaps every 3, 6 or 12 months. Appraisals are your opportunity to discuss the past, present and future. All discussion points and actions points should be noted in a formal document during an appraisal, and should begin to form part of an active development plan that you use and update constantly. Think carefully and prepare for every appraisal, as your input is just as valid as the things your supervisor has to say.

Gaining new knowledge and skills

Sharing discussions about your strengths and weaknesses and talking about your performance will help you and your supervisor or manager to identify gaps in your knowledge and skills. Before you leave your appraisal, agree a development plan with your supervisor; agree on the ways in which your success will be measured and the goals that they will be measured against; and, finally, agree on the date of your next review or formal appraisal. There are many sources open to you to improve your skills and knowledge; taking advantage of them will show clients and colleagues that you are a well-rounded professional expert. Potential sources include the following.

Your team members

Observing more skilled and experienced successful staff as they go about their day-to-day jobs will give you positive role models and will help you to learn.

Training nights

Your employer is likely to offer training of some kind every week, either as part of a weekly team meeting or during a pre-arranged 'model night', which typically takes the form of a demonstration or work session, or discussion and work session around certain techniques or themes. Make sure you grasp every opportunity to learn; pay attention and participate whenever possible.

Team meetings

These will usually take place in your salon on a weekly basis, and include information on new initiatives, products or procedures. Team meetings are also a good place to clarify how team members' roles interact and who is responsible for what.

Team events

Many employers offer team days, either inside or outside the salon environment, giving you the opportunity to be inspired, to learn something and to have a lot of fun, all in the same day. Be positive about attending these events, stay engaged and give them your full attention.

The internet

The internet is a rich source of information, with lots of hair-related sites that include everything from discussion forums to step-by-step technical tutorials.

Trade bodies

HABIA (Hair and Beauty Industry Authority) is responsible for the NVQ structure and holds all of the National Occupational Standards.

Knowing the standards by which your NVQ assessor will mark you is key to NVQ success. Check out the standards at www.habia.org – the site contains lots of other useful information about hairdressing, and is constantly updated with new industry information and guidelines that affect your job.

Industry events

Salon International Trade Exhibition, The Fellowship for British Hairdressing and countless private seminars all require a little investment, but they are a huge source of education and information for professionals seeking to improve their skills. Trade exhibitions are a great way to update and broaden your product knowledge, gain inspiration and see new techniques in action.

Trade magazines

Hairdressing trade magazines are available weekly, monthly and quarterly, and are rich in inspiration and information about the profession. The magazines are packed with seasonal hair collections, information and comment from notable figures in the industry.

Consumer magazines

The hair industry and the fashion industry have strong links, so stay informed about fashion by reading glossy magazines such as *Vogue* and *Elle*. Look out for seasonal 'edits' that occur twice a year, around November and April, and carry a summary of the following season's main trends. Being able to talk knowledgeably about the textures, shapes and colours that will keep your client's look on track will reinforce your expert status

Don't stop

Hairdressing is a privileged industry, with lots of opportunities for continuous professional development (CPD). CPD is a planned and sustained approach to improving and updating your skills. State colleges, private academies, product manufacturers and product wholesalers may all offer training that contributes to your CPD. Following the formal NVQ structure beyond Level 2 will help to sustain your structured learning, but with your appraisal document and the development goals you have set with your employer, you can seek out focused learning opportunities that will help you fulfil your need for career development.

Your tools

Contributing effectively to working relationships demands that you perform to the best of your ability and fulfil all the tasks within your job description. As an active and important team member, you are essential to the overall success of your salon, and there are a number of tools at your disposal to achieve that.

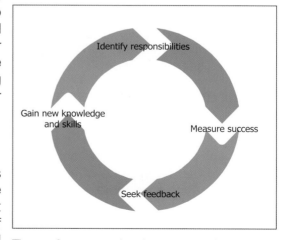

The performance development cycle

Appraisal notes

When you have agreed the outcomes of your appraisal, don't file your appraisal notes and never look at them again; refer to them regularly. Checking against the outcomes of the appraisal will be a constant reminder of the knowledge gaps you have committed to fill and the areas in which you need to improve. As you make progress, make notes of your progress, so that when your next review or appraisal comes round, you are ready.

Performance measurements

Your performance is going to be measured by your behaviour and your output. Your behaviour will be observed mostly by your colleagues, and will be discussed in informal reviews and formal appraisals. Your output will have specific targets and measures, such as the number of units of product sold, the number of new client requests and the percentage of days you arrived on time. Always ensure that measurements are given a timescale, so you know by what date or period of time you must achieve your targets.

Salon policies and procedures

Take time to understand all of your salon's guidelines on behaviour, conduct, timeliness, customer service, and so on. Always work within these guidelines.

Handling conflict

When people work together, there are bound to be differences in opinion and personality. Discovering a different perspective can be a great way to make positive changes, so differences aren't always a bad thing. If you have a misunderstanding, conflict or upset with a colleague, it is important to use good communication skills and clear steps to resolve the situation and move forward. When conflict arises, tackle it quickly and discreetly. Letting conflicts fester over time benefits no one, and having frank discussions in front of other colleagues and clients is inappropriate. Recognise immediately when working relationships are in crisis or struggling, and suggest a time and place where they can be discussed. The key steps of handling conflict are set out below.

Use neutral body language, facial expression and tone

Crossing your arms, averting your eyes and turning your body away are all signs of defensive body language. Try to keep your body and face relaxed and your tone of voice low and warm. The colleague you are speaking to is more likely to reflect your behaviour, so stay neutral.

Identify what happened

Clearly state and encourage your colleague to state what has happened. This will reveal both sides of the same story from each perspective, and will clarify why conflict should be avoided.

Find the root cause

Misunderstandings often occur when the original information is unclear. Use open questions and good listening skills to uncover the main source of the conflict – for example, how do you think this started? What more can you tell me about that?

Accept responsibility

If you find that you could have done something differently to avoid conflict, accept responsibility for your choices and apologise if necessary.

Plan a way forward

Work with your colleague to make a plan of how you can avoid repeating this conflict. This might include additional team meetings, checking for understanding, and clarifying roles and responsibilities.

Make a note and share it

Once you have agreed the way forward with your colleague, make a note of all the points and share it with your supervisor, salon manager and, if appropriate, your team members. Conflict can and does lead to improvements in policies and procedures, and might benefit more than just you and your colleague.

Do it and review it

Implement your plan for avoiding the conflict again and put in place a timescale to review it. If in a week or a month you find that your plan needs tweaking, work with your colleague again to make adjustments.

Activity Make a list of your strengths as you see them and then ask a colleague to do the same for you. Compare your lists.

Grievance procedures

Your salon will have a clear procedure on how to act in the case of a complaint or dispute with another employee. Check with your salon manager on the correct way to approach any personal or professional issues you have with a colleague.

Your employee rights are protected by a number of government laws. If you feel that your rights have been violated in some way and you wish to make a grievance against your employer, you should first check the laws. The Citizens Advice Bureau (www.citizensadvice. co.uk) is a good place to start; if you are a member of a professional body, you may also be entitled to free legal advice.

You and the law

Data Protection Act (1998) (see also Units G4 and G18)

All companies and organisations that hold any personal details about living people must register with the Information Commissioner.

> Data should be held safely and securely.
> Data should be fairly and lawfully processed for a defined and limited purpose.
> Data should be appropriate in content, depth and volume.
> Data should be kept in an accurate and timely manner.
> The keeping of data does not interfere with personal rights.

Trade Description Act (1968) (see also Unit G18)

The law requires that any descriptions of goods and services given by a person acting in the course of a trade or business should be accurate and not misleading. You may not:

> Apply a false or misleading description to goods by written or verbal means.
> Supply or offer to supply goods to which a false or misleading trade description is applied.

Equal opportunities and the law

The Equal Opportunities Commission has defined a number of acts which protect the rights of the individual against discrimination. You are obliged to offer equal opportunities to all clients and be offered equal opportunities by your employer. The main acts are outlined below.

Disability Discrimination Act (1995)

This Act outlaws discrimination based on disability in the areas of employment, education, access to goods, facilities and services, and in relation to land and property. The Act requires public bodies to promote equal opportunities for all individuals, regardless of ability. It also addresses the issue of equal access to public transportation, by setting minimum standards for ease of use by all passengers.

Sex Discrimination Act (1975)

This Act outlaws discrimination on grounds of sex, marital status or gender reassignment.

> Direct discrimination occurs when a person is treated less favourably because of his/her sex than a person of the other sex would be treated in the same circumstances.
> Indirect discrimination occurs when rules or circumstances are applied equally but clearly to the detriment of one of the sexes.
> Victimisation occurs as a result of an individual bringing a discrimination claim against their employer. Victimisation is

outlawed under the Sex Discrimination Act. Victimisation occurs if an individual is treated less favourably than someone who has not brought a discrimination claim.

Employment Equality (Age) Regulations (2006)

These regulations protect people against discrimination on grounds of age, and outlaws treating someone less favourably because of their age. This can include people of any age who are discriminated against, harassed or victimised.

Employment Rights Act (1996)

This Act deals with the minimum conditions and standards under which any employee should work, and includes the following.

> The right to receive an itemised wage slip.

> The right to be provided with a written statement of the main terms and conditions of employment within two months of commencing employment.

> The right to receive paid annual leave.

> The right for a female employee to receive statutory maternity pay and up to 52 weeks' maternity leave if she has worked for her employer for a continuous 26 weeks by the end of the 15th week before the baby's due date.

> The right to receive up to 13 weeks' unpaid parental leave for each child under the age of five.

> The right to receive National Minimum Wage at the recognised government rate.

> The right to receive statutory sick pay if off work for four consecutive days.

> Workers should not work longer than 48 hours in any one week.

> Part-time workers are entitled to the same contractual rights pro rata as full-time workers.

> An employee is entitled to at least one week's notice for each year of completed service and must have worked for their employer for at least two years to qualify for statutory redundancy pay.

Employment law is constantly subject to revision and change, so check www.direct.gov.uk for the latest information.

Note: Children and young people at work (safeguarding)

If you are under the minimum school leaving age of 16, you are classified in law as a child. If you are between the ages of 16 and 18, you are classified as a young person. Health and safety law, the Employment Act and the Children's Act (2004) will define the type of work you can do, the hours you are allowed to work, your minimum wage and the terms of your employment. Your employer is also obliged to safeguard your well-being, by protecting you from risks and monitoring your welfare. Ask your employer about their policies with regard to safeguarding and employing children and young people.

Activity

1 How many ways of improving your skills and knowledge can you name?
2 Name three steps in resolving conflict with your colleagues.
3 Describe positive body language.
4 What is an open question?
5 Which Act of law protects your rights as an employee? Name three points in the Act.
6 What should be included in a job description?
7 What should be included in an employment contract?

Summary

Developing effective working relationships is just as important to your career as your technical hairdressing skills. A harmonious and happy salon is a fantastic place to work, and that atmosphere is created by the people who spend the most time in the salon – and that includes you. Happy teams make happy clients, and this means a successful business; only successful businesses can offer you opportunities and choices that will give you a rewarding job on every level. As a trainee, you are on the threshold of a huge amount of choice: stage educator, trainer, stylist, art director, manager, NVQ assessor, session stylist, colour specialist, film and stage work – the list of potential industry roles isn't endless, but it is long. Cultivating good working relationships and remaining effective in your role will give you the knowledge, experience and support to sustain you through a fulfilling and rewarding career.

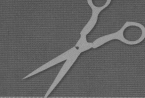

G18: Promote additional services or products to clients

In this chapter, you will learn:

> **how to identify and recommend services and products to clients**

> **your role in providing a full picture of your salon's scope of services and products**

> **the purpose and positive results that arise from promoting to clients.**

You will be assessed against your knowledge and ability to:

1 Understand your salon's processes and procedures in regard to promoting products and services.

2 Inform and update yourself regularly with the correct information about products and services as they become improved or updated.

3 Spot opportunities to share information about new products and services.

4 Understand and use all the communication tools available to you.

5 Communicate effectively with positive listening skills, body language and verbal communication.

6 Be sensitive to your client's communication and respond effectively.

7 Consider fresh approaches and ideas in promoting products and services in the salon.

8 Understand the role of promoting products and services in offering a full service to your clients.

9 Gain client commitment to purchasing products and services.

10 Refer clients to other sources of information or staff when appropriate.

We are bombarded by promotional messages during our every waking moment. From the brightly coloured images on our morning cereal box to the commercials on late-night TV, our daily lives have become a world of 'selling'. Your business is different because the sale does not have to be your focus; you are providing a professional service that is unique to 'the brand of you'. Your unique selling point (USP) includes the fact that you are a hair care expert; a trustworthy, reliable and knowledgeable source of information and advice. The client in your chair will be responding to the great communication and positive body language covered in Units G7 and G17. They will be experiencing the clear technical expertise shown in Units 8 to 15, and they will be enjoying the atmosphere created by a beautifully kept salon (see Units G20 and G4). The brand of you is how you grow your personal business as part of the overall salon business, to maximise your revenue, your commission and your clients' satisfaction.

How to create 'the brand of you'

> Be consistent, because your client wants a great standard of work and a fantastic experience every time.

> Be adaptable, because a client's needs change constantly.

> Be friendly and approachable, because it will encourage your client to share information that you can use to the advantage of both of you.

> Be open and honest. Sharing your opinion, with the basis of good reasoning, and protecting your client's interests will encourage them to return.

> Be service-centred, because while your client may not be able to spot the difference between good graduation and perfect graduation, they will spot the difference between good service and great service.

> Be trustworthy, because when a client trusts you, they are more likely to be motivated to action by your suggestions (e.g. 'This curl spray just came in and I immediately thought of you. With your hair texture, you should definitely plan to try it').

> Be curious, because you want to collect as much information about products/services and your clients as you can. That way you can match them all up intelligently.

> Be proactive. Think ahead and consider your client's needs and what's available before they visit, so you can plan conversations before they arrive.

> Be confident in your abilities and your knowledge, because confidence builds that all-important trust and relaxes clients.

> Be focused. You are there to serve the client *and* to build your business. Use the precious time you have with your client well. Strike a balance between friendly chit-chat and focused discussions about their hair that will seek out opportunities to add revenue, and give you the chance to go that extra mile to exceed their expectations.

> Be available. Don't let your client leave the salon without knowing how to contact you and tell their friends about you. Give your client your card, encourage them to call if they have questions or concerns about their hair and, above all, encourage them to give your card to their friends who might be looking for a hot tip on how to look their best.

Activity Make a list of your USPs – the qualities that make you stand out from your colleagues, the reasons why a client should choose to return only to you. Start with the statement: 'The brand of me is a great buy because…'

Why do we promote additional products and services?

In order to constantly maintain the commitment of existing clients and to encourage the interest of new ones, salons must review the services and products they offer. Communicating the key features and benefits of new items, or items that are new to a client, is the first step on the road to securing healthy financial returns on your time.

Features and benefits – what's the difference?

Benefits

This describes the ways in which a product or service satisfies a client's needs or improves their life in some way (e.g. fast, convenient, colour services in just ten minutes).

Features

These are the facts about a product or service and require the client to do all the thinking about how that fits in with their needs (e.g. ten-minute colour process).

Salons promote products and services to:

> broaden existing product ranges
> capture a new target market (e.g. ten-minute colour services to the lunchtime office crowd)
> meet a new need (e.g. fringe trims between visits)
> tap into a trend (e.g. tousled hair and the products to create it)
> build business (e.g. added-value services, such as head massage, to encourage rebooking)
> increase average bill (e.g. backwash treatments for shine or seasonal shades for colour)
> introduce new staff (e.g. adding a lower price band for 'graduate' stylists)
> offer a total and ever-changing hair-care service and encourage new business and client retention.

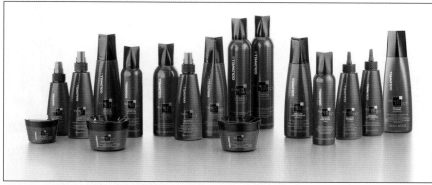

Know the difference between features and benefits

How do salons promote additional products and services?

Point-of-sale material

This may be in the form of small information cards that attach to the retail shelves, leaflets and tent cards (self-standing leaflets much like a greeting card). The idea is to inform at the point of sale, to be a visual prompt and source of information for clients.

Posters

Product manufacturers frequently provide professionally shot imagery and information to decorate the salon and inform clients.

Price lists

Probably the most used printed item in any salon, the price list is a good reference point for both clients and staff. Encourage clients to take newly printed price lists so that they are clear on charges and the scope of service and product brands on offer.

Showcards

These are small posters or upright leaflets which sit on the workstations where the client spends most of their time. Referring to them is a good way to open a conversation, and they can carry more information than posters because the client has plenty of time to look at them.

Window stickers

Sticky lettering that attaches to the inside of the front window is a good way to announce new products or services. As it faces out into the street, it also has more chance of attracting new clients and walk-ins than material inside the salon.

Website

The Web is the perfect place to flag news or new services. It also gives salons the opportunity to say more about the services they offer than can typically fit on a price list.

Advertising

Promotions such as deals and money off for new products and services can be added to advertising as 'a call to action'.

Staff!

As the professional experts, you and your colleagues will be the greatest tool in promoting any services or products available in the salon.

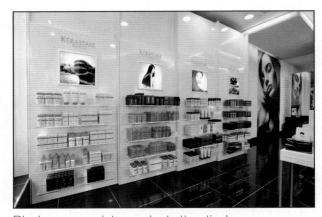

Display appropriate product attractively

How do *you* promote additional products and services?

Take responsibility

When your client is sitting in your styling chair, you are your salon's mouthpiece and one of its greatest assets, and it will be from you that they learn the most about the products and services on offer in your salon. Be proactive.

Inform yourself

> Lots of salons have team meetings, when new products and services will be presented and discussed. They may even revisit existing ones to refresh people's knowledge, so pay attention.

> The product manufacturer will have plenty of literature and usually offers great training about new products or new services, so sign up and make sure you take advantage of what is available.

> The Web is a huge source of information, so take the time to do a little research around benefits, features and fantastic ways to position a new product or service with the client.

> Listen to your colleagues and the type of information they are sharing – you might learn something!

> Read the trade press, in print and online. Hairdressing trade press will carry lots of information about trends for new services and new products available.

> Make suggestions if you come across a product or service that you believe would be good for your salon's clientele. It will keep your business competitive.

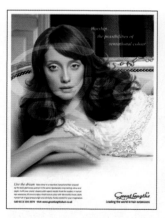 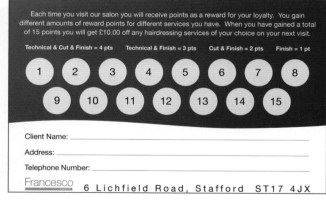 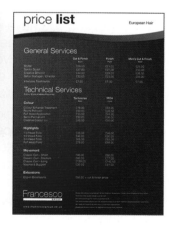

Common types of marketing material

Defer to the expert (don't miss the opportunity)

If there is a specialist product or service (e.g. new colour shades or extensions services) on offer that has peaked the interest of your client, don't risk losing potential revenue by bluffing it. Be upbeat about the fact that your salon has invested in specialists and introduce your client to them as promptly as possible. If there is ever any aspect about which you are unsure, ask your supervisor or salon manager to help. Your client will appreciate your sound judgement and your willingness to find out the information for them.

Communicate effectively

Communicate well and take the time to draw out your client's needs. Think about the ways in which you can help and discuss your ideas with them. The key steps to creating interest in a product or service are as follows:

> **A**sk questions. Open questions (see Unit G7 for more information), such as 'Tell me about your hair', or 'How do you care for your hair at home?' will draw out information about the challenges your client faces. Encourage your client to give you lots of information to work with. Nod attentively and maintain eye contact as you talk. Read the client's body language and the way in which they touch their own hair as they speak. Pay close attention and make mental notes throughout the conversation. Remember, your client is not sitting in your chair because they love their hair and everything about it is perfect; they have arrived with problems that you need to solve.

> **S**ummarise the problems. Repeat back to the client a short summary of the key points that you have heard which picks out the problems. This will achieve two things: it will show that you have listened and it will crystallise in the client's mind a real need for a solution (e.g. 'What I'm hearing you say is that your hair goes limp very quickly and often looks lifeless?').

> **I**dentify solutions. Here is your greatest opportunity to show your expertise. Only talk about products or services that are relevant to the problems you have identified. If you begin to talk about other things, you are in danger of losing the client's interest. If a client's hair is limp, talk about volumising with cutting techniques, colour to add bulk to the hair, care and styling products, or even added hair pieces. Stick to solutions for the problems that your client has expressed.

> **N**otify the client. Get specific about the possible solutions, involve other staff if you need to and gather necessary information leaflets, and even the products themselves for the client to handle.

Note: Appropriate communication is the key to all successful client interactions, and learning to uncover a client's problems is the key to promoting products and services. It would be **A SIN** not to! At every stage, give your client the opportunity to ask questions and openly ask, 'What further information can I give you at this time?'

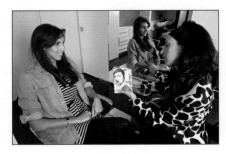

Appropriate communication is key

Engage the client's senses

Engage as many of the client's senses as you can, because different people absorb new information in different ways. Some will be interested in touching and smelling products or seeing the results in pictures or on other staff. Some will respond better to the facts and figures, such as formula ingredients. If you are introducing a new product, place the bottle in front of the client, show them how much they would use on their hair, encourage them to smell the scent and, if appropriate, show them how to apply it.

Use products and services yourself

Be an ambassador for any new services, such as colour shades, treatments or even added hair, by using them yourself. When suitable, there can be no better way for illustrating the results of a new product or service than showing it off yourself.

> **Activity** Role-play with your fellow students, your colleagues or your friends and family to uncover the 'problems' they experience with their hair. Use the **A SIN** process and practise matching products and services to their needs.

Case study
Service that sells

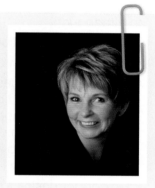

Julie Eldrett is an industry expert and customer care consultant who trains some of hairdressing's top salon names.

'When you keep your clients informed and up-to-date about the services and products that are right for them, you aren't selling them anything, you are fulfilling your obligations as their hair expert. I always say, "Information is power, but only when you share it", and I liken the client consultation to a doctor listening to a patient. Your client has arrived with problems and concerns which you need to listen out for. Typically a client will use words such as 'limp', 'fine' or 'frizzy' so when you talk about products or services link it back constantly to the place they are feeling pain – their problem. Using the same words as them will show you listened and giving them the opportunity to get a solution will show you care. In this way, recommending products and services can never be selling – if you surprise a client at reception with information about products then it's out of context and you've missed your chance.'

'Every time you touch a product or even a tool, share information, tell the client why and connect it to their problem. They aren't just paying for you to do their hair; they are paying for your time, your expertise and your advice. Salons often hold internal incentives and competitions to encourage staff to 'sell' new ranges or services but that doesn't mean you should put aside the core idea of customer service. Instead of talking to every client that comes through the door, call the clients for whom that product is relevant and tell them you have just the new thing for them – now that's great service! A great way to help close a business transaction is to write your clients a personal product prescription. That way they can carry it with them to reception and have time to decide if they would like to purchase or not without feeling any pressure. Remember that there are many, many reasons why a client will choose to make a purchase so don't take their decision personally, just give the right advice.'

Julie Eldrett, Julie Eldrett Consulting, www.julieeldrett.co.uk

When do you promote additional products or services?

> Don't hijack your client with information on new products and services. Remember to be both relevant and timely.

> Don't push your point. If your client begins to look uncomfortable, is visibly disinterested or even states that they are not interested, do not become defensive and do not take it personally. You are offering them information because it's part of your professional service. Lightly move on with the conversation or the service, and let them know that if they want more information at any time they just need to ask.

> The time to promote products and services is not during the consultation, at the backwash or at reception. It's *all the time*. Talking about everything that your business offers to your client is an integral part of your role and your service. It's not an add-on or an afterthought.

>> Use your consultation to help source 'problems'.

>> Listen attentively throughout the service to uncover 'problems'.

>> Anticipate challenges for your client (e.g. if they are investing in colour, recommend colour-protect services to help make their investment last longer). If they are preparing for a wedding, recommend a plan of treatments in the months prior to the wedding in order to improve the condition of their hair, so it's glowing on the day.

>> Link opportunities to the popular press, as celebrities are great conversation openers. For example, if you think your client would look great as a brunette and a celebrity has just gone for a big change to brunette, reference them in your conversation.

>> When your salon is running deals or promotions, such as buy one get one free (BOGOF) or gift with purchase (GWP), make sure you tell your client about the great deal. If it isn't right for their hair type, tell the client to 'tell their friends' who do have curly/dry/damaged hair, and so on.

> Never presume that your client won't be interested – it's not your place. Your place is to be consistent with your service levels and to prove your expert status and knowledge. Don't assume that your client cannot afford the product or service, or that they are not interested because they haven't asked. Sharing information may not encourage your client to spend more this time, but it may well help for their next visit.

> Many salons and product manufacturers provide 'prescription cards' that allow you to tick or highlight the products that your client should use to get the most from their hair. When your client comes towards the end of their service, make sure they have a copy of their personal prescription to take away with them.

> To close, you should always ask more questions: 'Which of the services and products we've discussed today can I give you more

information on?' Give them time to answer fully and then reassure them that they can drop in any time between visits to discuss any aspect of their hair.

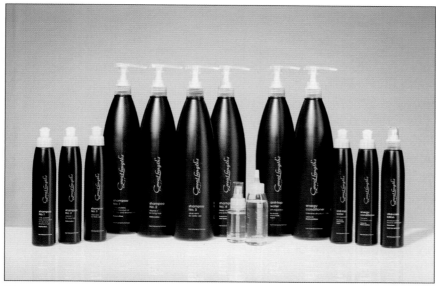

Never assume your client won't be interested

What do you do when your client is interested in products and services?

> If your client is interested in new services, walk them to reception and book the appointment with them.

> If they are interested in colour, recommend a skin test (see Unit G7) to check for any potential allergies before they leave the salon, so that there will be no delay when they return for the service.

> If they are interested in purchasing product, either inform the receptionist and hand them the client's personal prescription card or gather the products for the client yourself and place them at reception.

> If your client is interested, but not yet able to commit, gather information, website addresses, price lists, and so on, and tell them to call if they have any questions.

What might influence a client's decision to purchase?

Remember that talking about appropriate products and services that your client has yet to experience is your professional duty. Expert advice should be an integral part of the standard service – do not deny your clients! There are many factors that affect a client's purchasing decisions, and if you have built trust and rapport, none of them are your problem. Here are a few to consider.

> They just stocked up on product somewhere else.

> They don't have enough money.

Activity

1 Describe five ways that salons communicate about new products or services.

2 Name three potential reasons why a client will **not** purchase from you.

3 What process should you use to identify a client's potential needs for other products and services? Describe the process in detail.

4 Describe four 'hooks' you can use to introduce a product or service.

5 State the ways in which you can keep yourself informed about products and services.

> They don't have enough cash on them.
> They are rushing to pick up the children from school.
> They had colour once and it went wrong and they can't forget it!

The law

Data Protection Act (1998)

> Personal data shall be processed fairly and lawfully.
> Personal data shall be obtained only for one or more specified and lawful purposes, and shall not be further processed in any manner incompatible with that purpose or those purposes.
> Personal data shall be adequate, relevant and not excessive in relation to the purpose or purposes for which they are processed.
> Personal data shall be accurate and, where necessary, kept up to date.
> Personal data processed for any purpose or purposes shall not be kept for longer than is necessary for that purpose or those purposes.
> Personal data shall be processed in accordance with the rights of data subjects under this Act.
> The holder of the data can be prosecuted for misuse.
> Personal data shall not be transferred to a country or territory outside the European Economic Area unless that country or territory ensures an adequate level of protection for the rights and freedoms of data subjects in relation to the processing of personal data.
> The individual retains the right to access all information held about them.

For more information, you can see the Act in detail online at the Information Commissioner's Office (www.ico.gov.uk).

Trade Descriptions Act (1968)

The law requires that any descriptions of goods and services given by a person acting in the course of a trade or business should be accurate and not misleading. You may not:

> apply a false or misleading description to goods by written or verbal means
> supply or offer to supply goods to which a false or misleading trade description is applied.

Sale of Goods and Services Act (1980)

This Act protects the consumer's purchasing rights. In summary, it states that:

> The goods and services must be of an acceptable quality.
> The goods and services must be fit for purpose.

> The goods and services must be as described in marketing literature, advertising, labelling and by staff.

Supply of Goods and Services Act (1982)

This Act protects the consumer's rights when the goods or services are not fit for purpose. It states that:

> The consumer can claim back some or all of the purchase price paid if the goods or services are not in good condition.

> The consumer should be able to purchase services at a reasonable price and that are provided in a reasonable time frame with due care and attention.

Prices Act (1974)

This Act states that the price of goods should be clearly displayed, so that it cannot be misrepresented to the client.

Resale Prices Act (1964 and 1976)

This Act states the manufacturer can supply a recommended retail price (RRP), but that the retailer is not obliged by law to sell at this price.

Cosmetic Products (Safety) Regulations (2004)

These regulations state that all products supplied to the professional or the consumer in the UK must have undergone a safety assessment by a qualified person before they are made available on the market.

Summary

This chapter will bring you closer to providing a total service for your client, and taking responsibility for growing your revenue and that of the overall business. Product and service sales is a term that is now little used in the salon industry, as there is widespread recognition that the process is not one that 'pushes' goods and services at the client, but rather creates a 'pull' or need for them to be supplied. You are or will be working in a professional salon environment, where you and your colleagues will share a duty of care towards your clients, which includes keeping them up to date with any product or service that might be helpful or desirable to them.

Case study

Up and coming

Ross studied for his hairdressing NVQ at the Paul Falltrick salon in Romford. Falltricks is a combination salon and academy organisation where hairdressers can study for their NVQs in a real salon environment and for Ross this provided the perfect learning environment.

'Education is the base and while at the time some of the NVQ stuff seemed pointless, I now realise how valuable it is. Working on session and photographic work, I often have to call upon the techniques and skills I learned. And it's not just the practical skills, a lot of the business-orientated things I learned I'm now able to put into practice in my role as Assistant Manager. For example, I can remember having to design a salon as part of my course work and thought that it was a complete waste of time. Recently though what I learned about spacing and client flow helped me to create a new layout for the waiting area.'

'My advice for anyone studying hairdressing is to learn everything you can and set yourself goals. Your career can take you anywhere you want it to. And even when you have a bad day, remember that you're working in the greatest industry there is.'

A member of the 2009–2010 Fellowship Fame Team, Ross is now a principal in the Falltrick organisation, working in television, fashion shows and hairdressing education.

Ross Taylor, Paul Falltrick Hairdressing, Romford

Case study

A successful career choice

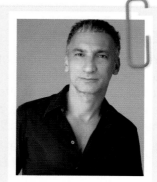

Akin Konizi has been awarded the highest accolade in UK hairdressing and has led his award-winning salon group and internationally acclaimed London Academy to achieve outstanding success.

'The most important element to succeeding in hairdressing is to continually learn and hone your skills. Education is the key to success and I strongly believe that by improving your technique, enhancing your ability and constantly learning and progressing, you will become a more skilled hairdresser and inevitably have greater professional success. All great hair professionals share one quality – they are strong communicators. Communication skills and the ability to really understand what the client wants, while blending this with expert advice on what is fashionable and suitable for them is key, whilst solid training will allow you to deliver exceptional hairdressing.'

'The best advice I give is to make sure you get the best training possible and always be open to learning more and expanding your own knowledge. The most successful, iconic hairdressers never stop learning. The training I had at the start of my career has given me solid foundations to build upon and surrounding myself with such talented, creative, supportive and driven people on a daily basis has been a huge factor in my personal success. It's also down to a lot of hard work, persistence and my unwavering commitment to excellence! The great thing about hairdressing is that it is constantly evolving and progressing forwards. My days are always so varied and the opportunities I get mean that I am always working on new and exciting projects, keeping me motivated, enthused and continually inspired by hairdressing and the industry.'

Akin Konizi, HOB Salons' International Creative Director and 2009 British Hairdresser of the Year

Best practice

You've chosen an interactive career, one that will require your energy and your input every day, so start as you mean to go on. Committed trainees make committed hair professionals, which leads to a successful and fulfilling working life. The key qualities of first-class hairdressing students include:

> An interest in hair! Get involved, read the trade magazines and websites and check out the seasonal edits in the monthly glossy magazines like *Vogue* and *Harpers Bazaar*.

> Being presentable and friendly. Think about the way you look, your body language and behaviour. Practise professional behaviour in the classroom as well as on the salon floor.

> Great communication skills. Remember that communicating isn't just about talking, it's about listening too. Make sure that you communicate clearly and appropriately as it's the foundation of every great hairdressing experience, and if there is something that you need help on, then ask!

> Being proactive and eager to learn. Make sure you are present for every lesson and work session, take every chance to observe qualified professionals and participate in all the model nights and work sessions you can.

> Taking responsibility for your portfolio. Whether you are storing your work on-line or in your evidence folder, make sure it is well thought out and organised. Your tutor or manager will offer you 'portfolio building' sessions where you will get guidance and support in building strong evidence of your growing skills, so make sure you attend them.

Moving on to the workplace and Level 3

Create a CV (curriculum vitae) with a personal statement summary of you, your attributes and your goals. List your achievements and technical abilities and your work experience. To help increase your experience during your course, seek out a Saturday job with a salon, and as you come to the end of your course your college will arrange Career Days and invite local hairdressing salons to attend to help you find a work placement. It's a great idea to continue your training and education with follow-on courses in subjects like 'hair-up'; it shows an on-going commitment to learning that employers will admire.

To be a successful NVQ Level 3 student, then, it's ideal that you should already be managing a column of clients, as much of the course content will focus on more advanced techniques such as colour correction. You will be required to show an even greater breadth of evidence for more complex work so make sure that you never stop those all-important model nights! And remember, wherever hairdressing takes you, enjoy the journey.

Special thanks to Martha Pountain.

Glossary

accelerator .... machine for speeding up the processing action of chemical services

acid perms .... perm lotion with an acid ph

aftercare .... the maintenance of a hairstyle by the client at home

alkaline perms .... perm lotion with an alkaline ph

allergy .... an immune response to a product or substance that produces irritation or illness

alpha keratin .... hair in its natural state

ammonium thioglycolate .... active ingredient in some perm lotions

androgenic alopecia .... male pattern baldness

angle .... the angle or direction at which hair is held to cut

anti-head shape .... a shape that accentuates or alters the perceived shape of the head

anti-oxidant .... product that helps restore the hair's natural ph level

applicator .... tool or bottle used to apply product

average bill .... the average amount a client spends in a salon, calculated by dividing turnover by the number of client visits

backbrushing .... pushing a hairbrush backward down the hair to create a matting effect

backcombing .... pushing a comb backward down the hair to create a matting effect

backwash .... shampoo unit where a client leans back into the basin and the hair is washed from behind

barbering .... men's hairdressing

barrier cream .... thick cream used to protect the skin

base .... the root area of a section or the barrier cream used before relaxing

base shade .... the depth shade of hair colour to which tone is added

baseline .... the perimeter or outside length

beta keratin .... hair that has been dried into a shape or style

bleach .... product that removes the colour pigment

blend .... the merging together of hair and sections

blow-drying .... drying hair with a hairdryer to create a style

book backs .... securing a booking for the next visit before a client leaves the salon

brickwork .... method of winding where the rollers are wound in offset rows like the bricks in a wall

brushing out .... brushing the hair after a set

chemical service .... hairdressing service that uses chemicals such as perming, colouring or highlighting

chipping-in .... texturising or pointing

client turnover .... the frequency with which clients do NOT return to the salon

clipper cutting .... cutting hair using clippers

clipper guard .... clipper attachment that regulates the cutting length

clippers .... electric haircutting tool

clippings .... pieces of cut hair

club cutting .... cutting the hair in a blunt line while held in the fingers

colour spectrum .... all the colours of the rainbow

combing through .... combing hair to remove tangles and to make it all go in the same direction

condition testing .... assessing the condition of the hair prior to a service

conditioner .... product used to smooth and repair the hair to improve the condition

consultation .... the discussion process with a client

contact dermatitis......................affliction of the skin (usually the hands) caused by exposure to chemicals and poor hand care

cornrows...............................plaits in rows along the scalp

cortex..................................the rope-like middle layer of the hair

counteracting.........................the process of using one colour tone to remove or counter another

cowlick................................a small section of hair that sticks up or grows in a different direction to the rest of the hair

crop....................................very short hair

cross-check............................holding the hair in the opposite way to how it was cut, to check for evenness

crown..................................highest point on the back of the head, usually where hair growth starts

cuticle.................................outside layer of the hair

cutthroat razor........................open-bladed razor for shaving

cutting collar..........................heavy plastic or rubber collar placed around the shoulders to stop hair going down the neck

dandruff...............................scalp condition that results in dead skin and scales on the scalp

density.................................thickness of the hair

depth..................................how light or dark the colour is

dermis.................................the second 'inner' layer of skin that holds and feeds the hair follicle

detergent..............................cleansing ingredient in shampoo

direction...............................the way the hair falls, is held or wound

dispensary.............................area in the salon for preparing, mixing and dispatching hair products

disulphide bonds......................bonds in the hair that are broken and reformed by perming

double crown..........................an unruly pattern of growth or crown with two growth patterns

dragging...............................winding the roller into the hair so that it sits behind its base (the roots)

dryer 1................................hand-held hairdryer

dryer 2................................mobile or static 'hood' dryer used for setting

edging.................................trimming and defining the perimeter of a haircut

effleurage.............................a shampoo technique of moving the fingers in one firm but smooth large circular action from the front to the back

elasticity..............................stretchiness of the hair or skin

electrical tools........................hairdryers, stylers, curling irons and other electrical hairdressing tools

elevation..............................lifting the hair

emulsify...............................adding water to hair colour on the head and massaging it prior to rinsing off

emulsion bleach.......................gel or oil bleach specially formulated for use on the scalp

end papers............................special papers used to keep the ends smooth during perming

ends...................................the tips or very ends of the hair

enhancements.........................wefts, extensions or hairpieces added to the hair to create a style

epidermis..............................the outer layer of the skin

eumelanin.............................the pigment in dark hair

exothermic perms.....................perm lotion that generates its own processing heat

extensions............................wefts of real or synthetic hair

faded line.............................line of a haircut that gradually gets shorter until it disappears

finger-dry.............................using the hands and fingers to push the hair into its style

finishing...............................adding final touches and product to a haircut

fish-hook ends........................ends of the hair that are permanently bent due to not being straight during the perming process

fishtail plait...........................type of plait that uses two pieces of hair

flat twists.............................way of twisting the hair on the scalp to create a style

flyaway .... hair that is light and hard to control
follicle .... a thin tube of cells and tissue that surrounds the root and provides the bed for hair growth
free-hand .... cutting hair without holding it in the fingers
French plait .... type of plait that uses three pieces of hair
French twist .... a hair-up style
fringe .... hair at the front of a haircut, on or over the forehead
frizz .... wiry, dry, unruly hair
frosting .... colouring the very tips of the hair with bleach or high-lift colour
full head .... colouring or treating all of the hair
gown .... protective cloak
graduation .... hair that gets either gradually longer or shorter
grey hair .... white hair or hair without pigment
guideline .... initial section of cut hair that is followed
hair shaft .... length of the hair
hair travel .... how hair falls in a certain way
hairline .... perimeter edge of hair growth
hairpiece .... false hairpiece added to enhance or create a style
harelip .... disfigured upperlip
henna .... vegetable natural hair colour product
highlights .... small sections of lighter colour added throughout the hair
hold .... strength of product or strength of hairstyle
hydrogen bonds .... bonds in the hair that are broken by water
hydrogen peroxide .... oxidising agent H_2O_2
hydroscopic porosity .... ability to absorb water
ICC .... International Colour Chart system
incompatibility test .... testing to see if the product is compatible with the hair
keratin .... fibrous protein that forms the main structure of hair
lanolin .... fatty oil from sheep, used in conditioner
layer .... section of hair cut to a length within the haircut
length .... overall length of a haircut or section
lowlights .... small sections of darker or richer colour added throughout the hair
manageable .... hair that can be combed or styled easily
medulla .... the central core of the hair
melanin .... the pigment in hair
metallic hair dye .... sulphide, reduction or progressive metallic hair dyes (such as Grecian 2000) that can interfere with chemical processes
mid-length .... the part of the hair that's between the roots and the ends
mousse .... styling product used to add hold and volume
moustache .... facial hair on the upper lip
movement .... curly or wavy texture
nape .... the back of the neck where the hair begins to grow
natural growth .... the natural way hair grows
natural parting .... where the hair naturally falls in two sides
neutraliser .... activator that reforms the disulphide bonds after a perm
non-permanent enhancements .... clip-in extensions or hairpieces
occipital bone .... protrusion at the back of the head
on base .... winding a roller so that it sits on the section's roots
one length .... hair cut to one perimeter length
over-angle .... holding the hair for cutting at more or less than 90°

panel..area or large section of the hair or head

para-dye.....................................compound in permanent colour products that changes the hair colour

parting..line or break in the hair

perimeter....................................outside line of the hairstyle

perm 1..permanent waving lotion

perm 2..service of perming

permanent colour.......................product that permanently changes the hair colour

permanent enhancements..........extensions that remain in the hair for longer than 24 hours

petrissage..................................a shampoo technique of moving the fingers in small massaging circular motions

ph..the acidity or alkalinity of a substance

pheomelanin..............................the pigment in blonde/red hair

pigment......................................colouring

pin curl.......................................small individual curl

plait..sections of hair woven together to create a style

pointing......................................cutting small pieces of the hair using the ends of the scissors

pomade......................................hair wax

porosity......................................the ability to absorb moisture

postiche.....................................the area of hairdressing that deals with wigs and hairpieces

PPD (para-phenylenediamine).....skin irritant found in some permanent hair colour

pre-damp....................................to add perm lotion to the hair before and during the perm winding

pre-treatment.............................a service or treatment carried out to prepare the hair for the main service such as a perm or a colour

process......................................the active stage of a chemical service when the hair is changed

processing time..........................the time it takes for the product to complete its action

psoriasis....................................affliction of the skin that causes dry flakes, redness and inflammation

pull test.....................................test to see if the hair can have extensions

quasi-permanent........................semi-permanent products with a small amount of chemical activator

receding hairline........................front hairline growth that has receded from where it used to start

recession line (1).......................point on the forehead where the hairline grows further back

recession line (2).......................the point at the temples where the hairline recedes

record card................................digital or hard copy form on which a client's personal information and service details are recorded.

re-growth (1).............................newly grown hair

re-growth (2).............................colouring the newly grown hair only

relaxing.....................................permanently straightening hair (not covered in this book)

retail..products sold to clients for home use

root..point at which the hair grows

round layer................................uniform layers of equal length around the head

scalp..skin of the head

scalp plaits................................another name for cornrows

scalp treatment.........................product used to treat the scalp

scissor over comb.....................cutting hair through the comb

sebaceous glands......................glands at the root of the hair that produce sebum (oil)

section (1).................................to divide the head into manageable working areas

section (2).................................a piece of hair to be cut or worked on

semi-permanent........................temporary, non-damaging colour

sensitivity test...........................testing to see if the skin will react to a product

serum..a hair-coating product to make the hair smooth and manageable

service.......................................a hairdressing procedure carried out for a paying client

session stylist............................hairdresser that works on fashion shows and on advertisement or film shoots
setting...................................drying hair in rollers to create a style
shade chart.............................book of colour swatches and samples
shampoo.................................product used to clean the hair
shape.....................................overall shape of a haircut
shaper....................................covered blade hand-held razor for shaping and cutting
shattered................................a broken or soft outside line
shoeshining.............................colouring the very tips of the hair with bleach or high-lift colour
sideburns...............................hair that grows on the cheeks below the hairline
side-wash...............................shampooing from the side
soften....................................remove weight or hardness
spot application........................product or colour applied to specific areas
staff turnover...........................the frequency with which staff leave
sterilise..................................remove bacteria and other living micro-organisms
stylers...................................electric tool for straightening or curling hair
styling....................................drying or finishing hair into a particular look or style
tapered..................................a gradual shortening or narrowing line
technique...............................skilled method of working
temples..................................the flat part of either side of the head between the forehead and ear
tension..................................degree of tightness at which hair is held when cutting
test curl (pre-perm)..................test carried out on a lock of hair to see how it reacts to the perm lotion
test curl (processing)...............test carried out to check how the perm has processed
texture (1)..............................the feel or appearance of the hair
texture (2)..............................choppy, broken or bitty finish to the hair
texturise................................to add a choppy, broken or bitty finish to the hair
thinning (1).............................hair that has become thinner due to hair loss
thinning (2).............................reducing the thickness of hair
tone ....the hair's colour properties
toner.....................................weak hair colour used to balance and even out coloured hair
traction alopecia......................baldness caused by excessive tension on the roots and scalp
treatment...............................product used to repair damaged hair
trichology...............................the branch of medicine that deals with the scalp and hair
trichosiderin............................a strong pigment found in rich, deep red hair
trimmers................................small, usually cordless clippers
turnover.................................the amount of money that a salon takes through the till
twists....................................way of twisting the hair to create a style
two-strand twist ....way of twisting two pieces of hair to create a style
uniform..................................even, balanced length or shape
unstructured...........................irregular shape or non-smooth, choppy finish
virgin hair...............................hair that has undergone no chemical process
volume ....body or fullness
washpoint..............................shampoo unit
wax......................................waxy hair-finishing product
weight..................................heaviness or length of a section of a haircut
widow's peak..........................a pointed and prominent front hairline
winding..................................rolling a roller into the hair
workstation.............................mirrored position (usually with a counter) where hairdressing services are carried out